Instrumental Methods and Scoring in Extrapyramidal Disorders

Springer
Berlin
Heidelberg
New York
Barcelona
Budapest
Hong Kong
London
Milan
Paris
Santa Clara
Singapore
Tokyo

H. Przuntek P.H. Kraus
P. Klotz A.D. Korczyn (Eds.)

Instrumental Methods and Scoring in Extrapyramidal Disorders

With 72 Figures and 25 Tables

Springer

Prof. Dr. Horst Przuntek
Dr. Peter H. Kraus
P. Klotz
Neurologische Universitätsklinik
St. Josef-Hospital
Gudrunstr. 56
44791 Bochum
Germany

Prof. Amos D. Korczyn
Tel-Aviv University
Sackler School of Medicine
Tel-Aviv 69978
Israel

Cover Illustration: Peter H. Kraus

ISBN 3-540-57875-7 Springer-Verlag Berlin Heidelberg New York

CIP-data applied for

Die Deutsche Bibliothek - CIP-Einheitsaufnahme
Instrumental methods and scoring in extrapyramidal disorders:
with 25 tables/H. Przuntek . . . (ed.). - Berlin; Heidelberg;
New York; Barcelona; Budapest; Hong Kong; London;
Milan; Paris; Tokyo: Springer, 1995
ISBN 3-540-57875-7
NE: Przuntek, Horst (Hrsg.)

Cover design: Springer-Verlag, Design & Production

Typesetting: Best-set Typesetter Ltd., Hong Kong

SPIN: 10081286 25/3134/SPS - 5 4 3 2 1 0 - Printed on acid-free paper

Preface

Many extrapyramidal motor diseases result from underlying neurodegenerative processes, which however are very advanced at the time the clinical diagnosis is made. From animal experiments it seems likely that we may soon have several substances that provide neuroprotective effects, but that their therapeutic use must be as early as possible. This fact was the starting point for the meeting, held at Chiemsee, that formed the basis of this book. The idea was to develop instrumental methods that, first, permit an earlier diagnosis by drawing on the experience of experts and, second, provide a better resolution of successful therapy than the currently used methods.

As early as 1886, Charcot tried to differentiate the tremor of polysclerosis and Parkinson patients by using a drum developed by Marey, a physiologist. Subsequently, many apparatuses were developed to better identify movement disorders, initially for diagnostic purposes. Most of these methods proved to be inferior to the skill of experienced observers. In the last two decades, however, both the technical advances made in measuring methods and the improvements achieved in methods of evaluation have led to marked advances in the quantification of motor disturbances. An objective of the symposium held at Chiemsee and of this book is to provide an overview of the procedures that are currently commonly used for extrapyramidal movement disorders, and to identify their potential and limitations.

Upon critical examination it becomes apparent that many of the methods are very capable of registering extrapyramidal motor disturbances when the illness is fully developed but have great problems when the disease is in its early stages. Furthermore, for many procedures results are only available for their capacity to distinguish different stages of the illness or to provide significant differences for comparisons between patients with clinically verified diagnosis and control persons. Yet since in this context early diagnosis means early differential diagnosis at a stage of clinically nonspecific symptoms, it is necessary for us to improve our ability to distinguish these symptoms.

In the studies in which technical methods and rating scales were used in parallel, it was shown that each of the procedures had its own advantages and disadvantages.

The future of the instrumental identification of extrapyramidal movement disorders will lie in the improvement of the early diagnosis of these illnesses and in the measurement of the effects of therapy even in early stages of the disease. This will be achieved by making the methods more specific and, above all, better validated.

We believe that the present book provides a good basis for the pursuit of these goals and wish to thank the firm ASTA Medica, Frankfurt am Main, for making it possible for us to conduct this symposium and publish this book.

Bochum, Germany/Tel-Aviv, Israel
August 1995

H. Przuntek
P.H. Kraus
P. Klotz
A.D. Korczyn

Contents

List of Active Contributors

Allum, J.H.J., Prof. Dr. biomed. Ing.
Uniklinik und Poliklinik für HNO-Krankheiten, Kantonsspital, Petersgraben 4, 4031 Basel, Switzerland

Bass, H., PD Dr.
Abteilung für Neurologie, Zentrum für Neurologie und Neurochirurgie, Klinikum der Universität Frankfurt, Schleosenweg 2-16, D-60528 Frankfurt, Germany

Bain, P.G., Dr.
MRC Human Movement & Balance Unit, Institute of Neurology, Queen Square, London WC1N 3BG, UK

Deuschl, G., Prof. Dr.
Neurologische Universitätsklinik Kiel, Niemannsweg 147, 24105 Kiel, Germany

Fahn, S., Prof.
College of Physicians and Surgeons of Columbia University, Presbyterian Hospital, Neurological Institute, 710 West 168th Street, New York, NY100032, USA

Findley, L.J., Dr.
National Hospital Institute of Neurology, Neurootol. Sect., Medical Research Council Human Movement and Balance Unit, Queen Square, London WC1N-3BG, UK

Flowers, K.A., Dr.
University of HULL, Human Performance Laboratories, Department of Psychology, North Humberside, HULL HU6 7RX, UK

Greulich, W., Prof. Dr.
Neurologische Klinik Hagen Ambrock, Ambrocker Weg, 58091 Hagen, Germany

Hallett, M., Dr.
Human Motor Control Section, Medical Neurology Branch, National Institute of Neurological Disorders and Stroke, NIH Building 10 Room 5N226, Bethesda MD20892, USA

Hefter, H., Dr.
Neurologische Klinik der Universität Düsseldorf, Moorenstr. 5, 40225 Düsseldorf, Germany

Hocherman, S., Dr.
Technion IIT, Faculty of Medicine, Efron Street, P.O.B. 9697, Haifa 31096, Israel

Hömberg, V., Dr.
Neurologisches Therapiecentrum, Hohensandweg 37, 40591 Düsseldorf, Germany

Inzelberg, R., Dr.
Departement of Neurology, Tel Aviv Sourasky Medical Center, 6 Weizman Street, Tel Aviv 64239, Israel

Klotz, P., Dipl.-Psych.
Neurologische Universitätsklinik im St. Josef-Hospital, Gudrunstr. 56, 44791 Bochum, Germany

Korczyn, A.D., Prof. Dr.
Sackler Faculty of Medicine, Tel Aviv University, Ramat Aviv 69978, Israel

Kraus, P.H., Dr.
Neurologische Universitätsklinik im St. Josef-Hospital, Gudrunstr. 56, 44791 Bochum, Germany

Lücking, C.H., Prof. Dr.
Neurologische Klinik der Universität Freiburg, Hansastr. 9a, 79104 Freiburg, Germany

Machetanz, J., Dr.
Neurol. Klinik und Poliklinik TU München, Möhlstr. 28, 81675 München, Germany

Müller, F., OA Dr.
Neurologische Klinik Bad Aibling, Kolbermoorer Str. 72, 83043 Bad Aibling, Germany

Olanow, W.C., Prof.
Dept. Neurology, Mount Sinai School of Medicine, One Gustave L. Levy Place, New York, NY100029-6574, USA

Panzer-Decius, V.P., Dr.
Associate Scientist, Oregon Health Sciences University, CROET L606 3181 S.W. Sam Jackson Park Road, Portland, OR 97201-3098, USA

Paulus, W., Prof. Dr.
Neurologische Klinik, Kliniken der Universität Göttingen, Robert-Koch Str. 40, 37075 Göttingen, Germany

Potvin, A.R., Prof. Dr.
Dean of Purdue University School of Engineering and Technology, Indiana University Purdue University, Indianapolis, ET 1219 799 West Michigan Street, Indianapolis, IN 46202-5160, USA

Przuntek, H., Prof. Dr.
Neurologische Universitätsklinik im St. Josef-Hospital, Gudrunstr. 56, 44791 Bochum, Germany

Rabey, J.M., Prof. Dr.
Dept. of Neurology, Tel Aviv Sourasky Medical Center, 6 Weizman St., Tel Aviv 64239, Israel

Rothwell, J.C., Prof. Dr.
National Hospital, Institute of Neurology Neurootol. Sect., Medical Research Council Human Movement and Balance Unit, Queen Square, London WC1N-3BG, UK

Ruß, M., Dipl.-Psych.
Abteilung für Neurologie, Zentrum für Neurologie und Neurochirurgie, Klinikum der Universität Frankfurt, Schleusenweg 2-16, 60528 Frankfurt, Germany

Steg, G.H., Prof. Dr.
Neurol. Dept., Sahlgren Hospital, 41345 Göteborg, Sweden

Spieker, S., Dr.
Universität Tübingen, Neurologische Klinik, Hoppe-Seyler-Str. 3, 72076 Tübingen, Germany

Struppler, A., Prof. em. Dr.
Klinikum rechts der Isar der TU München, Ismaninger Str. 22, 81675 München, Germany

Trenkwalder, C., Dr.
Max-Planck-Institut f. Psychiatrie, Klinisches Institut, Kraepelinstr. 10, 80804 München, Germany

Treves, T., Dr.
Sackler Faculty of Medicine, Tel Aviv University, Ramat Aviv 69978, Israel

Zeppenfeld, K., Dr.
Knappschaftskrankenhaus Universitätsklinik, Neurologische Klinik,
In der Schornau 23, 44892 Bochum, Germany

Theoretical Basics of Rating Scales

P.H. Kraus and P. Klotz

Developments in pharmacology demand high standards for therapy control. This is well documented by, for example, the history of rating and staging of Parkinson's disease: the character of one of the oldest approaches [5] was more a categorizing one, subsequently established scales focused more and more on quantifying the course of the disease with an increasing number of items [2,7], and newer scales also assess side effects of L-dopa therapy [3].

The theoretical basics of rating or testing are related to the theoretical basics of measurement theory: both methods are an assignment of objects or events to numbers following a certain rule. Rating scales are a special case, in which this projection is carried out by the subjective estimation of a rater. This rater can be an independent examiner or – in the case of self-rating – the examinee himself. Nearly all rating scales for neurological disorders supply ordinal or ranked information, but nonnumerical scales are also possible, for example the Kunin scale [1].

The specific aim of most rating scales established for assessment of motor disturbances is the control of therapeutic efficacy or of the course of the disease. In contrast, only a few scales are useful for diagnostic purposes. The following will give a short overview over basics of rating and testing, paying special attention to practical use.

Rating scales have to meet the main test criteria of objectivity, reliability, and validity. Objectivity means that different examiners arrive at the same result when rating the same patient. This is postulated for all steps of the test: implementation, evaluation, and interpretation.

Reliability means the formal precision of the assessment of a feature – independent of the question as to whether this feature should be measured at all. There are different kinds of reliability, including stability over time (test–retest reliability), equivalence with comparable tests, and internal consistency. These parameters can be different for the same scale. Reliability coefficients are more or less correlation coefficients. Stability is examined by retesting. It should be mentioned that the second rating may be influenced by the first. Furthermore, retest reliability cannot be achieved by assessment of time-dependent features, which occur in motor disturbances as fluctuations. Equivalence is measured by parallel use of different scales, and internal consistency by split half methods, for example.

Validity means the precision of assessment of the particular feature which has to be measured. Intrinsic validity means that the test directly represents the feature of interest. This is the kind of validity which underlies most scales for assessment of motor disturbances. Internal validity (construct validity) is given by correlation to similar tests. Criterion-oriented validation compares scores with an external variable considered to provide a direct measure of the feature in question. For most questions concerning assessment of motor disturbance, there is no real external criterion and therefore an external validation is not easily practicable. Because of the low resolution of rating scales into few discrete stages, the reliabilty of such scores is less a problem than validity.

A practical example may serve to clarify test criteria: If we try to estimate body weight by assessment of height, this is a procedure with very high reliability, but only limited validity.

For practical use, the economy of the test – one of the secondary test criteria (standardization, comparability, economy, usefulness; [6]) – is of special importance.

The following points have to be taken into consideration in compiling a new rating scale:

1. All instructions should be formulated unambiguously.
2. During the first step of creating a new scale in a preliminary design, many more items than are really necessary ought to be tested with a sample group.
3. These items should each only deal with one single feature (i.e., one dimension). All items together have to cover the whole spectrum of features of interest.
4. The defined stages for each item should differentiate between high and low intensity of this feature (symptom) and represent multiple degrees of intensity (i.e., adequate resolution).
5. For laying down the ideal number of stages, it has to be taken into consideration that verbal precision and subjective differentiation have limits. Experience shows that it is not useful to choose more than seven stages.
6. It makes a difference whether we have an unipolar- or a bipolar-expressed feature.
7. It is important whether the number of stages is even or not if we want to define a stage for average expression.
8. A subsequent item analysis has to be carried out to identify the best-fitting items for an effective and practicable one-dimensional scale. All items which do not contribute to information can be left out, and in choosing between similar items, the most meaningful should be kept (always considering that it is better not to use the fewest possible, but also to have some redundancy for confirmation).

Because most movement disorders represent complex syndromes (i.e., they are multidimensional), either the use of items with an integrative character or better use of a multidimensional (i.e., heterogeneous) test battery is necessary. In the first case, the rater gives a highly subjective overall impression (as, for example, for item 10 of the Webster rating scale, where independence has to be rated); in the second case, different items, each assessing one feature, cover the whole syndrome.

Simple addition of raw data of such a heterogeneous scale to a sum score produces a parameter of questionable benefit: In principle, an adequate summing of items to a homogeneous score improves the signal to noise ratio and therefore represents a better description of changes. However, by summing heterogeneous items, the dimensionality of the scale is projected to "1," taking into consideration neither the real dimensionality of the syndrome nor the different weights of the items. For example, in the Webster rating scale, we only have one single item concerned with tremor, so therapeutic changes in tremor-dominant Parkinsonian patients are not reflected sufficiently by the total score.

For an adequate evaluation, it is necessary to identify or construct one-dimensional test units consisting of items which together assess one feature of interest as homogeneously as possible.

For this problem factor analysis is a useful tool, which reduces the dimensionality of the raw data by weighted combination. However, here we have to remember that in most cases there are only ranked data and therefore use of parametric statistics is not allowed. On the other hand, the results of multivariate statistics data from a cross-section often are interpreted improperly as if they were longitudinal data.

Factors are "constructs" which have to be interpreted considering those items with high factor loading. This way of proceeding also helps to estimate the otherwise unknown relative weights of the items.

Based on our own examinations of scales for Parkinson's disease, data do not meet all the conditions for evaluation as a sum score. Table 1 shows the corrected item total correlation of the Webster rating scale items of 645 de novo Parkinsonian patients. Tremor is an outlier and cannot be used for calculation of a sum score.

Figure 1 shows an example of the same data set. Factor analysis of the Webster results gives two factors following the Eigenwert criterion (for identification of the best number of factors), which are mixed and cannot be interpreted in a simple way. However, using the Scree test, we gain a third factor and a more easily

Table 1. Reliability analysis of Webster rating scale items (n = 645 de novo parkinsonian patients)

Webster item	Mean	SD	Corrected item total correlation
1 Bradykinesia	1.38	0.65	0.58
2 Rigidity	1.24	0.65	0.45
3 Posture	0.81	0.66	0.56
4 Arms	1.49	0.83	0.48
5 Gait	0.83	0.71	0.60
6 Tremor	1.19	0.66	0.06[a]
7 Facies	1.10	0.62	0.55
8 Seborrhea	0.58	0.60	0.36
9 Speech	0.79	0.62	0.48
10 Independence	0.77	0.70	0.63

Cronbach's alpha = 0.80.
[a] The item "tremor" is an outlier.

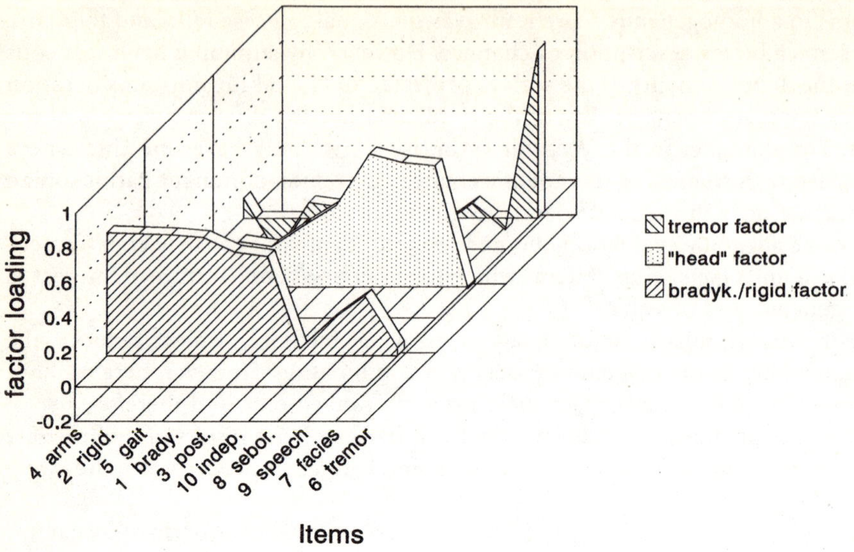

Fig. 1. Factor analysis of the Webster rating scale ($n = 645$ de novo patients). *arms*, arm swinging; *rigid.*, rigidity; *brady.*, bradykinesia; *post.*, posture; *indep.*, independence; *sebor.*, seborrhea

interpretable solution, with one factor describing akinesia and rigidity and another one for tremor only.

For the interpretation of multivariate analysis, it has to be taken into consideration that the data are clustered. Analogous to the clinical classification into the equivalence-type, akinesia–rigidity-type, and tremor-dominant type of Parkinson's disease, we find different data clouds, and one factor analysis for all patients is thus associated with fuzziness.

There are some further errors and disadvantages of the rating methods. The projection of symptoms is nonlinear for most items. Less-affected patients under a certain level of intensity are pressed into the lowest stage (floor effect), while those exceeding a certain high level are pressed into the highest stage (ceiling effect). Only the middle intensity is resolved sufficiently linearly into a few steps. Especially in the region of interest for studies with less-affected patients, we therefore find a reduced resolution. Following the classical testing theory, the error of the method should be constant for all stages. This is not given for extreme ratings, creating an additional problem for rating patients with very low expressed symptoms.

Another problem is concerned with selectivity, this includes on the one hand specificity (identification of subjects who *are* affected and avoidance of false-positive classification) and on the other hand sensitivity (correct identification of subjects who are *not* affected and avoidance of false-negative classification). For most rating scales, it is not clearly defined how to rate unspecific disturbance, e.g., that caused by multimorbidity. It is a topic of frequent debate on principles: can, for example, essential tremor be assessed by a rating scale for Parkinson's disease. Rating often is carried out only for specific symptomatology after subjective subtraction of the unspecific component and not for the total disability. This is a particular problem when a parkinsonian patient with additional depression has to be rated: because of the relatedness of the symptoms, it is impossible to separate the two syndromes and both parkinsonian rating and that of depression is biased. A similar problem is that of normal ageing: many features change during normal life, so what should be taken as the baseline for rating people of different ages.

In contrast to methods with a continuous distribution for a normal population, where deviation is defined by an arbitrary limit (e.g., 95%), most rating scales have only one stage for "not affected," which in most cases means a rating of "0". One-sided scales cannot contribute to diagnostic problems.

Several kinds of errors of observation can occur in rating; the halo effect is the phenomenon that assessment of several different features of a patient is dependent on an overall judgement. The leniency and severity error refers to a systematic shift of the subject's assessed stage to a higher or lower one. A central tendency occurs if extreme intensities are not adequately taken into consideration and the middle of the scale is preferred.

Rater–ratee interaction leads to a bias because of the rater's own position on the scale. A very important bias in the assessment of motor disturbances is the primacy–recency effect: judgment is influenced by earlier assessed patients with extreme intensity.

Evaluation of therapy effects or the course of a disease is a longitudinal method of examination. Most rating scales for movement disorders do not assess only the stage at a point of time, but also include items which rate over a recent time interval in a more anamnestic manner. These parts are not useful for fast, repetitive testing.

In principle, repetitive rating follows the sampling theorem: to receive an adequate resolution of changes over time, the number and the length of intervals have to be chosen under consideration of all time-dependent effects for the individual question.

In view of all these problems, how can rating be improved? One level where improvement is necessary is that of standardization: to improve objectivity, a detailed manual for each scale is required, as well as interrater training. All test criteria have to be met, with special attention being paid to validity.

Most of all, however, we need more intelligent methods of evaluation. Multivariate analysis with the help of linear statistical methods would constitute a first step in improving the assessment of multidimensional syndromes. Taking the nonlinearity of data distribution and scale ratio into consideration, multivariate, nonlinear methods such as the use of artificial neural nets could contribute to further improvement [4].

References

1. Butzin CA, Anderson NH (1973) Functional measurement of children's judgement. Child Dev 44:529–537

2. Duvoisin RC (1971) The evaluation of extrapyramidal disorders. In: Monoamines, noyaux gris centraux et syndrome de Parkinson: symposion Genève 1970. Masson, Paris, pp 313–325
3. Fahn S, Elton R et al. (1987) Unified Parkinson's disease rating scale. In: Fahn S, Marsden CD, Goldstein M, Calne DB (eds) Recent developments in Parkinson's disease, vol II. Macmillan Healthcare Information, Florham Park, pp 153–163
4. Fritsch T, Kraus PH, Przuntek H, Tran-Gia P (1995) Classification of Parkinson rating-scale-data using a self-organizing neural net. IEEE international conference on neural networks, 28 March 1993 (in press)
5. Hoehn MM, Yahr MD (1967) Parkinsonism: onset, progression, and mortality. Neurology 17:427–442
6. Lienert GA (1989) Testaufbau und Testanalyse, 4th edn. Psychologie Verlags-Union, Munich
7. Webster DD (1968) Critical analysis of the disability in Parkinson's disease. Mod Treatment 5:257–282

The Hoehn and Yahr Rating Scale for Parkinson's Disease

J.M. Rabey and A.D. Korczyn

Parkinson's disease (PD) is a complicated disease in which a number of theoretical and practical considerations on how best to assess the clinical deficit have been published [1–3]. In addition, the utilization of levodopa or dopamine agonists produces a large array of side effects which superimpose upon the motor fluctuations frequently seen in these patients, complicating even more the precise evaluation of disability. Since the introduction of levodopa, a number of clinical rating systems have been suggested and continue to be developed, suggesting that no single scale is completely satisfactory (Table 1). These scales attempt to measure symptoms, signs, and/or functional disability. Subjective methods of assessment of PD include: (a) clinical rating scale, (b) self-rating scale, and (c) functional disability. Simple objective methods include: (a) gait measurements, (b) finger movements, (c) reaction time (computerized), and (d) movement time (computerized). In the present paper, it is our purpose to review the Hoehn and Yahr scale [4], published in 1967, which is the most popular scale used worldwide for the staging of the functional disability associated with Parkinson's disease.

Hoehn and Yahr Scale

The Hoehn and Yahr scale [4] was elaborated in order to analyze the data of 802 patients bearing the diagnosis of PD who were seen at the Columbia Presbyterian Medical Center in New York from 1949 to 1964. These patients exhibited some or all of the accepted cardinal manifestations of PD, namely rest tremor, plastic rigidity, paucity or delayed initiation of movement, slowness, as well as impaired postural and righting reflexes. Review of this famous paper makes it clear that the main aim was not a publication of a new scale, but rather an attempt to classify the degree of disability found among the patients. The paper mainly analyzed epidemiological data on onset, progression, and mortality from PD. The popularity of this scale is manifested by the number of times it has been quoted in the medical literature (Fig. 1).

The Hoehn and Yahr scale (Table 2) was built according to four axes:

1. Unilateral versus bilateral functional impairment
2. Steadiness versus unsteadiness (postural balance) in standing and gait capacity

Discussion

Dr. Panzer: In your last slide, I think you ran out of time and you went over some complicated ideas very quickly. Could you explain it again?

Dr. Kraus: What we did is we examined in parallel the Webster rating scale and the Hoehn and Yahr scale and tried to make a kind of prediction. The multiple regression leads to a linear algorithm in which the Webster rating scale items are linearly combined to arrive at a function which describes the Hoehn and Yahr rating. The discriminant analysis uses planes in this multidimensional space of data to distinguish between the Hoehn and Yahr stages. Both methods are linear. The multiple regression is better in the middle of the distribution and discriminant analysis is better in the extremes. The neural network works out for every point a hyperplane to separate them, so it is much better for separation. Therefore, we have a very high recognition by the neural net.

Dr. Fahn: Let me just ask a question. On a theoretical basis of the ideal rating scale – do you think it could ever be achieved? A single scale? Could any single scale ever be the ideal scale?

Dr. Kraus: Existing scales – for Parkinson's disease, for example – assess really different parts of the disease. These parts don't change in the same way under therapy and therefore it is necessary to use a combined scale. We can prospectively create perhaps not the ideal scale, but a better one.

Dr. Fahn: I suspect we're going to end up concluding after 2 days that a number of scales are needed to cover everything and that certain scales are better for one particular feature and other scales for another.

Table 1. Clinical rating scales in Parkinson's disease

Scale
Karnofsky et al. [12]
Massachusetts General Hospital rating scale [13]
Northwestern University Disability Scale [14]
Hoehn and Yahr staging scale [4]
Webster rating scale [15]
New York University Rating Scale [16]
Klawans and Garvin [17]
Columbia University rating scale [18]
King's College Hospital rating scale [19]
Parkinson's Disease Information Center [20]
Rinne et al. [21]
Cornell weighted scale [22]
Anden et al. [23]
Parkinson weighted scale [24]
Birkmayer and Neumayer [25]
Potvin and Tourtellotte (unspecific) [26]
Lhermitte et al. [27]
UCLA disability score [28]
New York University Parkinson's disease scale [29]
Modified Hoehn and Yahr's scale [2]
Unified Parkinson's Disease Rating Scale [11]

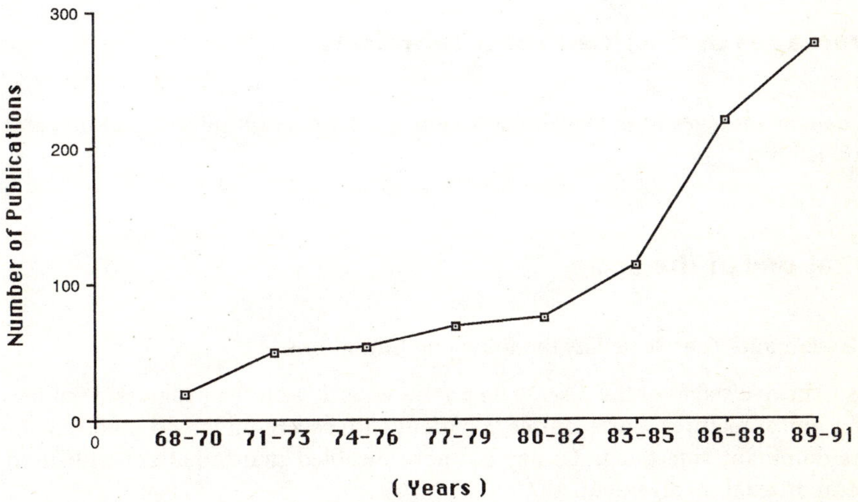

Fig. 1. The number of publications which have utilized the Hoehn and Yahr Scale (source: Citation Index) between 1968–1991

Table 2. Hoehn and Yahr Scale

Stage	Description
I	Unilateral involvement only, usually with minimal or no functional impairment
II	Bilateral or midline involvement without impairment of balance
III	First sign of impaired righting reflexes; this is evident by unsteadiness as the patient turns or is demonstrated when he is pushed from standing equilibrium with the feet together and eyes closed Functionally, the patient is somewhat restricted in his activities but may have some work potential depending upon the type of employment Patients are capable of leading independent lives and their disability is mild to moderate
IV	Fully developed, severely disabling disease The patient is still able to walk and stand unassisted, but is markedly incapacitated
V	Confinement of bed or wheelchair unless aided

3. Independence versus dependence in the activities of daily life
4. Degree of disease disability (mild to moderate versus severe)

According to the description of the different stages (Table 2), it is clear that axes 1 and 2 require a medical examination, while axes 3 and 4 are scored according to the history given by the patients and their caregivers.

Advantages of the Hoehn and Yahr Scale

The main advantages of the Hoehn and Yahr scale are its simplicity, rapidity, and reproducibility.

Limitations of the Scale

The Hoehn and Yahr scale has the following limitations:

1. The five stages of the disease do not necessarily reflect a progressive course of the clinical features. For example, a patient with severe unilateral involvement of the dominant side (stage I) may be more disabled than a patient with mild bilateral or axial involvement.

2. The five stages of the scale can give the wrong impression that patients with PD will initially present with stage I and will follow the other stages sequentially as the disease progresses. This is not the case, as it is well known that in many patients the disease may start at stage II or III.

3. Lack of linearity of the different stages of the disease is a major disadvantage. The difference between stage I and II, for example, is not similar to the

difference between stage III and IV, either in terms of disability or in the time it takes to progress from one stage to the next. In other words, the scale is nonparametric. Therefore, it is not justifiable to apply statistical methods employed for parametric data (for example, the mean of the group). The proper way to describe a given PD group utilizing this score is to calculate the median of the patients or more properly to describe numerically the distribution of the patients in each stage.

4. The scale was devised just before the introduction of levodopa. As a consequence, there is no consideration of the reaction of the patients to the treatment or the late complications so well known today, including motor fluctuations and dyskinesias [5–7] as well as hallucinations, etc.

5. Hoehn and Yahr's scale did not address the effects of therapy, i.e., whether patients are to be examined while on or off medication. This was of little significance at a time when anticholinergics were the only drug available. Their efficacy was limited and their effect on staging negligible. However, with the introduction of levodopa, and its dramatic effects, accommodations had to be made. A patient can be severely disabled while "off" medication and independent while "on." Since it is usually not possible to stop the treatment for staging purposes – at least in advanced cases – the rating today underestimates the true progression of the disease. The disability previously reflected disease progression; with levodopa, disease progression is masked. Hoehn and Yahr staging only reflects disability, and it should be clarified whether patients are examined "off" drugs or "on" and, in the latter case, how long after the administration of the last dose (or randomly), since disability may fluctuate during the day.

6. The scale did not consider at all the affective and cognitive status of the patients. Today it is quite clear that depression and dementia are relatively frequent features that may accompany the motor findings of PD patients and may have significant effects on their disability [8–10].

7. The scale is very generalized and does not allow proper characterization of the clinical status of the patients. Considering this point it is, however, important to stress the fact that this scale was not created to quantify the *motor disabilities*, but to give a general idea of the *functional performance* of the patients. The authors also included some physical characteristics which demand a neurological examination (axes 1 and 2) and have thus created some confusion, giving the impression that the scoring also implies an analysis of the motor performance.

Considering the clinical criteria for the staging of the patients, there are also two points which need clarification:

1. Most neurologists consider the impairment of postural reflexes as a prominent feature for the designation of patients as belonging to stage III. These postural reflexes however, are not standardized. They are usually examined by pushing or pulling the patient standing with the feet together and eyes closed. Hoehn and Yahr in their description (Table 2) stressed that a patient should be considered stage III if there is "unsteadiness as it turns while checking its walking characteristics or while it is pushed from a standing position." According to their concept,

patients with unsteady gait should be considered stage III even if their capacity to stand after a push is unaffected.

2. The other point which causes frequent confusion is that they consider a patient stage IV if he is still able to walk and stand unassisted, but is otherwise markedly incapacitated. In clinical practice, patients are usually considered stage IV only when they walk with help (even using a cane, a walker, or some support by a caregiver). Many patients should therefore be included in this stage instead of stage III if they have unstable gait *even* if they walk unassisted.

Complying with these two points, patients with gait impairment could be scored stage III or IV according to the subjective criteria of the investigator; their classification did not provide clear rules for differentiating between these two stages.

Modifications of the Hoehn and Yahr Scale

In 1983 Larsen et al. [2] published an article entitled "Theoretical and practical issues in assessment of deficits and therapy in Parkinsonism," wherein they included a modification of the original Hoehn and Yahr scale (Table 3). While adhering to the four axes mentioned above, they added some minor alterations which did not substantially change the basic classification published in 1967:

1. In the first stage they added: "Tremor at rest may be a prominent symptom and parkinsonism *may* be restricted to one side." Presumably they meant that stage I may also include patients with bilateral symptoms or signs.

2. In the description of stage III, Larsen et al. added that patients may be restricted in activities that require walking, dexterity, and rapid movements. Thus, they specify some motor functions that may be impaired in addition to gait.

Table 3. Stages of parkinsonism (modified Hoehn and Yahr scale)

Stage	Description
1	Minimal or no functional impairment Tremor at rest may be a prominent symptom and parkinsonism may be restricted to one side
2	Mild degree of disability with bilateral or midline involvement, but no impairment of balance
3	Moderate functional disability from parkinsonism Righting reflexes are impaired Patients may be restricted in activities that require walking dexterity and rapid movement
4	Fully developed, severely disabling disease Walking and standing are precarious, although some self-care is possible
5	Severe disability with inability to walk Other disabilities (e.g., rigid states, impairment of speech and feeding) may be prominent

3. In stage IV, they added that "some self-care by the patients is still possible," thus indicating a significantly worse functioning than the original description by Hoehn and Yahr, in which it was mentioned that the patient is still able to walk and stand unassisted.

4. In stage V, they added that the patient is not only unable to walk, but also "he may show a prominent rigid state, or impairment of speech and feeding." These modifications are somewhat more descriptive concerning the capacity of patients to cope with activities of daily life. Again, their staging does not allow proper characterization of the motor performance of the patients. In our opinion, the inclusion of some physical findings may confound an unaware physician, who may think that this modification allows quantification of the motor deficit, while their scoring actually classifies the degree of disability of PD patients.

The Unified Parkinson's Disease Rating Scale

The necessity for a standardized method of assessing PD prompted a group of clinical investigators led by David Marsden and Stanley Fahn to develop the Unified Parkinson's Disease Rating Scale (UPDRS). This scale has already been revised several times and one of the publications even included a statistical analysis of interrater reliability [11]. The fifth section of the UPDRS is basically a modification of the Hoehn and Yahr scale, including two new intermediate stages. Stage 1.5 indicates unilateral plus axial involvement. In this respect, it created a new problem, considering that stage II according to the original description includes patients "with bilateral *or* axial involvement." In this case, if a patient starts with only axial features, he would be classified stage II and later, when developing unilateral tremor or rigidity, he will be classified stage 1.5. A patient with unilateral *and* axial involvement is reduced from the original stage II to the new stage 1.5. However, depending on the severity of the symptoms, these patients, may be more incapacitated than stage II patients with mild bilateral symptomatology. Stage 2.5 of the UPDRS represents mild bilateral disease and mild postural instability with recovery (retropulsion but no falling) on the pull test, while in stage 3, patients fall on the pull test unless supported by the examiner.

Conclusions

The staging scale developed by Hoehn and Yahr is still the most popular and easy system developed for the evaluation of the disability of PD patients. Its success derives from its simplicity. Although it is not a useful tool for the quantification of motor deficits, it gives a good idea of the functional capacity of the patients and in this way also reflects their motor performance. Routine parametric statistical procedures should not be applied to data obtained with this scale. The modifications published to date are not useful, as they have not added information with significant clinical or therapeutic implications, and none of them have addressed the limitations mentioned above.

References

1. Marsden CD, Schachter M (1981) Assessment of extrapyramidal disorders. Br J Clin Pharmacol 11:129–151
2. Larsen AT, LeWitt PA, Calne DB (1983) Theoretical and practical issues in assessment of deficits and therapy in parkinsonism. In: Calne DB, Horowski R, McDonald RJ, Wittke W (eds) Lisuride and other dopamine agonists. Raven, New York, pp 363–373
3. Ward CD, Sanes JN, Dambriosia JM, Calne DB (1983) Methods for evaluating treatment in Parkinson's disease. In: Fahn S, Calne DB, Shoulson I (eds) Experimental therapeutics of movement disorders. Raven, New York, pp 1–7 (Advances in neurology, vol 37)
4. Hoehn MM, Yahr MD (1967) Parkinsonism: onset, progression and mortality. Neurology 17:427–442
5. Fahn S (1975) "On off" phenomenon with levodopa therapy in parkinsonism. Neurology (Minneapolis) 24:431–444
6. LeWitt PA, Chase TN (1983) "On off" effects: the new challenge in parkinsonism. TINS 6:1–4
7. Nausieda PA, Glantz R, Weber S, Baum R, Klawans HL (1984) Psychiatric complications of levodopa therapy of Parkinson's disease. In: Hassler RG, Christ JF (eds) Advances in neurology, vol 40. Raven, New York, pp 271–277
8. Korczyn AD, Inzelberg R, Treves M, Reider I, Rabey JM (1986) Dementia of Parkinson's disease. In: Yahr MD, Bergmann KJ (eds) Parkinson's disease. Raven, New York, pp 399–403 (Advances in neurology, vol 45)
9. Rabey JM, Scharf M, Oberman Z, Zohar M, Graff E (1990) Cortisol, ACTH and beta endorphin after dexamethasone administration in Parkinson's dementia. Biol Psychiatry 27:581–591
10. Mayeux R, Stern Y, Cote L, Williams JBW (1983) Clinical and biochemical features of depression in Parkinson's disease. Ann Neurol 14:135–136
11. Fahn S, Elton RL and members of the UPDRS development committee (1987) Unified Parkinson's disease rating scale. In: Fahn S, Marsden CD, Goldstein M, Calne DB (eds) Recent developments in Parkinson's disease, vol 2. Macmillan, New York, pp 153–163
12. Karnofsky DA, Burchenal JH, Armistead GC, Southam CM, Bernstein JL, Craver IF, Rhoads CP (1951) Triethylene nealamine in the treatment of neoplastic disease. Arch Intern Med 87:477–516
13. England AC, Schwab RS (1956) Postoperative evaluation of 26 selected patients with Parkinson's disease. J Am Geriatr Soc 4:1219–1232
14. Canter CJ, De la Torre R, Mier M (1961) A method of evaluating disability in patients with Parkinson's disease. J Nerv Ment Dis 133:143–147
15. Webster DD (1968) Critical analysis of the disability in Parkinson's disease. Mod Treatment 5:257–282
16. Alba A, Trainor FS, Ritter W, Dacso MM (1968) A clinical disability rating for parkinsonian patients. J Chronic Dis 21:507–522
17. Klawans HL, Garvin JS (1969) Treatment of parkinsonism with levodopa. Dis Nerv Syst 30:737–746
18. Duvoisin RC (1970) The evaluation of extrapyramidal disease. In: De Ajuriagerra J (ed) Monoamines, noyaux gris centraux et syndrome de Parkinson. Masson, Paris, pp 313–325
19. Parkes JD, Zilkha KJ, Calver DM, Knill-Jones RP (1970) Controlled trial of amantadine hydrochloride in Parkinson's disease. Lancet I:259–262
20. Cotzias GC, Papavasilou PS, Fehling C, Kaufman B, Mena I (1970) Similarities between neurologic effects of L-dopa and apomorphine. N Engl J Med 282:31–33

21. Rinne UK, Sonninen V, Sirtola J (1970) L-dopa treatment in Parkinson's disease. Eur Neurol 4:348–369
22. McDowell F, Lee JE, Swift T, Sweet RD, Ogsbury JS, Tesslet JT (1970) Treatment of Parkinson's syndrome with dihydroxyphenylalanine (L-dopa). Ann Intern Med 72:29–35
23. Anden NE, Carlsson A, Kerstell J, Magnusson T, Olsson R, Roose BE, Steen B, Steg G, Svangorg A, Thieme G, Werdinius B (1970) Oral L-dopa treatment of parkinsonism. Acta Med Scand 187:247–255
24. Treciokas LJ, Ansel RD, Markham CH (1971) One to two years' treatment of Parkinson's disease with levodopa. Calif Med 114:7–16
25. Birkmayer W, Neumayer E (1972) Die moderne medikamentöse Behandlung des Parkinsonismus. Z Neurol 202:257–264
26. Potvin AR, Tourtellotte WW (1975) The neurological examination: advancement in its quantification. Arch Phys Med Rehabil 56:425–437
27. Lhermitte F, Agid Y, Signoret JL (1978) Onset and end-of-dose levodopa induced dyskinesia. Possible treatment by increasing the daily dose of levodopa. Arch Neurol 35:261–263
28. Diamond DG, Markham CH, Treciokas LJ (1978) A double-blind comparison of levodopa, Madopar and Sinemet in Parkinson's disease. Ann Neurol 3:267–272
29. Lieberman A, Dziatolowski M, Gopinathan G, Kupersmith M, Neophytides A, Korein J (1980) Evaluation of Parkinson's disease. In: Goldstein M (ed) Ergot compounds and brain function: neuro-endocrine and neuropsychiatric aspects. Raven, New York, pp 277–286

Discussion

Dr. Fahn: I just want to point out a couple of statements here. First of all, this wasn't meant by Hoehn and Yahr to be a rating scale, but a staging scale to follow natural history; I think that's something that should be kept in mind. The other thing is that this paper was written pre-L-dopa; they didn't have L-dopa when they were doing this staging. So they didn't even have the effects of the drugs to consider, which is also a feature. I think one of the striking things about that paper, by the way, besides the Hoehn and Yahr staging scale that they published in it, is the data of the patients themselves and their severity in the natural history prior to L-dopa. That is still the gold standard: we have to go by the data with nothing like that sense because of the presence of L-dopa.

The other thing is in terms of your criticism and ambiguities, nevertheless as you pointed out it's so widely used. Maybe in use there are all slightly different definitions and I think the thing about a good scale is that it can grow in time and it can be honed down (that's not a pun!) and improved upon; I think all of us have done that and that's what's happened with some of these modifications as people have used it over time.

Dr. Olanow: First of all I thought you did a really nice job of reviewing the history of this. I enjoyed it, but I really want to emphasize some of the comments that Stan just made. If Melvin Yahr were here now, I think one of the things he would point out very quickly is this was never meant to be a scoring system, particularly in patients who were receiving levodopa. This was meant to be a staging of untreated Parkinson patients and, as such, really doesn't have applicability anymore in today's levodopa-treated era. He himself has often told me that he is somewhat amused by the fact that we continue to use this as a standard for evaluating treated patients, which we all do. Your points are, I think, very well made, but I think in fairness to Dr. Yahr and to Dr. Hoehn, they saw this as a staging pre-levodopa and never really intended it to be looked on as a means of evaluating response to therapy, for example.

Dr. Rabey: Generally speaking, you are right, like Professor Fahn, that this is staging of the disease. But then, how do you explain that in the later paper by Margaret Hoehn in 1983, when she's considering and analyzing the progression and mortality of the disease, she's comparing the staging (stages I–IV) before and after levodopa. So one of the branches of the group still considers their classification as a baseline and continued publishing new data about mortality in 1987. After the congress in New York, they have kept giving you the staging according to their classification. Maybe there is some message orally in-between, but when you look at the papers, they keep giving you their original classifications.

Dr. Fahn: It was interesting to see the definition that Larsen did to change what stage I meant. I don't know how many people actually use which definitions. I'd like to take a poll vote here. How many people would use stage I to mean unilateral findings as a definition of stage I rather than disability. How many use that as the criteria for spreading patients in stage I, no matter how disabled they are on that side? And how many would use disability as a feature for that staging? So I think that answers that. They are taking Hoehn and Yahr's first definition: this is unilateral disease and that's stage I, no matter how severe. That goes back to the last comment we had. It doesn't rate severity per se. It relates to progression along the parts of the body as well as loss of posture.

Dr. Korczyn: But even this is ambiguous, I think. For example, what happens to a person who had unilateral disease and on examination we find that on activation of one limb you can also see contralateral rigidity. Does this mean that this is now nearly stage II or is it still stage I? I think we've learned a lot since 1967 and we know a lot even about the progression of the disease. I think that the idea behind the Hoehn and Yahr staging scale was that patients start off by being in stage I and may end up in stage V, and we now know that this is not necessarily true. There are patients who begin with having equilibrium problems, who are falling, before they have these unilateral problems. So actually this is the whole point of having stage 1.5, which was later added. But by the same token, one could also speak about stage 0.5, of patients having midline disability prior to having unilateral signs. So as a functional test or disability test, too, it does not include some of the other things that we know are very important in the life of patients with Parkinson's disease, for example cognitive and affective changes.

Dr. Streifler: Actually, the Hoehn and Yahr scale was meant to be an overall assessment of the patient's stage and it was preparatory to assessing the effect of drugs and treatment upon the patient's condition. It was just the beginning of the levodopa therapy and we had other therapies and the question was: What are doctors, what is medicine actually doing to this disease? So it was not so much a function test, although if you go with it you may derive certain conclusions about functional approvement or deterioration, etc. But you should have this in mind when we talk of the Hoehn and Yahr scale. So to make out of it now a functional test for functional assessment is probably not correct and it was not originally meant to be one.

A Rational Basis for a New Scoring System Measuring Disability in Parkinson's Disease

H. Baas, K. Stecker, N. Bergemann, and P.A. Fischer

Introduction

For the quantitative assessment of disability in Parkinson's disease (PD), a number of rating scales (RS; Alba et al. [1], Birkmayer et al. [4], Canter et al. [6], Duvoisin [9], Gerstenbrand et al. [12], Hoehn et al. [15], Markham et al. [22], Schwab et al. [26], Webster [32], Yahr et al. [33]) have been introduced and are used just like the numerous apparative tests (AT; [7,8,13,17,19,20,23–25,30]). Each of them has its specific advantages, disadvantages, and limitations. In particular, the adequate use of RS is limited by the fact that they are restricted to the ordinal data level, permitting only nonparametric statistics, and by the large number of items and poor interrater reliability. In contrast, the use of AT is limited by higher costs, sometimes by the need of sophisticated technical equipment, the registration of only partial aspects of complex PD symptomatology, and time-consuming procedures.

Although the Unified Parkinson's Disease Rating Scale (UPDRS) has recently become the most frequently used RS worldwide [10], until today no generally accepted consensus has been achieved on the basic requirements for the construction of an universally applicable scoring system for PD. For this purpose, the following main topics have to be clarified:

1. Which parts of the complex PD symptomatology (in addition to the classical *trias* akinesia, tremor, and rigidity) have to be regarded as important/characteristic ("cardinal symptoms") and should be covered by such a scoring system? Up to now no clear definition of the so-called cardinal symptoms based on experimental data exists.
2. How should RS be constructed in order to measure complex symptomatology as comprehensively as possible, and how can the data obtained from those RS be adequately reduced by sum-scoring or subsum-scoring?
3. Can a universal scoring system be based exclusively on RS, or where and to what extent is the additional use of AT necessary?

In 1989, a multicenter group[1] was founded in Germany to establish a universal scoring system for PD suitable for clinical long-term and pharmaceutical trials.

---

[1] H. Baas, P.A. Fischer, K. Stecker, N. Bergemann (Frankfurt/M); G. Deuschl, J. Schulte-Mönting (Freiburg); P. Kraus, H. Przuntek (Bochum); W. Oertel (München); W. Poewe (Berlin); E. Scholz (Tübingen).

The data from the study presented here were derived from this work. Some aspects of this paper have already been published in detail [3] earlier. The data elaborated to serve as a rational basis for the construction of a new scoring system which, after completion, will be presented in detail elsewhere.

Material and Methods

A total of 354 PD patients were examined by a standardized procedure. All examinations were performed by an experienced investigator, and no re-examinations were done.

The following RS/AT were applied:

1. Questionnaire of ten items on basic data and history [3]
2. Questionnaire of 30 items on subjective complaints (SC; [3])
3. von Zerssen scale (Bfs) for self-rating of emotional status [31]
4. Hoehn and Yahr scale (HY; [15])
5. Columbia University Rating Scale (CURS) to assess motor disability [33]
6. Purdue pegboard (PP) for finger dexterity right/left [29]
7. Modified Webster step/second test (WSST) for gait disability [32]
8. Scale of 14 items for disability of daily living activities (ADL; [3])
9. Sandoz Clinical Assessment Geriatric scale (SCAG) for global psychic status [27]
10. "Leistungsprüfsystem von Horn No. 1/2, 3/4, 6, 7, 10" (LPS) for intellectual status [16]
11. "Wiener Determinationsgerät" (WDG) to determine complex reactions (Schuhfried Ltd., A-2340 Mödling Austria)
12. Orthostatic blood pressure on the tilt table [5]
13. Clinical assessment of dementia
14. Assessment of fluctuations/dyskinesias [2]

The data obtained from this battery were analyzed stepwise by the following procedure (Fig. 1):

1. Cronbach's alpha was calculated to measure the instrumental reliability of the RS which were applied.
2. A factor analysis - principal component analysis (PCA) with and without orthogonal varimax rotation - was performed for CURS, ADL, SCAG, and SC to obtain information on the possibilities of data reduction (sum-scoring/subsum-scoring).
3. The PCA with orthogonal rotation was performed for the entire data battery including all subscores from the RS (see above) and all raw data obtained from the AT. The objective aim of this analysis was to get information about symptom complexes which have to be regarded as clinically relevant (cardinal symptoms) in PD. In all PCA, only factors with an eigenvalue greater than 0.5 were considered for interpretation.

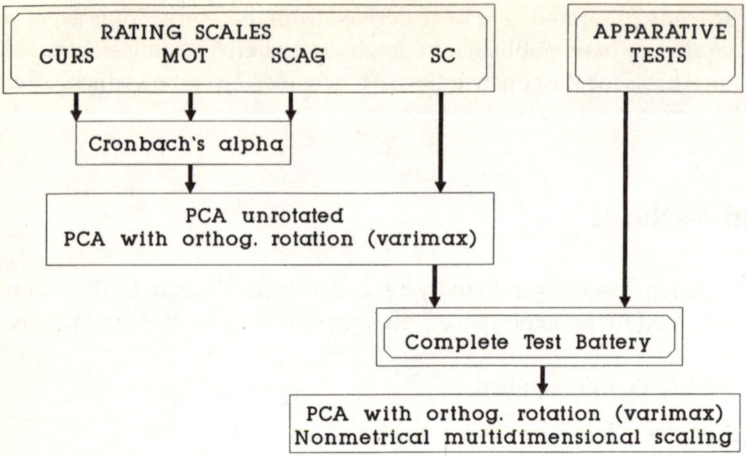

Fig. 1. Analytic procedure. Principal component analysis (PCA) was performed to test in RS and AT possibilities of data reduction by sum-scoring in rating scales and apparative tests. PCA and nonmetrical multidimensional scaling of the complete data were performed to identify cardinal symptoms. *CURS*, Columbia University rating scale; *SCAG*, Sandoz clinical assessment geratric scale; *SC*, subjective complaint. (See text for details)

4. The results of step 3 were verified by a different multivariate analysis procedure. For this purpose, a nonmetrical multidimensional scaling (NMDS) using the same data was performed [18].

Results

All three RS (CURS, ADL, SCAG) showed high instrumental reliability (Cronbach's alpha, 0.908, 0.893, and 0.921, respectively).

PCA of CURS

The PCA of the CURS without orthogonal rotation revealed two factors. One factor (loadings by CURS items 1,4, 10–25) could be interpreted as representing global motor disability. A second independent factor with loadings by CURS items 5–10 represented tremor.

After orthogonal rotation, the tremor factor remained unaffected, whereas the global factor could be divided into four subscores. According to their loadings they could be interpreted as gait disturbance, rigidity, dexterity of the right side, and dexterity of the left side.

From this PCA it is evident that sum-scoring and subsum-scoring of CURS items is possible if it is executed in accordance with above-mentioned factors. However, sum-scoring by summarizing all CURS items, as is frequently done, is not justified. Due to the similarities of the CURS with the motor part of the UPDRS, these results can probably be transposed to UPDRS without major modifications.

PCA of ADL

The PCA of the data from the ADL scale revealed a global score with loadings by all items (due to high intercorrelations between the items) with the exception of "impairment by pain," which formed an independent factor. After orthogonal rotation, "disability in writing" (ADL 9–11) was represented as an additional factor, and "pain" remained unchanged as an independent factor.

The structure of the ADL scale used in this analysis is very similar to most other well-established ADL scales. Due to high intercorrelations between the items on this scale some are obviously redundant and most ADL scales could be shortened without a major loss of information.

PCA of SCAG

The PCA of the SCAG without rotation again showed one global factor which represented global psychic impairment loaded by the majority of items (1–4, 6, 8, 9–16, 18). After orthogonal rotation, this global factor was differentiated into three factors which, due to their loading items, could be interpreted as "dementia" (1–4, 8, 12, 15, 16, 18), "depression" (5–7, 9, 11), and "alteration of patient's personality" (10, 14).

Therefore, the calculation of subsum scores is also possible for the SCAG. The structure of these scores is obviously different from scores that have been found for a population of normal elderly subjects [11,14].

PCA of SC

For the SC scale, only data analyzed by a PCA with orthogonal rotation are shown here, since, due to the obviously heterogeneous structure of the scale, no global factor was found. After rotation, a number of interpretable factors were found, mainly dealing with vegetative symptoms. Factor 1 represented orthostatic hypotension, factor 2, cardiac dysfunction, factor 3, subjective depressive symptoms, factor 4, exhaustion, factor 5, nausea, factor 7, sleep disturbances, factor 8, exogenous psychosis, factor 9, intestinal dysfunction, and factor 10, cardiac insufficiency. There was no reasonable interpretation for factor 6.

PCA of the Complete Test Battery

After orthogonal rotation, the PCA of the data of the complete test battery showed eight factors which could be interpreted meaningfully. The HY scale, all CURS subscores except tremor, ADL subscores except pain, the SCAG subscore for dementia, and the overall assessment of dementia showed high loadings on factor 1, which is therefore to be characterized as global impairment, mainly in the sense of motor disability, but also with some aspects of psychic alterations. Factor 2 showed loadings exclusively by the LPS data (LPS 1/2, 3/4, 6, 7, 10). It could therefore clearly be attributed to cognitive dysfunction. Factor 3 had loadings by the SCAG subscores for "depression" and "alterations of personality," as well as by "subjective depressive symptoms" and sleep "disturbances." Due to these loadings, it was likely to describe a depressive symptom complex. Results of some apparative motor tests were shown in factor 5 with loadings of PP right/left and WSST. WDG data were represented in an independent factor (factor 7). Orthostatic hypotension was also described by an independent factor (factor 6), with loadings by the tilt-table data and of "subjective orthostatic complaints." Factor 8 clearly described tremor, due to its exclusive loadings of the CURS subscore "tremor." Factor 10 was clearly related to pain, due to its isolated loadings by ADL pain data. For factors 4 and 9, no meaningful interpretation was possible. The remaining items of the test battery only showed loadings less than 0.5 to any of the factors. Summarizing this factor analysis, eight factors could be elaborated describing the following six major symptom complexes in PD:

1. Global (motor) impairment
2. Cognitive dysfunction
3. Depression
4. Orthostatic hypotension
5. Tremor
6. Painful sensations

Nonmetrical Multidimensional Scaling

An additional analysis of the same data by an NMDS led to similar, but slightly more detailed results. According to the stress values in this analysis (one dimension, 0.409; two dimensions, 0.207; three dimensions, 0.146; four dimensions; 0.106; five dimensions, 0.08) and the comparison with the corresponding stress value for random data (0.266; [28]), a three-dimensional graphic solution seemed to be adequate (Fig. 2). In the graph, a number of symptom clusters have been depicted. The first cluster was formed by HY, CURS subscores to gait, dexterity, and rigidity, PP right/left, WSST, some ADL subscores, and clinical assessment of dementia. This cluster obviously represented motor disability. The second cluster was formed by the SCAG depression score, the SCAG alterations in personality score, SC exhaustion, and SC exogenous psychosis. Therefore, it was likely to represent depression in PD. The third cluster was exclusively composed of items for assessment of fluctuations. Due to its formation by LPS and WDG scores, the fourth cluster could be identified as "cognitive dysfunction." The fifth cluster was formed by orthostatic dysregulation, indigestion, cardiac sensations and cardiac arrhythmia, nausea, sleep disturbances, and SC depression. This cluster could

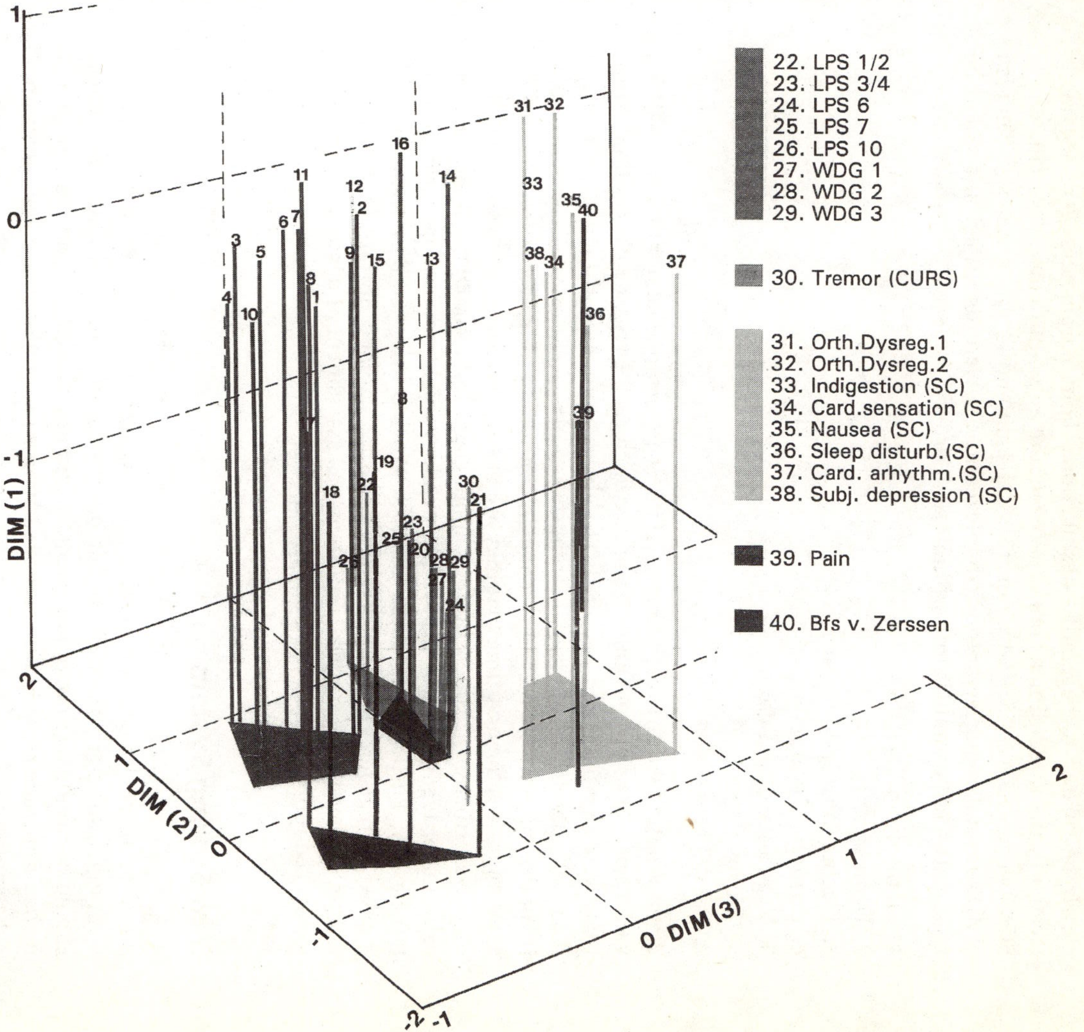

Fig. 2. Three-dimensional non-metrical multidimensional scaling soluton (stress = 0.146). Motor impairment, depression, dementia, tremor, pain, and vegetative dysfunctions are identified as major symptom complexes of Parkinson's disease (see text for details)

clearly be related to vegetative dysfunctions. Four parameters were separately located in the three-dimensional space without relation to any other cluster: (1) SCAG dementia, (2) CURS tremor, (3) ADL pain and (4) Bfs v. Zerssen. Thus, in NMDS the following symptom complexes in PD were described and could be regarded as important (listing without rank order):

1. Motor disability
2. Depression
3. Fluctuations/dyskinesias
4. Cognitive dysfunction
5. Vegetative dysfunction
6. Tremor
7. Painful sensations

By these latter two parts of the analysis (PCA with orthogonal rotation and NMDS), various main symptom complexes of PD which can be regarded as cardinal symptoms were identified and specified. The absence of major discrepancies between the results obtained from two different statistical procedures underlines the validity of the solution. To our knowledge, in contrast to other definitions of cardinal symptoms, it is the first time that they are based on an exact analysis of statistical data. Nevertheless, this description cannot claim to be complete, since, theoretically, major features of the PD symptomatology might not have been rated in our test battery. Furthermore, these analyses provide evidence that some methods applied to register PD symptoms are not adequate and do not lead to reliable results. Especially the simple, clinical, overall assessment of dementia seems to be influenced more by motor than by mental alterations.

New Scoring System

Based on these data, the development of the new scoring system to measure PD symptoms was started. On the one hand, the list of items of this scoring system should be minimal (time requirement, maximum 30 min), and on the other hand it should include reliable and valid measurements for all above-mentioned cardinal symptoms.

Since the development of the scoring system has not yet been completed, only its basic structure is demonstrated here. It consists of the following seven independent parts:

1. Basic data of history (13 items)
2. List of subjective complaints (36 items)
3. Rating scale of motor disability (19 items measuring akinesia, tremor and rigidity)
4. Rating scale of functional disability (9 items)
5. Scale to document fluctuations/dyskinesias (22 items)
6. Scale to measure dementia (DSM-III criteria; 13 items)

In each part of the scoring system, all items are constructed for strictly one-dimensional rating. The list of subjective complaints includes, in addition to other complaints, a number of vegetative dysfunctions. Intensity and frequency are rated separately. The rating scale of extrapyramidal motor symptoms is based on a one-dimensional 5-point scoring system and contains some additional integrative assessments. Otherwise, its basic construction is similar to part 3 of CURS/UPDRS. Functional disability in daily living activities is registered by a 5-point scoring system as well as by an integrative overall assessment of disability in a 0%–100% scale. Fluctuations/dyskinesias are also registered on a 5-point scoring system.

The fluctuations are qualitatively specified (wearing off, random on/off) and quantified with regard to the duration of off-periods (single-phased and cumulative). Dyskinesias are registered with regard to their intensity, duration, phenomenology, and distribution. For the assessment of dementia, a new scoring system based on anamnestic data closely following DSM-III criteria was developed, but the assessment of depression seems to be problematic. None of the methods used in the above-mentioned analysis fulfilled all the criteria for an adequate registration. Comparative examinations using various depression scales are planned to find out the most suitable instrument.

The application of the complete scoring system in the form presented here requires an overall examination time of more than 45 min per patient, which needs to be reduced to a maximum of 30 min for practicability reasons. Therefore, in a prephase the new scoring system will be tested for possibilities of data reduction by way of excluding redundant information. All individual parts will be tested for reliability and construct validity. It will be also tested whether the registration of some symptom complexes, e.g., vegetative symptoms, require additional apparative measurements.

Acknowledgment. This work was supported by the Bundesministerium für Forschung und Technologie, Germany.

References

1. Alba A, Trainor FS, Ritter W, Dacso MM (1968) A clinical disability rating for Parkinson patients. J Chronic Dis 21:507–522
2. Baas H, Fischer PA (1986) Fluktuationen der Beweglichkeit beim Parkinson-Syndrom. In: Fischer PA (ed) Spätsyndrome der Parkinson-Krankheit. Editiones Roche, Basel/Grenzach, pp 213–233
3. Baas H, Stecker K, Fischer PA (1993) Value and appropriate use of rating scales and apparative measurements in quantification of disability in Parkinson's disease. J Neural Transm Park Dement Sect 5:45–61
4. Birkmayer W, Neumayer E (1972) Die moderne medikamentöse Behandlung des Parkinsonismus. Z Neurol 202:257–280
5. Briebach T, Baas H, Fischer PA (1990) Orthostatische Regulationsstörung beim Parkinson-Syndrom. Nervenarzt 61:491–494
6. Canter GJ, de la Torre R, Mier M (1961) A method for evaluating disability in patients with Parkinson's disease. Nerv Ment Dis 133:143–147

7. Cassell K, Shaw K, Stern G (1973) A computerized tracking technique for the assessment of Parkinsonian motor disabilities. Brain 96:815–826
8. Cleeves L, Findley LJ, Gresty M (1986) Assessment of rest tremor in Parkinson's disease. Adv Neurol 45:349–352
9. Duvoisin RC (1970) The evaluation of extrapyramidal disease. In: Ajuriaguerra J (ed) Monoamines, noyeaux gris centraux et syndrome de Parkinson. Masson, Paris, pp 313–325
10. Fahn S, Elton RL, UPDRS Development Committee (1987) Unified Parkinson's disease rating scale. In: Fahn S, Marsden CD, Calne DB, Goldstein M (eds) Recent developments in Parkinson's disease. Macmillan Health Care Information, New York, pp 153–164
11. Gaitz CM, Varner RV, Overall JE (1977) Pharmacotherapy for organic brain syndrome in late life. Arch Gen Psychiatry 34:839–845
12. Gerstenbrand F, Klingler D, Poewe W, Schnaberth G (1986) Präsentation des Dokumentationsbogens für Parkinsonkranke der Österreichischen Parkinsongesellschaft. In: Schnaberth G, Auff E (eds) Das Parkinson-Syndrom. Editiones Roche, Vienna
13. Godwin-Austen RB, Tomlinson EB, Frears CC, Kok HWL (1969) Effects of L-dopa in Parkinson's disease. Lancet ii:165–168
14. Hamot HB, Patin RJ, Singer MJ (1984) Factor structure of the Sandoz Clinical Assessment Geriatric Scale (SCAG). Psychopharmacol Bull 20:142–150
15. Hoehn MM, Yahr MD (1967) Parkinsonism: onset, progression and mortality. Neurology 17:427–442
16. Horn W (1983) Leistungsprüfsystem (LPS) Handanweisung, 2nd edn. Hofgrefe, Göttingen
17. Jankovic J, Frosst JD (1980) Quantitative assessment of Parkinsonism and essential tremor: clinical application of triaxial accelerometry. Neurology 30:393
18. Kruskal JB (1964) Multidimensional scaling by optimizing goodness of fit to a non-metric hypothesis. Psychometrica 29:1–27
19. Lakke JPWF (1981) Classification of extrapyramidal disorders. J Neurol Sci 51:311–327
20. Larsen TA, Calne S, Calne DB (1984) Assessment of Parkinson's disease. Clin Neuropharmacol 7:165–169
21. Larsen TA, LeWitt PA, Calne DB (1983) Theoretical and practical issues in assessment of deficits and therapy in parkinsonism. In: Calne DB Horowski R, McDonald RJ, Wuttke W (eds) Lisuride and other dopamine agonists. Raven, New York, pp 363–373
22. Markham CH, Diamond SG (1981) Evidence to support early levodopa therapy in Parkinson's disease. Neurology 31:125–131
23. Parkes JD, Zilkha KJ, Calver DM, Knill-Jones RP (1970a) Controlled trial of amantadine hydrochloride in Parkinson's disease. Lancet i:259–262
24. Parkes JD, Zilkha KJ, Marsden CD, Baxter RCH, Knill-Jones RP (1970b) Amantadine dosage in treatment of Parkinson's disease. Lancet i:1130–1133
25. Potvin AR, Tourtellotte WW (1975) The neurological examination: advancements in its quantification. Arch Phys Med Rehabil 56:425–437
26. Schwab RS, England RC (1969) Projection technique for evaluating surgery in Parkinson's disease. In: Gillingham FJ, Donaldson MC (eds) 3rd symposium on Parkinson's disease. Livingstone, Edinburgh
27. Shader RI, Harmatz JS, Salzman C (1974) A new scale for clinical assessment on geriatric populations: SANDOZ Clinical Assessment Geriatric (SCAG). J Am Geriat Soc 22:107–113
28. Spence I (1979) A simple approximation for random ranking stress values. Multivariate Behav Res 14:355–356
29. Tiffin J (1979) Purdue Pegboard. Examiner Manual. Lafayette Instruments Company, Reorder no 7-435. Lafayette 2
30. Velasco F, Velasco M (1973) A quantitative evaluation of the effects of L-dopa on Parkinson's disease. Neuropharmacology 12:89–99
31. von Zerssen D, Koeller DM, Rey ER (1970) Die Befindlichkeits-Skala. Ein einfaches Instrument zur Objektivierung von Befindlichkeitstörungen, insbesondere im Rahmen von Längsschnittuntersuchungen. Arzneimittelforschung/Drug Res 20:915–918

32. Webster DD (1968) Critical analysis of the disability in Parkinson's disease. Mod Treatment 5:257–282
33. Yahr MD, Duvoisin RC, Schear MJ, Barrett RE, Hoehn MM (1969) Treatment of parkinsonism with levodopa. Arch Neurol 21:343–354

Discussion

Dr. Rabey: I realize that you put dementia factor in different columns, but I didn't understand what the interpretation of this was in the final evaluation.

Dr. Baas: The dementia was measured in different ways. Once we measured one clinical assessment. The rater, who was quite experienced, said the patient is demented or not demented. Also we checked this by some tests and what we found is that the result of the rating of the investigator was much more related to motor disability than to the results of these psychometric tests. Our interpretation of this is that it is obviously not possible to assess clinically, only clinically, dementia in parkinsonian patients. Motor disability probably gives the wrong impression. Many patients are probably rated by the global clinical impression as demented when they are not, because of motor disability. The same might also happen here for the SCAG dementia score. Above all, the SCAG scale did not lead to very impressive results. We also think that the SCAG scale is probably not sufficient to rate either dementia or depression in Parkinson's disease. This has to be replaced by another instrument, by another scale.

Dr. Rabey: But we're told that dementia is usually a clinical diagnosis according to DSM-III, but later on when you go on to score dementia, you use these items, which are not weighted in the same way. You diagnosed dementia by clinical functions. The measures you are using usually score the amount of dementia. But dementia and depression are clinical diagnoses according to DSM-III. It doesn't matter what the criteria are, but this is a clinical diagnosis. Of course you can't put the same weight on scoring the dementia, which is the next step after the diagnosis of dementia.

Dr. Baas: Anyway, if we really measure dementia by this clinical impression, it should be anywhere in this bright green area. Our results and our impressions should relate in some way to these results – but they don't.

Dr. Rabey: But the second point is that I would like to see what the advantage is of using this instead of, for example, the Folstein mini-mental score or the Hamilton or the Zung score. So if we have good methodology for scoring the amount of dementia or depression, why do we need to go back to another system? What are we adding to the methods we use?

Dr. Baas: I don't say that this is the optimal method. This evaluation just has to be done to identify some symptom complexes, just to tell you that you have to measure dementia. What the appropriate method to measure dementia is is another question. I don't want to comment on this. I don't say this is the best way to measure dementia. I'm just saying that this is not sufficient and this is probably not sufficient either. That's the next step. We have to compare different rating scales or any simple psychometric tests to see which is the best one to measure dementia in Parkinson's disease. For instance, we have done this for the mini-mental state; I don't have the data with me, but the results were quite bad because the mini-mental state doesn't measure slight dementia properly. You can only use it for moderate or severe dementia; here it's quite good, but it misses all those patients who are affected by a slight dementia. We very frequently see early stages of dementia in parkinsonian patients.

Dr. Fahn: That's why we all pass the test. Slight dementia isn't picked up by that.

Dr. Rabey: That's true, but we have the Wechsler Memory Scale, which was developed even before the Folstein mini-mental state and which is better and would take up all the modifications.

Dr. Baas: Yes, but it takes a lot of time.

Dr. Machetanz: It's on the same point. I have a question: isn't it possible that you don't measure dementia, but that you measure your specific test conditions and that your multidimensional scaling and your factor analysis does not identify what you believe it measures?

Dr. Baas: OK, that's always a problem with this sort of analysis. Sometimes you get some apparative factors that just reflect part of the measurements. But I think it's quite well validated that the LPS measures some cognitive dysfunctions; I think it does indeed measure something like dementia. But this is a question of interpretation, I must admit.

Dr. Machetanz: But you have completely different test environments and it could be that the NMDS and the factor analysis do not tell you what exactly responded in your test. It only shows you they're similar somehow, and so it could be that you just test the test condition, not the dementia.

Dr. Baas: I think that's a matter of the interpretation of what you do. I mean it's very difficult. How do you want to get more information, how do you want to get more precise information for the construction of a new rating scale? Most of the other rating scales have just been built up by personal experience of all those people who have created the rating scale; we at least tried to base it on some empirical data.

Dr. Korczyn: Is it possible that your dementia complex is actually a pseudo-dementia? I see that it overlaps very highly with the depression score.

Dr. Baas: It just overlaps here at the base, but you have to look at the three-dimensional space. Here the dementia score only goes up to this level, here in dimension 1, whereas the depression goes up much higher here in this first dimension.

Dr. Korczyn: But that's still consistent, I think, with the possibility that what you call dementia is pseudo-dementia, the manifestations of dementia which are related to an underlying depression.

Dr. Baas: Not according to this data. That's the reason to build it up in this three-dimensional space. Also, you have to look at the bottom of these bars and also at the top and I think there's quite a big difference.

Depression Inventories in Parkinson's Disease

T.A. Treves, D. Paleacu, J.M. Rabey, and A.D. Korczyn

Introduction

Although Parkinson's disease (PD) is primarily a motor disorder, increased attention has been directed towards other manifestations of the disease. Depression has been reported to occur in 32%–51% of patients with PD [1,2]. Recognition of affective changes is important, since it has therapeutic implications. The assessment of depression is based upon clinical impression, while its quantitative evaluation is expressed as scores obtained on "depression inventories," which were originally constructed for patients with endogeneous depression, but not validated for patients who suffer from organic, debilitating conditions. Most of the popular inventories, e.g., Hamilton's [3] and Beck's [4], contain items which refer to symptoms that can also be explained by the accompanying motor and/or mental impairment. Therefore, it is important to establish the reliability of such tests in PD. Also, it is possible that certain questions, not included in the depression inventories mentioned above, could apply more specifically to the depression of PD. The subjective nature of the depressive symptoms stresses the importance of patients' own evaluations of their affective state, as well as that of the caregiver. In the present study, we have compared the affective status assessed by the physician with the assessment made by patients and their caregivers.

Subjects and Methods

The motor, cognitive, and affective states of 105 consecutive PD patients referred to the Movement Disorder Clinic or the Department of Neurology of the Tel Aviv Medical Center were assessed by a senior neurologist (T.A. Treves or J.M. Rabey). The diagnosis of PD was made if at least three of the four cardinal signs of the disease were present, provided that there was no other etiology (such as medication, normopressive hydrocephalus, progressive supranuclear palsy, or Creutzfeldt-Jakob disease) that could be related to the symptomatology. The Hoehn and Yahr scale [5] was used to define motor severity, the mental status was quantified as the score obtained in the Hebrew version of a short mental test (SMT) [6], and presence of depression was evaluated by the physician using DSM-III-R criteria for major depressive episodes or dysthymia [7]. Another physician, D.

Paleacu, without knowing the diagnosis of depression made by the senior neurologist, asked the patient to indicate his affective state on a visual analog scale of 0–100 [8], where 0 means "no depression" and 100 "the worst state of depression one could have." Independently, the next of kin or the caregiver of the patient, whenever available ($n = 68$), were also asked to evaluate the affective state of the patient using the same clinimetric method. The same physician also submitted the Hamilton and Beck depression inventory (HDI, BDI, respectively; Appendices A, B), as well as five additional items, a priori expected to reflect depressive symptomatology (ADI, Appendix C).

For the sake of comparison between the physician's and the patients' or caregivers' evaluations of depression, the physician (senior neurologist) also translated the severity of depression on a visual analog scale. Depression severity was defined as none (for marks measuring 0%–9%), mild (10%–29%), moderate (30%–69%), or severe (70% or more). The distributions of such evaluations were analyzed and compared using chi-square test. Kappa index [9] was used to test agreement between the physician's, patients', and caregivers' evaluations of depression.

The HDI and BDI were each subdivided: items thought to be directly affected by the somatic aspects of PD (HDI-S, BDI-S) and "purely" affective items (HDI-A, BDI-A) were grouped separately, as indicated in Appendices A and B. Analysis of correlations between the scores obtained in the depression inventories (HDI, BDI, ADI), as well as their subscales, and the physician's, patients', and caregivers' evaluations were performed. Regression analysis was used to examine whether motor disability or cognitive state correlate with evaluation of depression and stepwise linear regression to identify which of the items included in the HDI, BDI, or ADI were best predictors of depression.

Results

Men ($n = 64$) and women ($n = 41$) had similar age, motor, and mental state distribution (Table 1) and were analyzed together. As indicated in Table 2, the physician (using DSM-III-R criteria) judged depression to be present in about half of the patients (mostly dysthymia). However, 9% of the patients were judged to be severely depressed (major depression type). In the evaluations of the patients themselves or of the caregivers, the frequency of depression was close to that calculated from the physician's evaluations; these evaluations rated 39%–47% of the patients as nondepressed and 12%–25% as mildly depressed (Table 2). Agreement between the physician and the patients and between the physician and the caregivers evaluations were good ($K = 0.81$ and 0.85, respectively). Patients with affective changes (DSM-III-R criteria) had higher depression inventories scores (mean HDI = 18; mean BDI = 38; mean ADI = 6) than those without (mean HDI = 12; mean BDI = 33; mean ADI = 2; $p < 0.001$). The scores cumulated in the different depression inventories correlated well with those obtained on their subscales

Table 1. Patients' characteristics

	Males	Females	Total
Number	64	41	105
Mean age ± SD (years)	72.4 ± 9.2	68.2 ± 9.9	70.7 ± 9.6
Stage Hoehn and Yahr I	2	2	4
Stage II	22	20	42
Stage III	27	15	42
Stage IV	12	2	14
Stage V	1	2	3
Mean SMT ± SD (%)	81.5 ± 15.7	79.3 ± 14.7	80.5 ± 15.3

SMT, short mental test; SD, standard deviation.

Table 2. Clinical evaluation of depression by physician, patients, and caregivers

Depression	DSM-III-R	Patients	Caregivers	
			(*n*)	(%)[a]
None	41	41	32	49
Mild	26	19	8	21
Moderate	29	39	23	20
Severe	9	6	5	10
Missing information	0	0	37	–
Total	105	105	105	100

Chi-square = 7.9 (degree of freedom, df = 6).
DSM-III-R, revised third edition of the Diagnostic and Statistical Manual of Mental Disorders [7].
[a] Frequency adjusted to total available information.

(Table 3). There were also good correlations between the physician's evaluation and the HDI, the BDI, and particularly the ADI, for which it was stronger (Table 4). Regardless of severity of motor impairment, "somatic" items of the HDI (HDI-S) and BDI (BDI-S) maintained a significant correlation with the existence of depression rated according to the DSM-III-R (Table 5), although this correlation was lower than that observed between the DSM-III-R rating and the "affective" items (HDI-A and BDI-A, respectively). The severity of depression (DSM-III-R criteria) was not affected by the motor impairment ($r = -0.07$, $p = 0.25$) nor by the mental status ($r = -0.12$, $p = 0.15$) of the patients. However, there was a trend toward higher rating of depression by the patients who had lower scores on the short mental test (SMT) and increased motor impairment ($r = 0.17$, $p = 0.08$, and $r = 0.15$, $p = 0.07$, respectively).

Table 3. Correlations between scores obtained in the different depression inventories in Parkinson's disease[a]

	HDI	HDI-A	HDI-S	BDI	BDI-A	BDI-S
HDI-A	0.96					
HDI-S	0.90	0.74				
BDI	0.79	0.77	0.67			
BDI-A	0.74	0.74	0.62	0.97		
BDI-S	0.71	0.68	0.65	0.84	0.67	
ADI	0.50	0.50	0.43	0.55	0.57	0.39

HDI, Hamilton depression inventory; BDI, Beck's depression inventory; ADI, additional items; –A, affective items; –S, somatic items.
$p < 0.001$ for all correlations.
[a] The numbers in cells are Pearson correlation coefficients.

Table 4. Correlations between clinical evaluations and depression inventories

	DSM-III	Pt	CG
ADI	0.68	0.69	0.69
HDI	0.59	0.61	0.67
BDI	0.45	0.48	0.56

The numbers in the cells correspond to Pearson correlation coefficients; for all of them $p \leq 0.002$.
Pt, patients; CG, caregivers; HDI, Hamilton depression inventory; BDI, Beck's depression inventory; ADI, additional items.

Table 5. Correlations between DSM-III-R evaluation and depression inventories by motor severity

	HDI	HDI-A	HDI-S	BDI	BDI-A	BDI-S	ADI
HY-I	0.68	0.72	0.46	0.72	0.42	0.83*	0.41
HY-II	0.46*	0.57**	0.28*	0.46*	0.50*	0.29*	0.74**
HY-III	0.59**	0.72**	0.34*	0.45*	0.49**	0.30*	0.67**
HY-IV and V	0.64*	0.68*	0.44	0.66*	0.47	0.83**	0.28
All Pts	0.59**	0.64**	0.35*	0.45*	0.49**	0.38*	0.68**

HY, Hoehn and Yahr scale; Pts, patients; HDI, Hamilton depression inventory; BDI, Beck's depression inventory; ADI, additional items; –A, affective items; –S, somatic items.
*$p \leq 0.05$ and **$p \leq 0.001$ for Pearson correlation coefficients that appear in the cells.

The items with greater capacity of predicting diagnosis of depression, based on DSM-III-R criteria, are presented in Table 6. The first item of the HDI (evaluation of mood) was also the one that accounted for most of the variance in similar regression analysis based on the patients and their caregivers ratings.

Table 6. Best predictors of diagnosis of depression in Parkinson's disease (DSM-III-R)[a]

Rank	Item	Symptom category	R square
1	HDI-1	Depressed mood	0.42
2	ADI-5	Overreaction	0.50
3	HDI-3	Suicide	0.54
4	HDI-20	Paranoid symptoms	0.56
5	HDI-18	Diurnal variation	0.58
6	BDI-5	Guilt feeling	0.59
7	BDI-8	Self-accusations	0.61
8	BDI-13	Indecisiveness	0.63
9	ADI-4	Interest in hobbies	0.64
10	BDI-14	Body image	0.65

HDI, Hamilton depression inventory; BDI, Beck's depression inventory; ADI, additional items.
[a] After stepwise linear regression analysis. R square reflects the variance associated with the use of the factor under consideration. Only the first ten discriminatory items are shown.

Discussion

The distribution of depression in our PD population was similar to that found in other PD studies [10–13]. Depression is a common feature in PD, and it may result from several factors. Neurotransmitters thought to be decreased in endogeneous depression may also be abnormally low in PD [2,10,14]. Also, it has been shown that patients with PD frequently report a history of "psychoneurosis" or depression several years prior to the onset of extrapyramidal symptomatology [15–17]. Secondly, any progressive incapacitating disease is likely to result in reactive depression [18,19]; however, depression in PD patients was found to be more prevalent than in other elderly chronically disabled subjects [19,20]. It is also possible that cultural factors can affect the prevalence of depression in PD, since in China only 4.6% of PD patients were found to be depressed [21]. Thus, there seems to be a complex relationship between PD and depression.

Patients' and caregivers' evaluations were similar to the physician's diagnosis. This was not surprising, since the clinical diagnosis depends mainly on information provided by the patient or caregiver. The recognition of depression may be complicated, because some of its features are also present in PD. These include hypomimia, bradykinesia, bradyphrenia, and impairment in daily activities. However, it is important to diagnose depression in PD, since drug therapy may reverse the affective changes. In addition to clinical evaluation, rating scales are useful in the follow-up of patients and in assessing the efficacy of treatment.

Our results seem to confirm the validity of the common depression inventories in PD. The correlation between the scores obtained in the HDI and the BDI was high, as previously observed for patients with primary affective disorder [22,23]; this was not unexpected, because of the overlap in several items of these questionnaires. The correlations between the clinical evaluation of depression on one hand and the scores of the HDI, BDI, and ADI on the other hand were good, thus validating these scales in the evaluation of depression in PD. The correlation between the diagnosis of depression according to the DSM-III-R and the "affective" subscales was slightly higher than for the global depression inventories (HDI, BDI). The satisfactory correlations with the "affective" subscales (Table 5) suggests that the inventories employed by us reflect the depression present in PD and, as was already mentioned for BDI [24], somatic items do not detract from their validity. As in other studies [12,13], PD patients with advanced physical disability did not necessarily have significantly higher depression scores. Huber et al. [25] found an association between the "somatic symptoms" of the BDI and the motor impairment of the patients, while the "affective symptoms" did not differ between mildly disabled and more advanced cases; such a trend was not obvious in our results (Table 5).

From the large number of items included in the inventories studied, those correlated best with the clinical diagnosis of depression in PD are listed in Table 6. Most of these items are not expected to be directly affected by the somatic aspects of the disease (Appendices A, B), which may suggest that in depression of PD, symptoms expressing "purely" affective state have heavier clinical weight than those resulting from the motor disability.

In conclusion, clinimetric methods, as presented here, were shown to be valid for the evaluations of depression in PD. Although the symptoms of the disease may bias the evaluation of depression on the one hand, and the depression inventories are strongly related to somatic-related items on the other hand, these depression inventories still correlated better with the affective-related items. However, selection of the most predictive items of depression may restrict "somatic" contamination in the measurement of depression in PD.

Appendix A. Hamilton rating scale for depression (HDI)

1. Depressed mood
2. Feeling of guilt
3. Suicide
4. Insomnia, early
5. Insomnia, middle
6. Insomnia, late
7.[1] Loss of work and interests
8.[1] Retardation
9. Agitation
10.[1] Anxiety, psychic
11.[1] Anxiety, somatic
12.[1] Loss of appetite
13.[1] Somatic symptoms, general
14. Loss of libido
15. Hypochondriasis
16. Loss of insight
17.[1] Loss of weight
18. Diurnal variation
19. Depersonalization and loss of sense of reality
20. Paranoid symptoms
21. Obsessional and compulsive symptoms

[1]Somatic items.

Appendix B. Beck depression inventory (BDI): symptom–attitude categories

A	Mood	L	Social withdrawal
B	Pessimism	M	Indecisiveness
C	Sense of failure	N	Body image
D	Lack of satisfaction	O[1]	Work inhibition
E	Guilty feeling	P[1]	Sleep disturbance
F	Sense of punishment	Q[1]	Fatiguability
G	Self-hate	R[1]	Loss of appetite
H	Self-accusations	S[1]	Weight loss
I	Self-punitive wishes	T[1]	Somatic preoccupations
J	Crying spells	U	Loss of libido
K	Irritability		

Appendix C. Additional depression inventory (ADI)

1. Do you feel you are less inclined to enjoy yourself and laugh at jokes than you once did? (score 0–2) ——
2. Are you less careful about your outward appearance than you once were? (score 0–2) ——
3. Do you feel indifferent or less involved in what is happening around you? (Score 0–2) ——
4. Do you feel that you have less interest in hobbies (such as reading, watching TV, or others) than you once had? (score 0–2) ——
5. Do you feel irritable and that you overreact to minor nuisances? (score 0–2) ——

References

1. Santamaria J, Tolosa E, Valles A (1986) Parkinson's disease with depression: a possible subgroup of idiopathic Parkinsonism. Neurology 36:1130–1133
2. Mayeux R, Stern Y, Sano M, Rosenstein R, Williams JHW, Cote LJ (1987) Coexisting dementia and depression in Parkinson's disease: "double trouble." Ann Neurol 22:134
3. Hamilton M (1967) Development of a rating scale for primary depressive illness. Br J Soc Clin Psychol 6:278–296
4. Beck AT, Ward C, Mendelson M, Mock J, Erbaugh J (1961) An inventory for measuring depression. Arch Gen Psychiatry 4:561–571
5. Hoehn MM, Yahr MD (1967) Parkinsonism: onset, progression and mortality. Neurology 17:427–442
6. Treves TA, Ragolsky M, Gelernter I, Korczyn AD (1990) Evaluation of a short mental test for the diagnosis of dementia. Dementia 1:102–108

[1]Somatic items.

7. American Psychiatric Association (1987) Diagnostic and statistical manual of mental disorders, 3rd edn, revised. Washington DC, pp 213–233
8. Aitken RCB (1969) Measurement of feelings using visual analogue scales. Proc R Soc Med 62:989–993
9. Feinstein AR (1985) Statistical indexes of association. In: Feinstein AR (ed) Clinical epidemiology: the architecture of clinical research. Saunders, Philadelphia, pp 170–190
10. Mayeux R, Stern Y, Williams JHW, Sano M, Cote LJ (1986) Depression and Parkinson's disease. Adv Neurol 45:451–455
11. Celesia GG, Wanamaker MM (1972) Psychiatric disturbances in Parkinson's disease. Dis Nerv Syst 33:577–583
12. Starkstein SE, Preziosi TJ, Bolduc PL, Robinson RG (1990) Depression in Parkinson's disease. J Nerv Ment Dis 178:27–31
13. Mayeux R, Stern Y, Rosen J, Leventhal J (1981) Depression, intellectual impairment and Parkinson's disease. Neurology 31:645–650
14. Wolfe N, Katz DI, Albert, ML, Almozlino A, Durso R, Smith MC, Volicer L (1990) Neuropsychological profile linked to low dopamine: in Alzheimer's disease, major depression, and Parkinson's disease. J Neurol Neurosurg Psychiatry 53:915–917
15. Rajput AH, Offord KP, Beard CM, Kurland LT (1987) A case-control study of smoking habits, dementia, and other illnesses in idiopathic Parkinson's disease. Neurology 37:226–232
16. Todes CJ, Lees AJ (1985) The pre-morbid personality of patients with Parkinson's disease. J Neurol Neurosurg Psychiatry 48:97–100
17. Treves TA, Rabey JM, Korczyn AD (1990) Case-control study with use of temporal approach for evaluation of risk factors for Parkinson's disease. Mov Disord 5[Suppl 1]:11 (abstract)
18. Gotham AM, Brown RG, Marsden CD (1986) Depression in Parkinson's disease: a quantitative and qualitative analysis. J Neurol Neurosurg Psychiatry 49:381–389
19. Koenig HG, Meador KG, Cohen HJ, Blazer DG (1988) Depression in elderly hospitalized patients with medical illness. Arch Intern Med 148:1929–1936
20. Robins AH (1976) Depression in patients with Parkinsonism. Br J Psychiatry 128:141–145
21. Chen RC (1989) Clinical profile of Parkinson's disease among Chinese in Taiwan. Abstracts of XIVth world congress on neurology, New Dehli. Neurology India 37[Suppl]:270 (abstract)
22. Bailey J, Coppen A (1976) A comparison between the Hamilton rating scale and the Beck inventory in measurement of depression. Br J Psychiatry 128:486–489
23. Faravelli C, Albanesi G, Poli E (1986) Assessment of depression: a comparison of rating scales. J Affective Disord 11:245–253
24. Levin BE, Llabre MM, Weiner WJ (1988) Parkinson's disease and depression: psychometric properties of the Beck Depression Inventory. J Neurol Neurosurg Psychiatry 51:1401–1404
25. Huber SJ, Freidenberg DL, Paulson GW, Shuttleworth EC, Christy JA (1990) The pattern of depressive symptoms varies with progression of Parkinson's disease. J Neurol Neurosurg Psychiatry 53:275–278

Round Table Discussion 1: Scoring

Dr. Hallett: We have been hearing historical aspects of a number of different features, which have all been very interesting. One of the parameters that we heard about in relation to the DATATOP study is the moment required for L-dopa to be begun in a particular patient. I wonder whether that particular parameter has ever been judged against any of the other ones that we have talked about. What is the history of that particular parameter and has it ever been validated in any other way compared to any of these other scores?

Dr. Fahn: This was an evolution – more a revolution I guess – a development. And how to judge this? It can only be used by people who feel that they don't start levodopa on any other basic other than disability. So if you're going to start on the day of diagnosis, obviously this is not a good rating scale. As a rating scale for disability, that's a different story, and that's how this was used. So you had investigators who were willing to say they're disabled enough to the point that they need to do something about it and that's how the concept came about. It hasn't been validated against anything else, but if you want you can compare it with UPDRS in this sense, because we have seen it compares very favorably. Actually, it may even be more sensitive. I think the *p* value – I don't think that's a measure of sensitivity, but nevertheless – the *p* value – was greater than it would be for differences in the UPDRS scale at the time of endpoint. Basically, what it amounts to is that the big advantage in having an endpoint is that it tells you "all or nothing"; in other words, that patients die or the patients live. It's a very simple kind of endpoint for statisticians to use for evaluation compared to parametric and nonparametric tests. And that's of course, a global judgement; two physicians may interpret a patient's needs differently. On the other hand, when you don't know what the patients are on whether – placebo or drug – it's still your judgement on that particular patient. The other problem with this as a single scale comparing one person with another is the fact that some people are young, are working, and have to be on the factory line and thus can't have any slowness, whereas others are retired. So again, in any population you have to have the same kind of patients to make valid comparisons. So it is not good in that sense either. As far as how it turned out – although there were doubts about it being included by the NIH reviewers and everything – it turned out to be a very simple thing, because what ends up happening in Parkinson's disease (and I hadn't seen this reported anywhere, but the DATATOP investigators have been aware of it) is that just before reaching that endpoint the patient seems to go off the edge; they can no longer continue what they're doing the way they've been doing it and they reach endpoint. It's very dramatic. It's like a sudden worsening. Everything collapses. All their compensation factors have now crumbled. Now they need the drug. So it's not that difficult to judge. That's an interesting feature, too, in the disease by itself. So that kind of endpoint is pretty easy to use.

Dr. Hallett: Was it compared to the Schwab and England part of the scale?

Dr. Fahn: For the other choices – what other choices should we have. One of the proposals was you have to reach a Schwab and England of 70 or 60 or 65, then that's your endpoint. It turns out that most people didn't reach that. They wanted treatment before they got the Schwab and England 70, it turns out.

Dr. Korczyn: So who decided that, the patient or the physician?

Dr. Fahn: This was the physician's decision, not the patient's. A lot of patients wanted to continue. They want to hold out, but the physicians decided in each case on the final endpoint in DATATOP: the physician's decision that you need to be on medication, you're too disabled, or your disability's imminent.

Dr. Korczyn: Could it happen the other way round, that the patient says he wants to go on medication and the physician says no?

Dr. Fahn: Yes, if the patient wants to go on medicine because they don't want to hold off any more and the physician feels that they are not ready, they can go on medicine but then they are removed from the study. You can't stop them from going on medicine. We had a few terminations, a small number of people, mostly because they had to leave, because they moved to a different city. There are some patients who said, "Look here, I don't want to do this any more, I want to be on medicine." So there are those, even though they weren't considered disabled by the doctor.

Dr. Rabey: Two points. First, I think that one of the ways to answer this question is to put the delta of the total disability scale in each patient and to check the delta for each when he needs the rescue drug.

Dr. Fahn: That is one of the things that's extremely interesting. If you look at the Unified Parkinson's Disease Rating Scale (UPDRS) at the time of endpoint for the deprenyl group and the non-deprenyl group, it was about the same. But it took 9 months to 1 year longer to reach it. No one knew what they were on. That is what is so striking about it. It was very consistent.

Dr. Rabey: But then there is some contradiction between that and what you mentioned before, that before they ask for the drug you suddenly realized that they were doing very badly. So something is missing there.

Dr. Fahn: This is the endpoint score. What I just gave you was: "What were they like at that time? What were their total scores?" Whether they were in the deprenyl group or the placebo group, the scores were the same in the end. It just took that much longer to get there.

Dr. Klotz: I would like to hear some comments about the problem of selectivity. When I have a patient who has broken a joint and I have to rate his gait, I have problems. How could we solve this problem?

Dr. Fahn: That's a big problem. We have lots of patients who have broken a hip or have arthritis. Obviously, if you can't rate it, you just leave it blank, unrateable at that stage of the disease. The same thing is true if you have a man who's lost an arm. You can't rate tremor or bradykinesia in that arm. That's true with everything, even if you wanted to do quantitative rating scales of the right hand. You just can't use the right hand.

Dr. Klotz: But the problem is that if I do that, I have a big loss of data and so I might not be able to use my data for any statistical analysis.

Dr. Fahn: If you were doing a quantitative study, for example of drug trials, you would probably have to exclude patients like that who you can't rate. I don't think you can include them in a study.

Dr. Potvin: I wonder if we might at least begin to see if there is any consensus forming here or if we're eternally divided. The issue is (taking Parkinson's disease as an example) one of using rating scales and then doing a nonparametric data analysis: should we add or average or use parametric statistical tests. I wonder whether anyone in the room would speak in favor of doing parametric analysis on rating scales? Are we divided on this or are we reaching a consensus? I think it's an important issue.

Dr. Fahn: The question is whether we should start to use parametric analysis for these kinds of nonparametric data.

Dr. Korczyn: Ray Watts said it all. You should use it only if you want to publish in the *New England Journal of Medicine* or in the *Lancet*. But if you want to be scientific, you can't use it.

Dr. Fahn: Are you saying you can't publish in any other journal?

Dr. Korczyn: *Movement Disorders* doesn't accept papers that have been incorrectly statistically analyzed.

Dr. Klotz: The problem is that if I take a look at other scales constructed after Likert 1932, parametric analysis is allowed; for some questions it should be possible to use parametric statistics, but for other cases, if I have problems with multidimensionality, I think I shouldn't use them.

Dr. Korczyn: Can you give an example?

Dr. Klotz: If we take the Webster rating scale, it's really problematic to add up tremor and the other items to one sum score and then to make parametric statistics. I don't think that's allowed. But to take the other nine items, which are about one dimension, I could say the sum score is something about a Likert scale which I could use.

Dr. Korczyn: I really don't see how you can do that, because it's nonlinear and there is no way that you could use a *t* test for that, or say that mean and standard deviation has any meaning.

Dr. Klotz: There is also the question of whether we have an ordered metric or only a ranked scale. It's true that there are some nonlinearities, but if I take enough items that can be partialized out, I could use it, but I always have to use it carefully.

Dr. Korczyn: I don't think I agree. Perhaps we should leave it at that: I am not a statistician.

Dr. Fahn: I think we need a panel of statisticians to discuss this. I don't know how many of us feel competent to handle the question Dr. Potvin raised.

Dr. Korczyn: If we had such a panel, there's another question I would raise. I would ask how you analyze statistically the UPDRS. If you have a patient whose score is mainly because of tremor and another person who gets the same number of points because of bradykinesia or whatever, you cannot put them together.

Dr. Klotz: That's true; I cannot put different symptoms together. But if I accentuate four extremities on the one hand, and on the other hand I take an overall look at a symptom, I have different weights, which causes problems.

Dr. Hallett: I have another question for Dr. Korczyn. We heard earlier – and it's certainly true – that motivation plays a big role in motor performance. It certainly seems to be true that depression would have some influence on motivation. Yet you found a very poor correlation between depression and motor scores. Why is that the case? Why shouldn't there be more of an effect by depression on motor performance?

Dr. Korczyn: Firstly, it could work both ways. You could also say that people who are more severely impaired, with a Hoehn and Yahr scale of IV, should be more depressed because they are more severely sick than those patients who only have a score of I or II and are still functioning. Basically, I think what you've said about the influence of motivation on functioning is absolutely true, but it's even truer if you measure something than if you ask for historical data. The Hoehn and Yahr scale mainly deals with functioning at home. Probably patients who are severely depressed could be reduced from Hoehn and Yahr scale IV–V to III–IV; we did not rule out this possibility, but just did not find a correlation. So maybe if we had a much larger population, if we had a lot more patients who are severely depressed, it could have been shown, but in our population we did not find it.

Dr. Rabey: There was a paper by Lang in *Brain* about 3 years ago about a correlation between depression, Parkinson's disease, and movement time. He found that patients with depression were very bradykinetic. They have a relatively high grade of bradykinesia that has got nothing to do with Parkinson's disease. Conversely, there were parkinsonians who were not depressed, but who showed some items of depression.

Dr. Spieker: I think there is another big problem. How do you assess treatment effects in very mildly affected patients who have scores of 1 in most items before treatment and are very much better after treatment, but still do not have a score of 0? I think that's a problem with de novo studies.

Dr. Fahn: Do you mean mildly affected patients who just don't go down from 1 to 0?

Dr. Spieker: Who don't go down completely to 0, so you have almost the same scores and the same sum scores on your rating scale, although they report that they are very much better.

Dr. Fahn: When I held my talk, I didn't mention the fact that if you can't decide between a score of I and a II, it's 1.5. The same thing is true between a 0 and a I. In fact, if I only can detect rigidity by reinforcement maneuver, I personally give it a score of 0.5 automatically. Again, this is not stated in any text or definition, but you begin to use these things. So there are possible ways to hone it down a little bit.

Dr. Korczyn: I think the answer to your question is that if you can't rate it clinically, you have to use an instrument.

Selecting Neurologic Function Tests for Parkinson's Disease: A Primer

A.R. Potvin, W.W. Tourtellotte, G.V. Kondraske,
K. Syndulko, and J.H. Potvin

Introduction

Recent advances in quantitative procedures have greatly enhanced the sensitivity, objectivity, and reliability of neurologic evaluation and diagnosis. Innovative electrophysiologic, radiologic, and biochemical laboratory procedures have proven useful to the clinician, whose traditional evaluation of the patient has been based on inference and indirect evidence of disease processes and pathologies.

However, a continuing problem in neurologic evaluation has been the lack of widely available devices to obtain sensitive, objective, and reliable measures of neurologic functions or performance associated with sensory and motor activities. The problem is serious for investigators who wish to evaluate the efficacy of neuropharmacologic drugs or other therapy in patients physically handicapped by neurologic or muscular disease or trauma.

In recent years, several quantitative approaches have evolved to measure neurologic functions. In addition to electrophysiologic, electroneuromyographic, and cognitive neuropsychologic methods, six approaches have been used clinically: (1) the classic neurologic examination, (2) coded examinations of neurologic function (rating scales), (3) motion picture ratings, (4) instrumented activities of daily living tests, (5) instrumented non-computerized neurologic function tests, and (6) computer-automated neurologic function tests.

Since the availability of effective pharmacologic treatment for Parkinson's disease (PD) in the late 1960s, investigators have developed and used these quantitative approaches to measure changes in motor functions over time and in clinical trials. The scope of tests has ranged from the crude and amateurish to the sophisitication of space-age technology. The literature, today, includes numerous studies, some equivocal, but also a good number of sound investigations. Several investigators have evaluated the functions of their patients for a decade or more.

Based on past experiences in developing and using tests for PD [1–3,18,19,21,23–25,30,31,33,34,38–40,42,43] and for other patient and normal subject groups [4,6,7,10,11–17,20,22,24,26–29,32,35,36,38,41], we believe that criteria can be established for selecting and evaluating tests and for improving the design and conduct of clinical studies. It is our objective in this report to propose such criteria and to recommend tests for specific studies in PD. Figure 1 shows the main requirements for and applications of instrumented tests in PD.

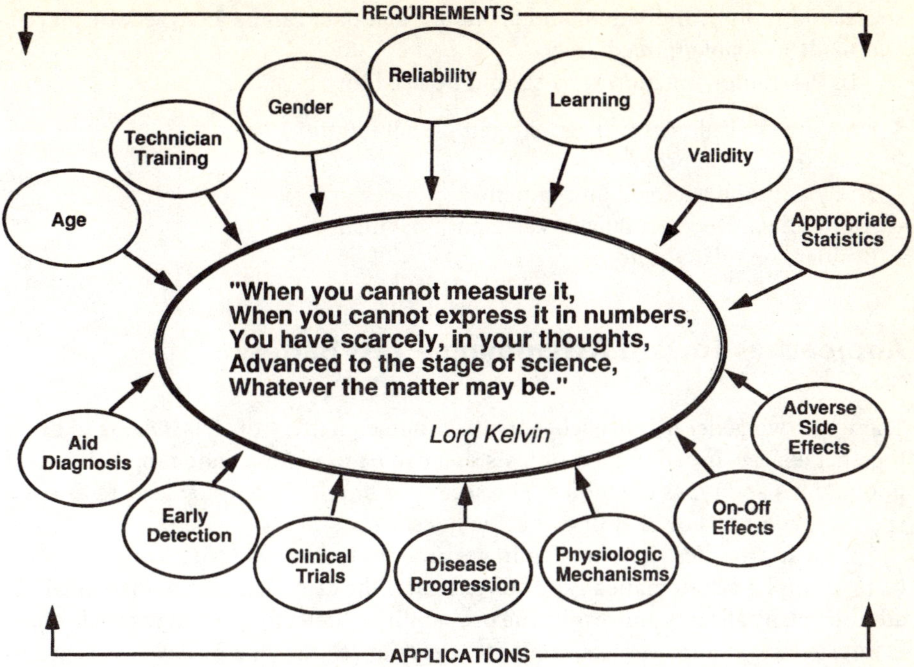

Fig. 1. Rationale for using instrumented tests in Parkinson's disease, key evaluation studies, and major areas of application

Motor Function Tests and Their Areas of Application

The purpose of motor function tests in PD is to follow modest to large improvements or worsenings in function that occur over time with and without treatment. Tests are used in clinical trials and in clinical practice to follow disease progression. The major types of motor functions include strength, reactions, speed and coordination of movement, tracking, muscle tone, steadiness, range of motion, gait, postural sway, and activities of daily living. Sensations such as two-point discrimination, temperature, vibration sense, vision, and audition are often excluded because PD does not affect sensory systems.

Tests of motor function may be in the form of rating scales, motion picture ratings, or instrumented tests with or without inclusion of a computer. Motion picture ratings are exceedingly time-consuming and for this reason are seldom used. Rating scales are the least expensive and the most quickly completed, and, for these reasons, are the most widely used. However, even in the best of designs, rating scales lack sensitivity, reproducibility, and reliability [10]. Instrumented tests are the most sensitive and, if evaluated appropriately, can be demonstrated to be reproducible, reliable, and valid. Computer-automated instrumented tests are preferred over instrumented tests without the computer because they save time, space, and money. Individual and group patient data can be analyzed, displayed, and made available immediately.

In PD, motor function tests should be used to:

- Evaluate clinical trials (drugs, surgery, rehabilitation)
- Evaluate disease progression
- Study pathophysiologic mechanisms
- Aid in diagnosis, particularly early parkinsonism
- Evaluate on–off symptoms

Approaches Toward Assembling a Test Battery

There are two general approaches to assembling a battery of tests. One is to bring together a large, broad battery of tests that can be used for a wide range of patient populations and types of studies. The second is to tailor a few key tests to assess a specific hypothesis or answer a specific question.

Both approaches present advantages and disadvantages. With a broad battery of tests applied systematically to all patients, the technician remains skilled in administering all tests uniformly; the probability of detecting an adverse side effect is improved; patients who subsequently experience a trauma or develop a second disease affecting different neurologic functions have a quantitative medical record; and a substantial patient data base for each test is rapidly developed. Disadvantages include capital costs, time to administer tests, and the volume of data analysis, display, and storage. With a small test battery, capital costs are lower, technician training is easier, less time is required to administer tests, and data analysis, display, and storage are easier to manage. The disadvantages are that important tests may be inadvertently omitted, adverse side effects are less likely to be detected, and a smaller data base is developed.

When selecting tests for a specific study, the investigator should carefully balance the advantages and disadvantages discussed above, along with all the important questions and application areas that are foreseeable. Clearly, it is preferable to include a few too many rather than too few tests. The costs of repeating a study far outweigh the savings of a few minutes testing time per patient.

An important consideration in assembling a test battery is the utility of a computer for automation of test sequencing and data collection, analysis, display, storage, and retrieval. With modern, low-cost yet powerful personal computers, the advantages of computer automation are enormous, even for a small five-test battery.

Criteria for Accepting a Test

The major criteria for selection, acceptance, and use of neurologic function tests are as follows:

1. Test is easy for:
   - Patient to understand
   - Technician to administer and obtain measure
   - Investigator to interpret and use
2. Device is small size, reproducible, economical
3. Test preparation and duration are short (<5–10 min)
4. Test has demonstrated reliability and reproducibility
5. Test has validity for patient diagnosis, monitoring, and treatment
6. Effects of age, gender, learning, and handedness are known
7. Test can be done by all patients with function ranging from normal to severe loss
8. Device can be interfaced to low-cost computer for automated testing and data management

Clinical investigators are advised to seek the assistance of a senior biostatistician to design studies to evaluate each test under consideration. Potvin and Tourtellotte [16] provide experimental designs and examples.

A particularly important criterion is the evaluation for reliability. In clinical settings, reliability data are both widely used and abused. It is, of course, easy to obtain high values for the Pearson product moment correlation coefficient, r. The investigator need only include patients with functions ranging from normal to severe loss and conduct a study with a test–retest interval that is very short, perhaps less than 1 min. Resulting values for r can exceed 0.95, but such a study is both meaningless and misleading.

Recognizing that the purpose of many clinical studies and the goal of physician and patient is restoration of function to normal, studies for reliability should be done by testing normal subjects. Because the range of function for normal subjects is quite narrow compared with that for patients, such a study presents a rigorous assessment of reliability. The normal subjects should be age- and gender-matched to applicable patient group(s), the test–retest interval should be comparable to that in a clinical trial, and the test protocol should be the same as that for a clinical trial. For a test to be acceptable as reliable, r should be at least 0.70, accounting for about 50% of variability.

Then, the investigator should assure that tests are reliable over the broad range of performance from normal to severe loss. Patients should be selected whose functions are stable over the test–retest interval. For acceptance, r should be higher, perhaps 0.90 or greater.

A better measure than the Pearson product moment correlation coefficient is the reliability coefficient [45]. The correlation coefficient is based on analysis of variance for repeated measures, allows for more than one retest, and compensates for learning. We have used this measure in normal and patient studies [2,3].

When rating scales are evaluated for reliability, patients with near normal to severe loss of function should be evaluated, providing that their functions are stable over the testing interval. Other guidelines remain the same. However, instead of using the Pearson product moment correlation coefficient as is often observed in the literature, a nonparametric statistic, such as the Spearman rank correlation coefficient, should be used.

Rigorous evaluation studies are essential for credibility when using quantitative approaches for measuring neurologic functions. Over the past three decades, our group has been surprised on more than one occasion because objective studies demonstrated that devices, procedures, and measures that appeared to be satisfactory were, in fact, unsatisfactory [16]. Appearances can be deceiving!

What a waste of time and what a shame it is to carry out a modestly large, long-term clinical trial with a battery of motor function tests only to find out later that the results lack credibility. Key reasons for equivocal results include the following: (a) the technician was not trained to obtain data reproducibly; (b) tests were not reliable or valid; (c) learning effects were not controlled or accounted for; (d) results are confounded because the effects of age, gender, or handedness were unknown or could not be accounted for.

The clinical investigator may feel that it is a formidable task to design and complete studies fulfilling the criteria listed above, and it indeed may be. However, it is not necessary that each investigator carry out a complete set of evaluation studies. If a large multicenter clinical trial is planned, only one center need carry out the studies, providing that all assessments of functions are to be carried out in similar environments and all technicians are trained and objectively evaluated in their ability to obtain reproducible data. Also, as commercial companies begin to manufacture and make available batteries of neurologic function tests, it is in their best interest to do these evaluations in an appropriate clinical setting and to provide assurance at each center that technicians are appropriately trained.

Total Quality Management

Total quality management (TQM) is a practice, some say an obsession, developed and refined in recent decades by the Japanese in private industry [5,8]. Today, it is rapidly being instituted in American and European industry in an attempt to re-establish and sustain competitiveness in our rapidly developing single world economy.

The fundamental principles of TQM to continually improve products and processes should be considered seriously by investigators as they address major problems in management of patients with PD. Neurologists increasingly recognize that continued progress is difficult to achieve. Sensitive, specific instrumented tests are likely necessary for early diagnosis, improved understanding of pathophysiologic mechanisms, and identification of different subsets of patients with PD. Instrumented tests are also needed to objectively evaluate alternative treatments. However, with few exceptions, instrumented tests, clinical trial processes, and patient management practices are far below what they could be if world-class expertise, technology, and practices were employed.

Likely, it will take world-class investigators to make important discoveries and contributions that substantially improve quality of life for PD patients. Leading investigators should direct their efforts so as to attract the best engineers, statisticians, pharmacologists, and others toward research in parkinsonism. Conference chairs and journal editors should strive for reports that employ appropriate experimental designs, evaluations of tests, and use of statistics. Continuous improvement and TQM have the potential to greatly accelerate improvements in the management of patients with PD.

Recommendations for Test Batteries

For specific studies, it may not be practical to test patients in a broad battery of coded and instrumented tests of neurologic functions such as the one that our group developed. Based on the hypothesis to be tested or the question(s) asked, the investigator may choose from an inventory of tests. Doing so places limitations on a study that should be recognized at the outset. In this section, we recommend a few key tests for consideration in carrying out different types of studies in PD.

Early Diagnosis

Today, a patient is ordinarily diagnosed as parkinsonian well past disease onset or even initial presentation of one or more symptoms. If patients were diagnosed earlier, it could be that existing or new treatments would significantly improve management of the course of the disease. Of course, the purported benefit of earlier treatment cannot be determined unless methods are developed to achieve early diagnosis. Eventually, DNA probes and biochemical markers may exist for early diagnosis. Today, sensitive instrumented tests of neurologic functions thought to be affected at early stages may prove to be useful. Early markers are believed to be tremor and bradykinesia, especially delay to initiation of movement.

For use in early diagnosis, four types of tests should be considered:

1. Simple electromyogram (EMG) analysis of muscles that drive the characteristic "pill-rolling" hand tremor. The investigator should analyze the amplitude of 4 Hz to 6 Hz frequency content [1]. An abnormally high amplitude may exist, even when the hand appears steady.
2. Measurement of delay to initiation of movement in a multichoice hand reaction and movement time test, as developed by our group [16 pp. 98–99] or by Watts [44]. As the number of choices increases from two to four or more, the reaction time in early parkinsonism may increase disproportionately, compared to age- and gender-matched normal subjects.
3. Arm progressive tracking (or the critical tracking test) as developed initially for NASA astronauts and Air Force pilots by Jex et al. [9] and modified for patients by our group [16]. This is one of the most sensitive tests that we have used in

parkinsonism and multiple sclerosis drug studies [4,21,37,39,40,43] and one that patients with slight-to-moderate disability enjoy performing. The task resembles that of a truck driver traveling down a winding hill with no brakes. As the driver progresses down the hill, the speed of the truck increases, and it becomes more and more difficult to remain on the road. The increasing test difficulty stresses the patient's functional capacity. The measure corresponds to the effective time delay between the position of the stick on the visual display and the patient's corrective movement of the position stick. A patient who can respond quickly (a small effective time delay) can manage the task for a longer time duration and thus achieve a better score. Data do not relate to data from reaction time tests.

Another tracking task that may provide early detection is step tracking. Like progressive tracking, it is easy to understand and fun to do. Results from our studies suggest the tests are sensitive to changes in function [11,12,22,25,27,30,31,34,37,39,40,42].

4. A multiple simultaneous task, such as performing the early phase of test 3 above, while simultaneously performing test 2 above. This task provides a measure of delay to initiation of movement while further stressing functional capacity, which diminishes in parkinsonism.

In addition to the general issues associated with test evaluation discussed earlier, other issues include the requirement to eventually carry out longitudinal studies for validation of test sensitivity and specificity for use in early diagnosis, costs associated with a large population study, and the demonstration of effective therapy for early parkinsonism. Also, there are likely other markers and tests that may help identify patients earlier, but they may not become known without using a larger, more inclusive test battery. The investigator should consider the positron emission tomograph (PET) and biochemical tests to aid with early confirmation.

Pathophysiologic Mechanisms

The same tests suggested for early diagnosis may be used to improve understanding of pathophysiologic mechanisms. Cognitive tests, especially those that stress functional capacity, should also be considered. Other specific tests should be included as appropriate, depending on the hypotheses being tested. A small number of patients may be all that is needed, and testing may be done for greater durations or more frequent repeat testing sessions than ordinarily done in a clinical trial study.

Clinical Trials and Disease Progression

The number of instrumented tests should be greater for evaluating therapy in clinical trials and disease progression than for early diagnosis. The patient's symptoms and signs are broader in mild and advanced disease and at least the key symptoms should be quantified. In addition to the tests suggested for early diagnosis, the investigator should also consider including about five instrumented activities of daily living tests of those functions that the PD patient wants improved. These include speech, speed and coordination of the upper extremities, tracking or following a target, and dexterity. Tests for the lower extremities should include stability of station and speed of walking. To reduce test variance, we recommend the use of a patient-actuated timer to start–stop each test instead of a stopwatch actuated by the technician administrator [16]. Other tests include cognitive/mental state tests, tracking tests (especially step tracking), rigidity of distal joints, and possibly postural sway/gait [12,16]. To enhance validity and obtain measures of functions that are not easily instrumented, we recommend including a coded examination of neurologic functions using four to six rating levels, such as the Unified Parkinson's Disease Rating Scale (UPDRS) and the modified Hoehn and Yahr scale. Quality of life can be assessed by using a minimal record of disability, as has been developed for multiple sclerosis [14,35]. As always, analysis of rating scale data should *not* include addition, averaging, or use of parametric statistical tools.

Comments

Especially for following disease progression, investigators should consider contracting with a commercial firm to develop a simple test battery with automated scoring that could be done routinely at home, with a TV set. Such a self-testing process for PD patients could provide great value for improving patient management over years.

Because PD is a disease of the elderly, it is extremely important that data analysis be adjusted for age, gender, and learning effects [18,19,23,26,28,29]. With instrumented tests, the effects of normal aging are pronounced between the young and the elderly, and changes are most pronounced after 60 years of age. Women perform both significantly better and worse than men, depending on the function measured. Learning effects are greatly reduced in the elderly compared with young adults, after practice trials. Because of these effects, our group has developed and used the measure of "percentage of normal function adjusted for age and gender" and Z-scores [12,16]. We recommend its adoption more generally for evaluating studies in PD.

Evaluation of On–Off Symptoms

A relatively simple way to assess on–off symptoms is to use a real-time activity recorder, similar to a Holter monitor for cardiac arrhythmias. A built-in motion detector provides a quantitative measure of patient activity in real time. The patient also conducts a self-evaluation of symptoms with rating scales whenever change is observed and indicates when medication is taken. Data are keyed into the activity recorder, which includes a real-time clock. Data can be quickly and automatically analyzed and displayed with an "activity analyzer" in the physician's office, during routine visits.

Conclusion

We believe that an important next step in advancing the management of PD is to bring leading investigators from around the world together to discuss and agree to one or more specific test batteries. Once agreement is reached, the group of investigators may contract with a commercial firm to build low-cost, effective test batteries and to have the tests evaluated extensively prior to delivery to clinical research centers.

References

1. Albers JW, Potvin AR, Tourtellotte WW, Pew RW, Stribley RF (1973) Quantification of hand tremor in the clinical neurological examination. IEEE Trans Biomed Eng 20:27–37
2. Behbehani K, Kondraske GV, Richmond JR (1988) Investigation of upper extremity visuomotor control performance measures. IEEE Trans Biomed Eng BME-35(7):518–525
3. Behbehani K, Kondraske GV, Tintner R, Tindall RAS, Imrhan SN (1990) Evaluation of quantitative measures of upper extremity speed and coordination in healthy persons and in three patient populations. Arch Phys Med 71(2):106–111
4. Domino EF, Albers JW, Potvin AR, Repa BS, Tourtellotte WW (1972) Effects of amphetamine on quantitative measures of motor performance. Clin Pharmacol Ther 13(2):251–257
5. Goldratt EM, Cox J (1986) The goal: a process of ongoing improvement. North River, New York
6. Henderson WG, Tourtellotte WW, Potvin AR (1975) Training examiners to administer a quantitative neurological examination for a multicenter clinical trial. Arch Phys Med Rehabil 56:289–295
7. Henderson WG, Tourtellotte WW, Potvin AR, Rose AS (1978) Methodology for analyzing clinical neurological data: ACTH in multiple sclerosis. Clin Pharmacol Ther 24(2):146–153
8. Imai M (1986) Kaisen: the key to Japan's competitive success. Random House, New York
9. Jex HR, McDonnell JD, Phatak AV (1966) A critical tracking task for manual control research. IEEE Trans Hum Fac Eng 7:138
10. Kelman HR, Willner A (1962) Problems in measurement and evaluation of rehabilitation. Arch Phys Med Rehabil 43:172
11. Kondraske GV (1982) Design, construction, and evaluation of an automated computer-based system for quantification of neurologic function. Thesis, University of Texas, Arlington, Texas
12. Kondraske GV (1990) A PC-based performance measurement laboratory system. J Clin Eng 15(6):467–478
13. Kuzma JW, Tourtellotte WW, Remington RD (1965) Quantitative clinical neurological testing. II. Some statistical considerations of a battery of tests. J Chronic Dis 18:305
14. LaRocca NG, Scheinberg LC, Slater RN, in collaboration with Giesser B, Smith CR, Traugott U, Schapiro RT, Paty DW, Franklin GM, Cobble N, Petejan JH, Kraft GH, Frankel D, Catanzaro M, Poser CM, Tourtellotte WW, Baumhefner RW (1985) Field testing of a minimal record of disability in multiple sclerosis: the United States and Canada. Acta Neurol Scand 70[Suppl 101]:126–138
15. Potvin AR, Tourtellotte WW (1975) The neurological examination: advancements in its quantification. Arch Phys Med Rehabil 56(10):425–437
16. Potvin AR, Tourtellotte WW (1985) Quantitative examination of neurologic functions, vol. I and vol. II CRC Press, Boca Raton, Florida

17. Potvin AR, Tourtellotte WW, Dailey JS, Walker JE, Albers JW, Henderson WG, Snyder DN (1972) Simulated activities of daily living examination. Arch Phys Med Rehabil 53:476–487
18. Potvin AR, Tourtellotte WW, Pew RW, Albers JW, Henderson WG, Snyder DN (1973a) The importance of age effects on performance in the assessment of clinical trials. J Chronic Dis 26:699–717
19. Potvin AR, Tourtellotte WW, Pew RW, Albers JW, Henderson WG, Snyder DN (1973b) Motivation and learning in the quantitative examination of neurological function. Arch Phys Med Rehabil 54:432–440
20. Potvin AR, Albers JW, Repa BS, Henderson WG, Walker JE, Stribley RF, Pew RW, Tourtellotte WW (1974) Quantitative evaluation of neuropharmacological trials. Clin Pharmacol Ther 15:229–241
21. Potvin AR, Albers JW, Stribley RF, Tourtellotte WW, Pew RW (1975a) A battery of tests for evaluating steadiness in clinical trials. Med Biol Eng 13:914–922
22. Potvin AR, Salamy JG, Crosier WG, Jones KW, Doerr JA (1975b) Effects of secobarbitol on performance upon arousal from stage 4 sleep. Appl Neurophysiol 38:240–250
23. Potvin AR, Tourtellotte WW, Henderson WG, Snyder DN (1975c) Quantitative examination of neurological function: reliability and learning effects. Arch Phys Med Rehabil 56(10):438–442
24. Potvin AR, Tourtellotte WW, Snyder DN, Henderson WG, Albers JW (1975d) Validity of quantitative tests measuring tremor. Am J Phys Med 54(5):243–252
25. Potvin AR, Doerr JA, Estes JT, Tourtellotte WW (1977) A portable clinical tracking task instrument. Med Biol Eng Comput 15:391–397
26. Potvin AR, Syndulko K, Tourtellotte WW, Lemmon JA, Potvin JH (1980a) Human neurologic function and the aging process. J Am Geriatr Soc 28(1):1–9
27. Potvin AR, Tourtellotte WW, Syndulko K, Potvin JH, Baumhefner RW (1980b) Multiple sclerosis clinical trials: a comprehensive system for the measurement and evaluation of neurologic function. In: Bauer HJ, Poser S, Ritter G (eds) Progress in multiple sclerosis research. Springer, Berlin Heidelberg New York, pp 603–625
28. Potvin AR, Syndulko K, Tourtellotte WW, Goldberg Z, Potvin JH, Hansch EC (1981a) Quantitative evaluation of normal age-related changes in neurologic function. In: Maletta GJ, Pirozlo FJ (eds) Advances in neurogerontology, vol 2. Praeger, New York, chap 2, pp 13–57
29. Potvin AR, Tourtellotte WW, Syndulko K, Potvin JH (1981b) Quantitative methods in assessment of neurologic function. CRC Crit Rev Bioeng 6(3):177–224
30. Repa BS, Albers JW, Potvin AR, Tourtellotte WW (1971) The use of a battery of tracking tests in the quantitative evaluation of neurological function. In: Proceedings of the 7th annual NASA-University conference on manual control, University of Southern California, NASA-SP, 281: 119–123
31. Repa BS, Albers JW, Pew RW, Tourtellotte WW (1972) Clinical applications of tracking. In: Proceedings of the 8th annual University of Michigan-NASA conference on manual control
32. Rose AS, Kuzma JW, Kurtzke JF, Sibley WA, Tourtellotte WW (1968, 1970) Cooperative study in the evaluation of therapy in multiple sclerosis: ACTH vs placebo in acute exacerbations. Preliminary report: Neurology 18(6); final report: Neurology 20(5):Part 2, 1
33. Stribley RF, Albers JW, Tourtellotte WW, Cockrell JL (1974) A quantitative study of stance in normal subjects. Arch Phys Med Rehabil 55:74
34. Syndulko K, Tourtellotte WW (1989) Use of a quantitative test battery for long-term evaluation of clinical efficacy in Parkinson's disease. In: Davis R, Kondraske GV, Tourtellotte WW (eds) Physical medicine and rehabilitation, vol 3/2. Hanley and Belfus, Philadelphia, pp 168–176
35. Tourtellotte WW (1985) Minimal record of disability for multiple sclerosis. National Multiple Sclerosis Society, April 1985
36. Tourtellotte WW, Haerer AF, Simpson JF, Kuzma JW, Sikorski J (1965) Quantitative clinical neurological testing. I. A study of a battery of tests designed to evaluate in part the neurological function of patients with multiple sclerosis and its use in a therapeutic trial. NY Acad Sci 122:480
37. Tourtellotte WW, Potvin AR, Costanza AM, Hirsch SB, Syndulko K (1978) Cyclobenzaprine: a new type of anti-parkinsonian drug. Prog Neuropsychopharmacol 2(5/6):553–578
38. Tourtellotte WW, Potvin AR, Mendez M, Baumhefner RW, Potvin JH, Ma BI, Syndulko K (1980a) Failure of intravenous and intrathecal cytarabine to modify central nervous system IgG synthesis in multiple sclerosis. Ann Neurol 8:402–408

39. Tourtellotte WW, Syndulko K, Potvin AR, Hirsch SB, Potvin JH (1980b) Increased ratio of carbidopa to levodopa in treatment of Parkinson's disease. Arch Neurol 37:723–726
40. Tourtellotte WW, Potvin AR, Syndulko K, Hirsch SB, Gilden ER, Potvin JH, Hansch EC (1982) Parkinson's disease: Cogentin with Sinemet, a better response. Prog Neuropsychopharmacol Biol Psychiatry 6:51–55
41. Tourtellotte WW, Syndulko K, Baumhefner RW, Potvin AR (1986) Neuroimmunologic pharmacology of multiple sclerosis. I. A comprehensive protocol for preliminary clinical trials in MS. In: Hommes OR, Mertin J, Tourtellotte WW (eds) Proceedings on immunosuppressive treatment in multiple sclerosis, pp 219–225
42. Walker JE, Albers JW, Tourtellotte WW, Henderson WG, Potvin AR, Smith A (1972a) A qualitative and quantitative evaluation of amantadine in the treatment of Parkinson's disease. J Chronic Dis 25(1):149–182
43. Walker JE, Potvin AR, Tourtellotte WW, Albers JW, Repa BS, Henderson WG, Snyder DN (1972b) Amantadine and levodopa in the treatment of Parkinson's disease. Clin Pharmacol Ther 13(1):28–36
44. Watts R (1992) An electrophysiological test battery to aid in the early diagnosis of Parkinsonism. Oral presentation at Second International Congress of Movement Disorders: Satellite Symposium Instrumental methods and scoring in diagnosis and quantification of extrapyramidal disorders, Prien/Chiemsee June 21–22, 1992
45. Winer BJ (1962) Statistical principles in experimental design. McGraw-Hill, New York

Discussion

Dr. Horstink: I don't think you discussed the question of whether you test specificity, and I don't think that you can differentiate between multiple sclerosis and parkinsonian hypokinesia.

Dr. Potvin: We have never used our tests to help diagnose a patient's disease. That's not to say that you couldn't do so. I don't want to advocate that these tests can or should be used for diagnosis. I think neurologists do a very good job with diagnosis. We use these tests as an adjunct to clinical assessment to quantify functions in an objective kind of way, to primarily follow disease progression as well as to evaluate putative treatments in clinical trials.

Dr. Inzelberg: I think one of the problems which occurs in everyday life is the large amount of data that you collect. The more sophisticated the technique, the greater the amount of data which has to be analyzed, interpreted, and kept in the memory of the computer.

Dr. Potvin: That's a comment I fully agree with and I think I have a slide that addressed the three different approaches that we have looked at for data reduction; it's something that we are continuing to work on. You have to understand that we've got a large test space, about 125 measures by now, but we don't run any one patient through all 125 test measures. So Parkinson patients undergo a subset of tests, and multiple sclerosis patients a subset of tests. If we're looking at the effects of, say, amphetamine in normal individuals, the set of tests is very small. So we take this broad test battery and hone it down to the few tests that make sense for the question being asked and for the subjects' health. Then we go through the appropriate data reduction; we have made a lot of progress in data reduction. I didn't have time today to show you in the presentation how we reduce and present the data.

Measurement of Muscle Tone — Demarcation Between Spasticity and Rigidity

A. Struppler and C. Jakob

Posture and movement are the two extremes of our motor performances. However, postural components contribute to every motor task.

What is Muscle Tone?

Muscle tone, the postural component of our motor performance, can be clinically observed as a resistance to passive stretch of the muscles around the joint of a limb, under relaxed and activated states. The physical correlate to the clinical phenomenon of tone is resistance against passive displacement, defined as "stiffness" (dF/dx), or its reciprocal value "compliance" (dx/dF).

Apart from inertia, stretch resistance of the limb is determined by inherent mechanical properties of connective tissues and muscle fibers as well as the effects of innervation. These factors are mutually related, as indicated in Fig. 1.

Changes in one of the factors will modify the other one consequently. For example, stiffness of the intrafusal muscle fibers can modulate the threshold of the muscle spindle with subsequent effects on the functional stretch reflex. Because of this feedback, muscle stiffness is not a fixed parameter, but is time dependent on its history.

General Approaches to Assessing Muscle Tone

In man, skeletal muscle tone can be assessed by measuring the resistance of a limb against mechanical perturbation. Here we are not able to measure the stiffness of a single muscle, but rather the joint stiffness. Synergistic and antagonistic muscles as well as soft tissues contribute to joint stiffness.

There are two approaches to evaluate joint stiffness:

1. To apply a defined torque and measure the displacement; torque pulses, steps, and ramps are often used.
2. To apply a defined displacement and measure the induced torque; ramp or sinusoidal movements are generally used.

Stiffness depends on the experimental conditions under which it is measured, i.e., motor task and kind of perturbation.

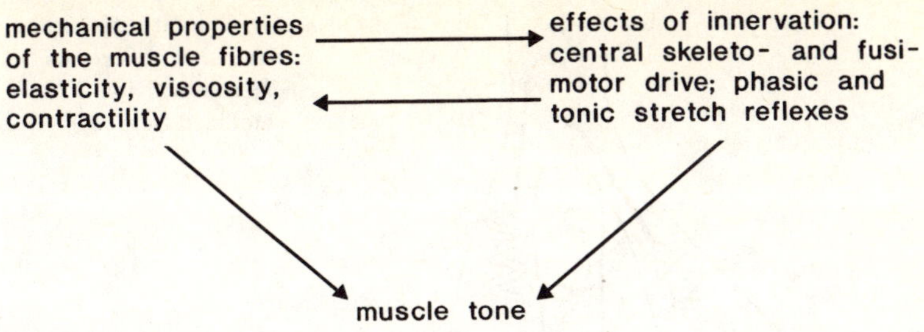

Fig. 1. Relationship between mechanical properties, effects of innervation, and muscle tone

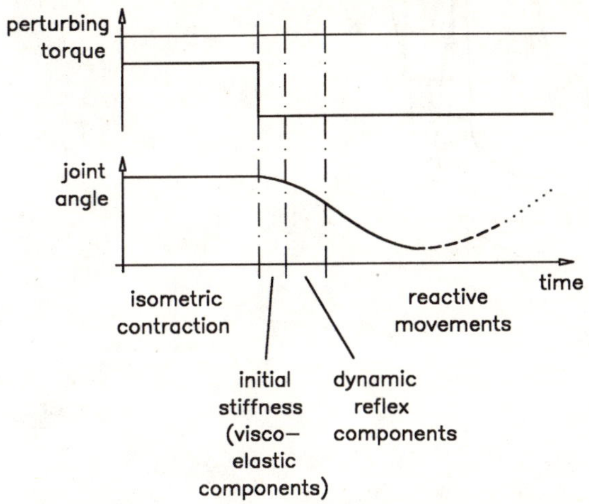

Fig. 2. Time intervals of occurring stiffness components following a torque step

The motor task can modify the initial stiffness preceding the dynamic reflex response and the reflex stiffness, depending on whether the perturbation is expected or unexpected. The applied stimuli, necessary for measuring muscle tone, modify the stiffness following the perturbation via the functional stretch reflex, as well as shortening and unloading responses.

Figure 2 symbolizes the time intervals of the occurring stiffness components following a torque step.

The position of the limb can be controlled by two different strategies (see Fig. 3):

1. Cocontractions of flexors and extensors increases joint stiffness in order to reduce displacement in the case of unexpected external perturbations.
2. Reciprocal innervation of flexors and extensors is a more economic strategy to stabilize the joint. Adequate load compensation requires, however, information about the direction, amount, and timing of the perturbation.

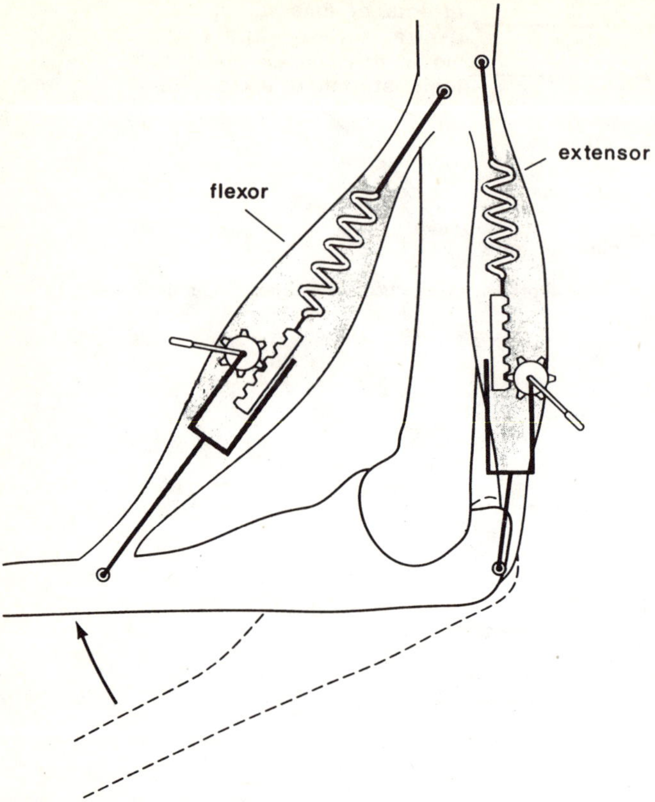

Fig. 3. Joint stiffness as a function of flexor and extensor activity. (Modified from [6])

Methods

Our investigations of muscle tone are focused on the forearm flexors and extensors and the finger flexors. In the proximal limb muscles (the forearm flexors and extensors), we test a system involved in body balance, postural tone of the proximal limbs, and force-controlled movements. In the finger flexors, however, which are predominantly longitudinally controlled distal muscles for skilled movements, the postural component is lower.

The experimental conditions, especially the mechanical stimuli, should be such that they remain within physiological ranges as far as possible. In order to optimize the conditions for generating adequate stimuli, in cooperation with the "Institut für elektrische Maschinen und Geräte (Prof. Lorenzen)" of the Technical University in Munich, different types of torque motors were developed. Each of them is adapted to evaluate a special range of properties contributing to muscle tone. The main differences are maximum torque, rise time, displacement range, and moment of inertia. We record the mechanical parameters (force, displacement, acceleration) simultaneously with the electromyogram (EMG) of agonistic and antagonistic muscles.

Results

Investigations on Finger Flexors

By means of the torque motor, we investigate the postural component of the finger flexors during isometric contractions (Fig. 4). The maximum torque (2 Nm) can be produced within 5 ms. Maximum displacement is ± 1°, i.e., 10 mm. Since the inertia of the fingers is low, its contribution to stretch resistance is small. During isometric contraction of the finger flexors against a defined standing torque (2 N), we applied additional forces (3 N). The average displacement and acceleration were recorded simultaneously with the EMG of the deep flexor muscles of the finger. These components should be separated, because resistance against stretch consists not only of elasticity, but also of inertia and viscosity. Since the stretch of the muscle is small, these components can be assumed to be constant. Therefore, muscle stiffness can be calculated on the basis of a linear model at various time intervals. This analysis method allows us to distinguish between initial stiffness and stiffness during the short- and long-latency stretch reflex components (Fig. 5).

This method allows us to investigate how conditioning maneuvers such as extension or contraction preceding the perturbation modify the ongoing sustained activity and the stretch reflex components.

Figure 6 shows the effect of a preceding conditioning with active isometric contraction of 25% of the maximal voluntary force (on the left) of a passive stretch

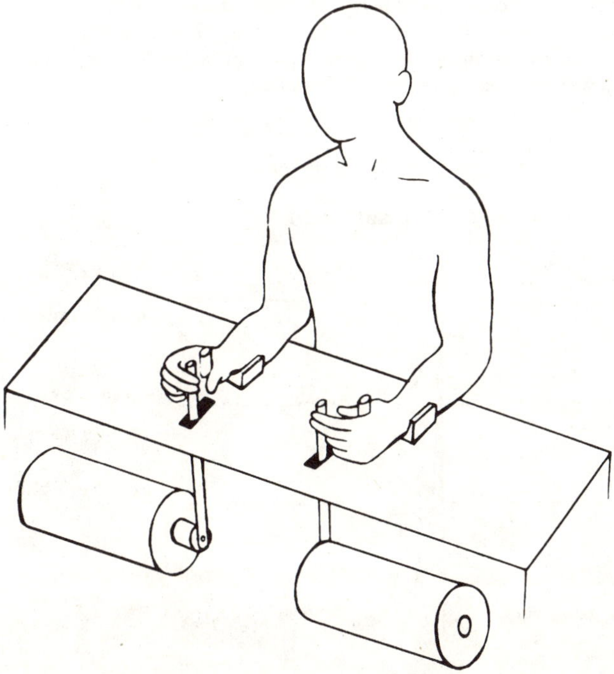

Fig. 4. Torque motor (see text for details)

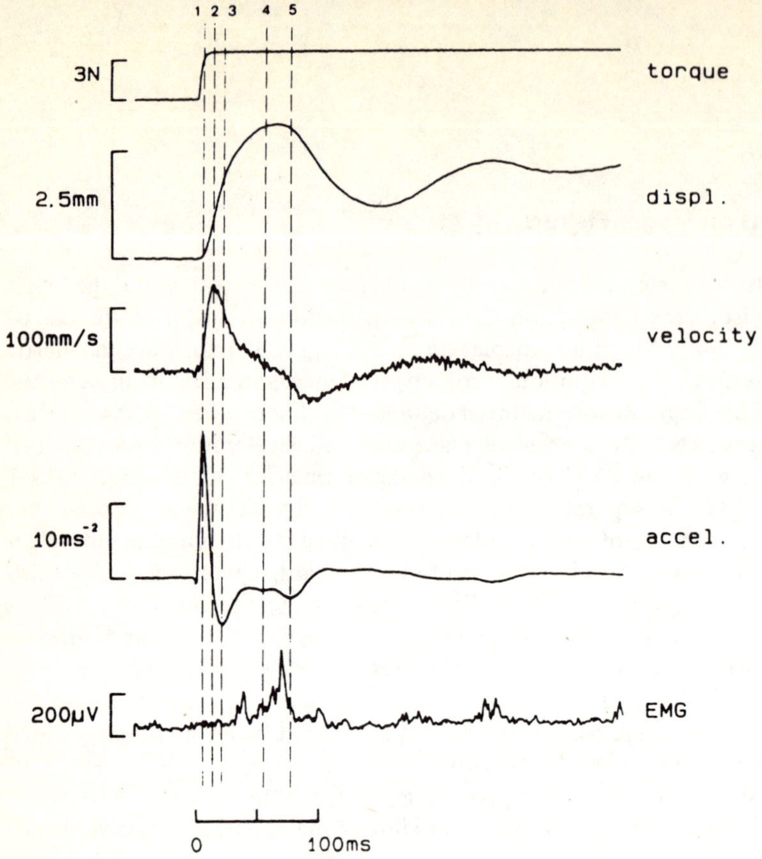

Fig. 5. Time courses of torque pulse, displacement, and acceleration of the finger tips (from *top* to *bottom*). The velocity is calculated from the displacement. The *bottom* trace shows the rectified and averaged surface electromyogram (*EMG*) of the finger flexors. The initial stiffness is calculated from the mechanics 1, 2, and 3, and the reflex stiffness includes 4 and 5 (from [23])

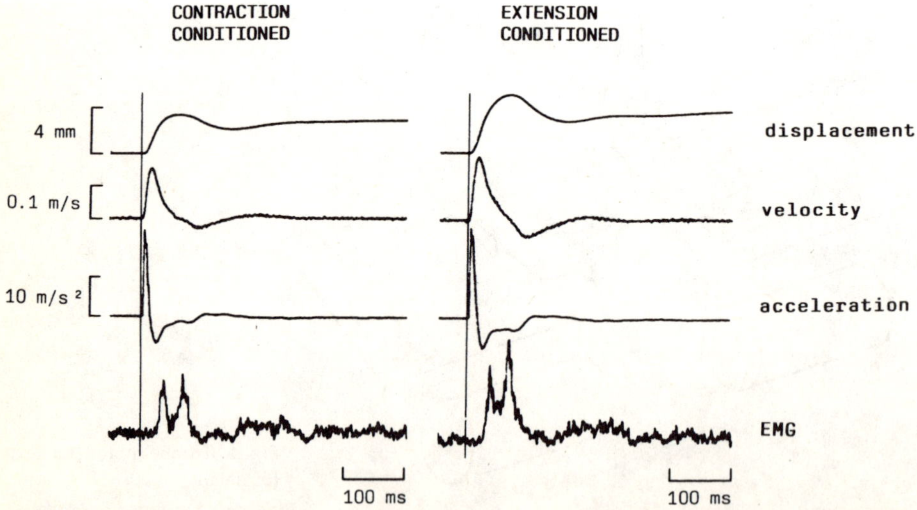

Fig. 6. Overall average time courses for five normal subjects (15–20 single trials). From *top* to *bottom* as in Fig. 5. The standing torque was 3%, the additional torque 4%, of the individual maximal voluntary force (from [23]). *EMG*, electromyogram

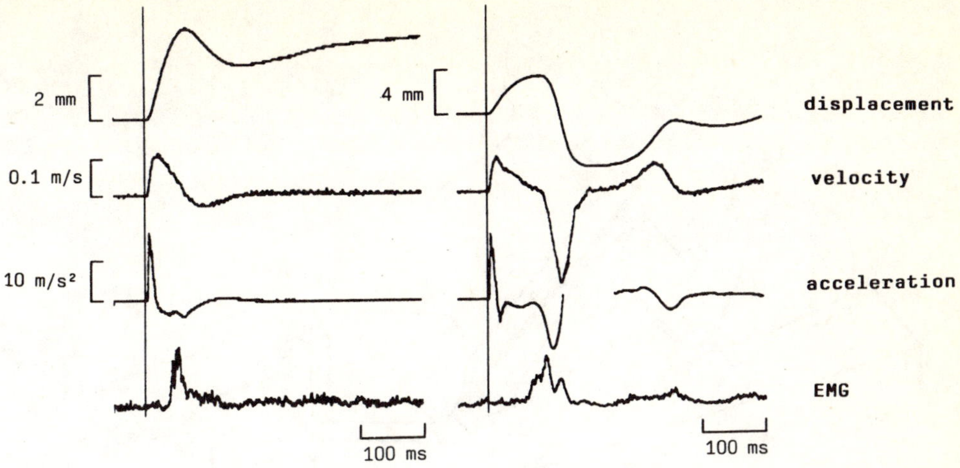

Fig. 7 Comparison between the mechanics and electromyogram (*EMG*) for spasticity (*left*) and parkinsonian rigidity (*right*). See text for details. (From [23])

of the relaxed muscle (on the right). The maximal displacement and the velocity of the displacement following passive stretch was greater than when compared with a preceding contraction. More detailed analysis showed that not only the initial, but also the reflex stiffness was diminished. It was assumed that the conditioning maneuver modifies the viscoelastic behavior of the extra- and intrafusal muscle fibers [8].

Figure 7 illustrates how spasticity (on the left) is reflected in the mechanics and EMG under these experimental conditions as compared to parkinsonian rigidity (on the right). In the spastic subject, there is a very pronounced short-latency reflex response in the EMG, associated with a considerable deceleration peak in the accelerogram with a latency of approximate 50 ms. In the rigid patient, however, the same torque perturbation elicits only an exaggerated late reflex component, which is associated with a pronounced deceleration peak after approximately 80 ms (note that the right EMG was plotted with a lower magnification factor). Furthermore, maximum velocity (second trace) was lower in rigidity than spasticity, indicating an increased viscous resistance in rigidity. The exaggerated long-latency reflex response caused a marked drawback (notice the uppermost position trace on the right, which was plotted on a larger vertical scale than that on the left).

Investigations on the Forearm Flexors and Extensors

The torque motor shown in Fig. 8 is adapted to generate up to 12 Nm to the forearm. The horizontal axis of the motor makes an optimal fixation of the arm at the elbow joint possible, which helps to minimize cocontraction even at high force levels. The low inertia of the motor together with the short rise time (7 ms) make it possible to evaluate the initial stiffness of the forearm flexors [24].

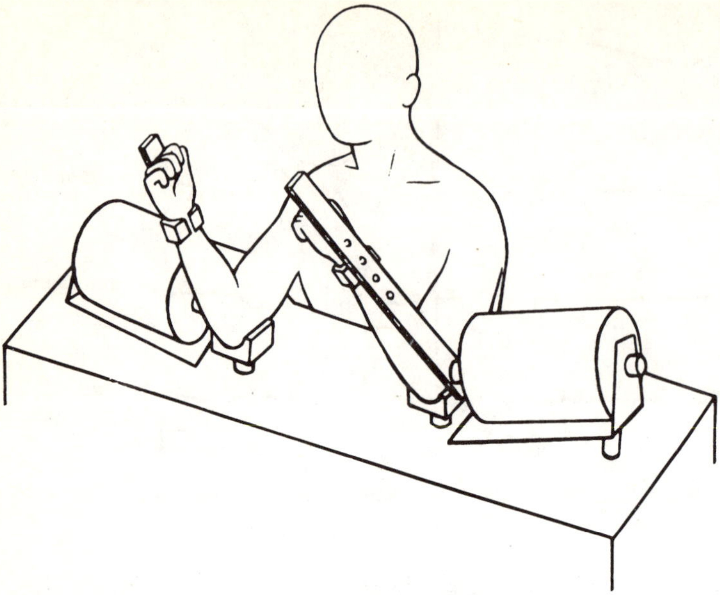

Fig. 8. Use of torque motor to investigate forearm muscles. See text for details

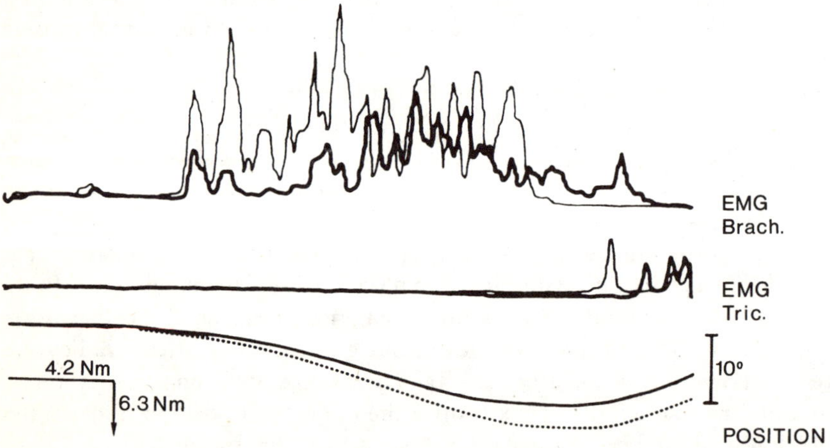

Fig. 9. Responses obtained at "resist" instruction, taken from one subject. Electromyogram (*EMG*) activity rectified and averaged ($n = 8$; from [16])

Figure 9 shows one example of the quantification of muscle tone before and after application of antispastic drugs. During isometric contraction of forearm flexors and extensors, respectively, additional loads were applied and the displacements of the forearm were measured. Simultaneously, the EMG from brachial and triceps muscle were recorded with wire electrodes (thin lines).

Following Tizanidin E (1 mg i.m.), there is a larger displacement (dotted line) as well as a reduction in the short and late components of the proprioceptive

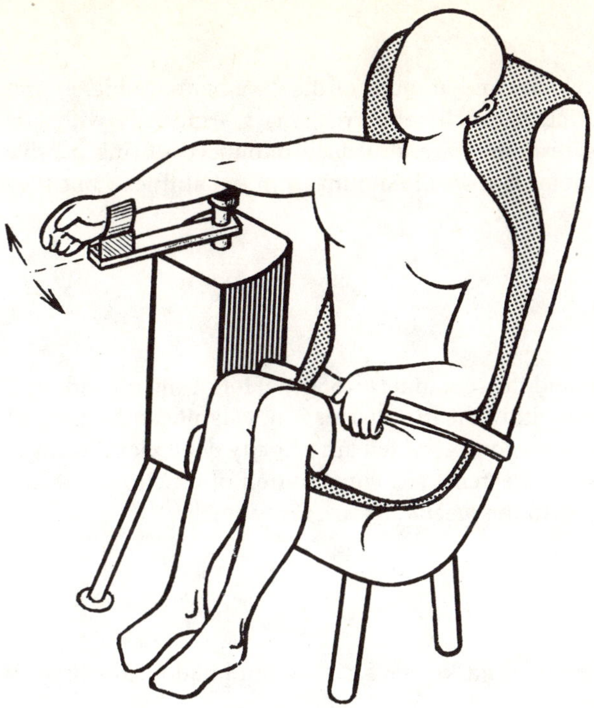

Fig. 10. Force- and length-controlled motor (see text for details)

reflexes in the stretched muscles (thick lines). This method seems to be sensitive enough to reveal changes in stiffness even following small dosages of myotonolytic drugs.

The recently developed motor shown in Fig. 10 is force and length controlled. As the motor axis is vertical, gravity is compensated by the lever, and stimuli can be applied during a relaxation or even during sleep. This motor can produce accurate, slow movements as well as high torques up to 20 Nm in a rotation range of 120°. Intrinsic viscoelastic properties of the muscle, such as thixotropy, and long-lasting tonic responses can be investigated under various conditions.

The following two examples may demonstrate approaches for evaluation and quantification of spasticity and rigidity on the forearm flexors and extensors. We apply torque stimuli during relaxation (passive extension) and isometric contraction (combined rebound, i.e., extension followed by unloading). We record the elbow joint angle, the force between the lever of the motor and the forearm, and the EMG of biceps and triceps muscles. The limb stiffness is calculated at different time intervals following the stimulus.

The evaluation of spasticity and rigidity in the forearm flexors and extensors may be presented in each of the following examples.

Spastic Hemiparesis

The patient was 61 years old and female and had been suffering from spastic hemiparesis for 6 months.

Passive Extension (Fig. 11)

Within the first 100 ms, the velocity and amount of displacement are higher and the stiffness is less than normal. Stretch reflex responses, especially with late components, and shortening responses are already pronounced during passive extension. They can contribute only a small amount to initial stiffness, but they may accelerate the drawback.

Combined Rebound (Fig. 12)

The displacement ($t = 100$ ms) and the rebound ($t = 350$ ms) following unloading is more pronounced, but stiffness within the first 250 ms is not significantly changed compared to normal. The reflex responses, which are velocity dependent, seem to only add to the rebound to a small extent. The contribution of functional stretch reflexes or unloading responses to the mechanics are fairly small.

Hemirigidity

The patient, a 48-year-old man, had Parkinson's disease and had been suffering from heminrigidity for 2 years.

Passive Extension (Fig. 13)

During relaxation, the displacement is shorter and the stiffness greater than normal. The EMG makes no obvious contributions to the mechanics. However, in rigidity "activity at rest" is often not manifested in surface EMG.

Combined Rebound (Fig. 14)

Whereas the initial displacement ($t = 100$ ms) is the same as normal, the rebound ($t = 350$ ms) is much smaller in the rigid patient, probably due to increased late stretch reflex components ("braking effect").

Differences between Rigidity and Spasticity

In summary, following a perturbation during isometric contraction, there are no pronounced differences in stiffness between the normal and the affected side in either spasticity or rigidity. However, during passive extension in the relaxed state, initial stiffness differs in both compared to normal. Whereas the rigid patient shows increased initial stiffness, in spasticity it is clearly decreased (Fig. 15).

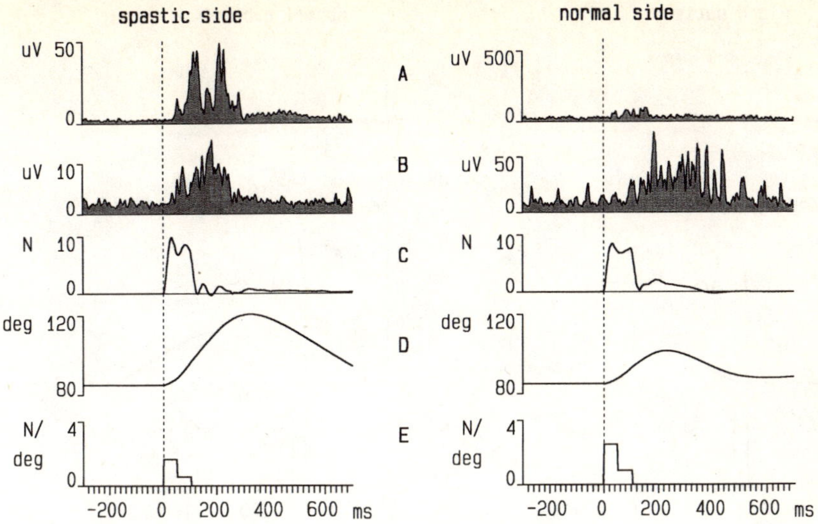

Fig. 11. Spastic hemiparesis: passive extension

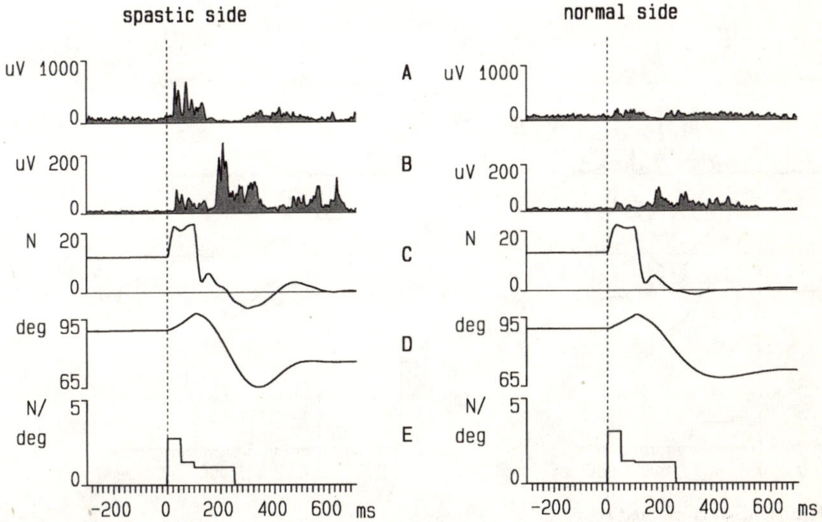

Fig. 12. Spastic hemiparesis: combined rebound

Figs. 11–14A–E. In each of the figures, average data from six trials are shown (see text for details). Within one paradigm (passive extension or combined rebound), each electromyogram (*EMG*) channel is scaled to equal background activity level. The absolute scales are indicated on the *y-axes*; they are NOT equal. Within one paradigm, each mechanical data channel is scaled equally. **A** Rectified surface EMG of biceps muscle; **B** Rectified surface EMG of triceps muscle; **C** Tangential force, measured at the wrist, approximately 25 cm distal to the elbow; **D** Elbow angle (180°, total extension); **E** Total stiffness, calculated in the time intervals 0–50 ms, 50–100 ms and in the paradigm "combined rebound" 100–250 ms. Note that inertia contribution has not been removed. The *hatched vertical lines* indicate the onset of the mechanical stimulus

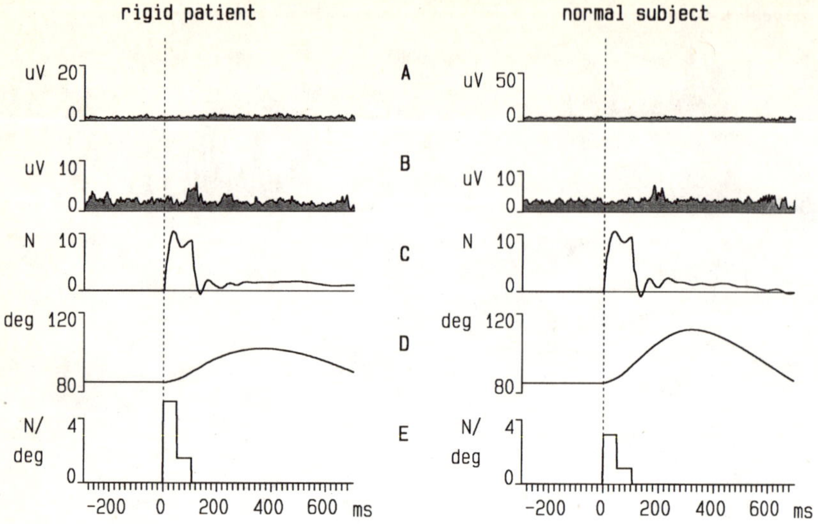

Figs. 13. Hemirigidity: passive extension

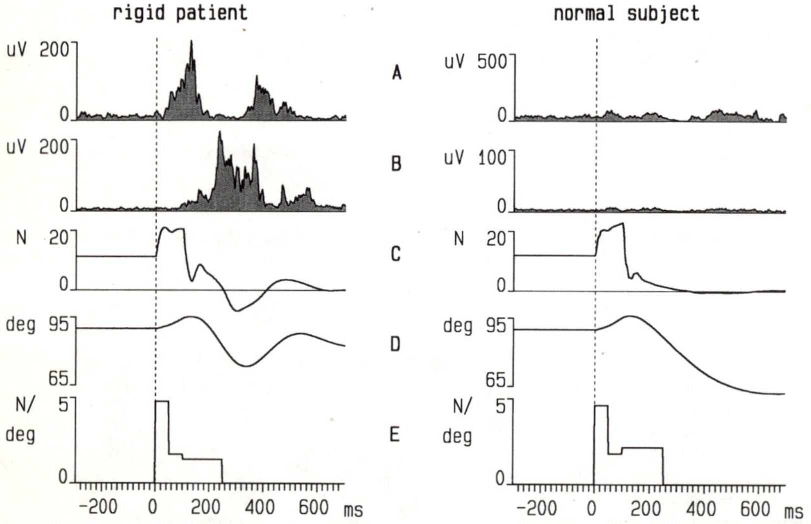

Figs. 14. Hemirigidity: combined rebound

Using the length-controlled mode of the motor, we apply ramp stretches at different angles and measure the relationship between elbow torque and imposed angle. Calculating the time course of the stiffness during each ramp stretch, the thixotropic effect can be evaluated (see Fig. 13).

Another way of presenting this data is to plot the force against the elbow angle. The resulting hysteresis curve is a measurement of static stiffness as well as of energy absorbed during one movement cycle.

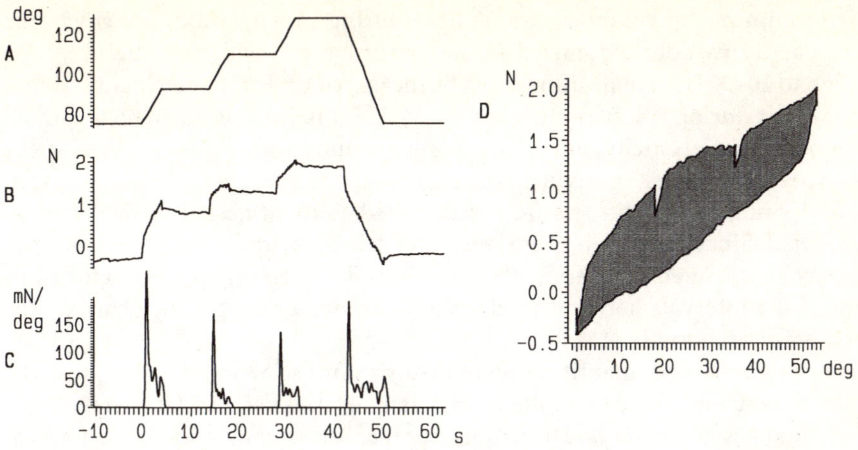

Fig. 15. One trial of a slow ramp stretch sequence of the relaxed forearm of a healthy subject. **A** Elbow angle (angular velocities were 0°/s, + 4.5°/s or − 6.2° /s, respectively). **B** Tangential force, measured at the wrist approximately 25 cm distal to the elbow. **C** Total stiffness, calculated from **A** and **B** (note that inertia contribution has not been removed). **D** Tangential force plotted against the elbow angle. The *shaded area* corresponds to the energy absorbed by the arm during the movement sequence. The first derivative of the curves correspond to the total stiffness

Discussion

Evaluation and Quantification of Muscle Tone

Our goal was to elaborate methods for investigating separately various components contributing to muscle tone in the upper extremity.

To minimize influences of the mechanical stimuli on muscle tone, we applied single perturbations during relaxation and isometric contraction.

The wide range of perturbation amplitude allow the application of our methods to patients with various degrees of hyper- and hypotonia.

For evaluation of muscle stiffness in the upper extremity, various methodological approaches are described, which differ mainly in motor task and kind of perturbation. The aim of most of the investigations was to analyze mechanisms contributing to muscle tone [3,5].

The various perturbation methods can be separated in three groups: (1) oscillation, (2) stochastic, and (3) transient perturbation. To generate oscillatory movements of joints, periodic [13] or single-pulse perturbations [7,12] can be induced. From the measurement of amplitude, resonance frequency, and damping, the total stiffness can be evaluated and separated in elasticity and viscosity. With this method, nonlinearity in mechanical properties such as thixotropy and fatigue-induced changes were investigated. However, initial and reflex components of stiffness cannot be separated.

To minimize the voluntary component during investigation, the stochastic methods apply pseudorandomized torque perturbations with maximal frequencies of up to 10–50 Hz. Total stiffness can be measured under isometric contraction [10] as well as during voluntary movement [1]. The total stiffness can be separated continuously into elasticity and viscosity. As dynamic stimuli applied during the whole experiment, reflex components cannot be separated from the initial stiffness.

To separate initial stiffness from reflex-mediated stiffness, transient stimuli were applied. Since in disorders of skeletal muscle tone, various stiffness components may be modified independently, this method is currently preferred for clinical use. If the intervals between single stimuli are long enough, they can also be applied pseudorandomly [11].

For evaluation and quantification of disturbed muscle tone, e.g., in spasticity, one has to consider the concomitant paresis and weakness. In later stages, additional changes in tissue and neuronal compensation may contribute to joint stiffness.

The degree of paresis should be investigated to choose adequate perturbation ranges and also be considered in evaluating the results.

Demarcation Between Spasticity and Rigidity

In spasticity, during relaxation or slight activation we found decreased initial stiffness in both the finger flexors and the forearm flexors and extensors, probably due to the concomitant weakness, whereas in the finger flexors the short-latency reflex response is increased, in the forearm flexors and extensors the long-latency reflex responses are magnified.

In rigidity, during relaxation in both the finger flexors and the forearm flexors and extensors the initial stiffness is increased. This could be explained by spontaneous tonic activity and larger viscous resistance. During isometric contraction, the late reflex components are enlarged in both finger flexors and forearm flexors and extensors. Remarkably, under isometric contraction there is no obvious difference to normals in initial stiffness in either spasticity or rigidity. According to our observations, the main difference between spasticity and rigidity relevant for muscle tone is obvious in stiffness during relaxation.

Our findings concerning the stretch reflex activity in spasticity during relaxation confirm the interpretation by Thilmann et al. [29] as a pathological increase in stretch reflex gain in the passive limb. In spasticity, however, there is some controversy concerning the role of reflex activity for muscle stiffness during active movement [30]. Dietz et al. [4] have suggested that pathological change in the muscle fibers themselves is a major cause of spastic hypertonia in the leg, rather than activation. Measuring the muscle stiffness in spastic hemiparesis within the first 200 ms following the stimulus, we could not find significantly increased joint stiffness on the spastic side, and the late stretch reflex components are even magnified. This is in analogy to the findings of Lee et al. [15], Powers et al. [18], and Sinkjær et al. [20].

Concerning rigidity, our results are almost in line with previous findings [2,17,28]. It is not surprising that not all investigations reveal clear correlations between amplitude of the long-latency reflexes and muscle tone, especially under voluntary activity [9,14,19]. One can suppose that in rigidity, the current level of ongoing spontaneous activity modulates the amount of late reflex components. In this case, the muscle stiffness during relaxation or slight voluntary activation is increased, whereas muscle stiffness during isometric contraction remains nearly the same.

Conclusion

Dynamic perturbations permit the evaluation and quantification of initial and dynamic reflex components of muscle stiffness. Slow movement with large displacement of limbs during relaxation or low activity enables us to measure long-lasting tonic responses as well as intrinsic factors such as static stiffness and thixotropy. Investigations of the intrinsic mechanical behavior of muscle might provide more insight into the role of intrafusal muscle fibers modifying alpha motor unit activity and muscle tone.

It is only the mechanics (displacement and/or stiffness) that enable us to evaluate and quantify the postural components of our motor tasks. Simultaneous EMG recordings (superficial EMG of the underlying muscles) show the timing of the contributing reflex responses. However, there is little information about force and stiffness, especially under dynamic conditions. On the basis of our experience with the described experiments, we are developing a universal torque motor for standardized measurements of muscle tone in patients. This method should allow us to evaluate initial stiffness and dynamic mechanical behavior as well as thixotropic and long-lasting tonic phenomena.

References

1. Bennett DJ, Hollerbach JM, Xu Y, Hunter IW (1992) Time-varying stiffness of human elbow joint during cyclic voluntary movement. Exp Brain Res 88(2):433–442
2. Berardelli A, Sabra AF, Hallett M (1983) Physiological mechanisms of rigidity in Parkinson's disease. J Neurol Neurosurg Psychiatry 46:45–53
3. Carter RR, Crago PE, Keith MW (1990) Stiffness regulation by reflex action in the normal human hand. J Neurophysiol 64:105–118
4. Dietz V, Quintern J, Berger W (1981) Electrophysiological studies of gain in spasticity and rigidity. Evidence that altered mechanical properties of muscle contribute to hypertonia. Brain 104:431–449
5. Doemges F, Rack PMH (1992) Task-dependent changes in the response of human wrist joints to mechanical disturbance. J Physiol (Lond) 447:575–585
6. Ghez C (1991) Muscles: effectors of the motor systems. In: Kandel ER, Schwartz JH, Jessell TM (eds) Principles of neural science, 3rd edn. Elsevier, New York, pp 548–563
7. Gurfinkel VS, Ivanenko YP, Levik YS (1989) Dissipative protsessy V passivnoi skeletnoi myshtse cheloveka. Biofizika 34:499–503 (with English abstract)

8. Jahnke MT, Proske U, Struppler A (1989) Measurement of muscle stiffness, the electromyogram and activity in single muscle spindles of human flexor muscles following conditioning by passive stretch or contraction. Brain Res 493:103–112
9. Keidel M, Klein W, Struppler A (1990) Stretch reflex modifications by subthalamotomy: a follow up study in parkinsonian patients. J Psychophysiol 4:103–114
10. Kirsch RF, Rymer WZ (1992) Neural compensation for fatigue-induced changes in muscle stiffness during perturbations of elbow angle in human. J Neurophysiol 68(2):449–470
11. Lacquaniti F (1990) Quantitative assessment of somatic muscle tone. Funct Neurol 5(3):209–215
12. Lakie M, Robson LG (1988) Thixotropic changes in human muscle stiffness and the effects of fatigue. Q J Exp Physiol 73:487–500
13. Lakie M, Walsh EG, Wright GW (1984) Resonance at the wrist demonstrated by the use of a torque motor: an instrumental analysis of muscle tone in man. J Physiol (Lond) 353:265–285
14. Latash M, Neyman I, Nicholas J (1992) Changes in joint compliance with age and Parkinson's disease. Mov Disord 7[Suppl]: 335
15. Lee WA, Bughton A, Rymer WZ (1987) Absence of stretch reflex gain enhancement in voluntarily activated spastic muscle. Exp Neurol 98:317–335
16. Mackel R, Brink EE, Nakajima Y (1984) Action of tizynidine on responses of forearm flexors and extensors to torque disturbances. J Neurol Neurosurg Psychiatry 47:1109–1116
17. Mortimer JA, Webster DD (1979) Evidence for a quantitative association between EMG stretch responses and parkinsonian rigidity. Brain Res 162:169–173
18. Powers RK, Marder-Meyer J, Rymer WZ (1988) Quantitative relations between hypertonia and stretch reflex threshold in spastic hemi-paresis. Ann Neurol 23:115–124
19. Rothwell JC, Obeso JA, Traub MM, Marsden CD (1983) The behaviour of the long latency stretch reflex in patients with parkinsonian disease. J Neurol Neurosurg Psychiatry 46:35–44
20. Sinkjær T, Toft E, Larsen K, Andreassen S, Hansen HJ (1993) Non-reflex and reflex mediated ankle joint stiffness in multiple sclerosis patients with spasticity. Muscle Nerve 16:69–76
21. Struppler A (1990) Feedback mechanisms controlling skeletal muscle tone. In: Deecke L, Eccles JC, Mountcastle VB (eds) From neuron to action. An appraisal of fundamental and clinical research. Springer, Berlin Heidelberg New York, pp 71–80
22. Struppler A, Jahnke MT (1989) Sensomotorische Kontrolle am Beispiel der Arm- und Fingermotorik. In: Hippius H, Rüther E, Schmauß M (eds) Katatone und dyskinetische Syndrome. Springer, Berlin Heidelberg New York, pp 13–26
23. Struppler A, Jahnke MT (1990) Some aspects of reflex and non-reflex muscle stiffness. In: Dengler R (ed) The motor unit: physiology, diseases, regeneration. Urban and Schwarzenberg, Munich, pp 43–47
24. Struppler A, Riescher H, Lorenzen HW, Grueter HP, Schaller J, Chen XZ (1986) Torque motors for investigation of functional stretch reflex. Proc Intern Electr Machines (ICEM) Munich, part 3, pp 940–943
25. Struppler A, Jahnke MT, Riescher H (1989a) Electrophysiological assessment of spasticity. In: Emre M, Benecke R (eds) Spasticity. The current status of research and treatment. Parthenon Publishing Group, Carnforth, UK, pp 81–95
26. Struppler A, Jahnke MT, Riescher H (1989b) Assessment of spasticity: changes in muscle mechanical properties as related to the EMG. Abstract for the international congress on epidural spinal cord stimulation in movement and vascular disorders. Groningen, the Netherlands, 1–3 June 1989
27. Struppler A, Jahnke MT, Riescher H (1989c) Quantification of parkinsonian rigidity: changes in prereflex and reflex stiffness. In: Basal ganglia 1989, 3rd triennial meeting, Capo Boi-Cagliary, Italy, 10–13 June, abstract book, p 168
28. Tatton WG, Lee RG (1975) Evidence for abnormal long-loop reflexes in rigid parkinsonian patients. Brain Res 100:671–676
29. Thilmann AF, Fellows SJ, Garms E (1991) The mechanism of spastic muscle hypertonus. Variation in reflex gain over the time course of spasticity. Brain 114:233–244
30. Wiesendanger M, Palmieri A, Corboz M (1990) Some pathophysiological considerations about muscle tone and spasticity. In: Benecke R, Emre M, Davidoff RA (eds) The origin and treatment of spasticity. Partenon, Casterton, pp 15–27

Discussion

Dr. Hallett: You use both electromyography (EMG) and force measurements; following up the last point that you made you, if were setting up a relatively simple instrumental method for quantifying spasticity or rigidity, would you prefer to use EMG or force or do you think that you'd have to use both?

Dr. Struppler: I think we have to use both. When we're discussing muscle tone I think we have to use both, because the EMG gives no information about muscle tone. It gives information about motor unit activity, but you have no chance to say anything about the mechanics which are developed by the motor units. Therefore, I think we have to measure mechanics. The point is the discrimination between viscosity and elasticity, which is not simple.

Dr. Rabey: In your presentation you discriminate between spasticity and rigidity. Maybe I didn't understand what you said about deceleration properly.

Dr. Struppler: Deceleration is the first paradigm, We are only interested in the so-called short-range stiffness, i.e., stiffness in isometric contraction – when the tonic reflex is involved, of course, but preceding the shortest dynamic reflex response. Under sustained isometric contraction in spasticity, you usually have a decrease in muscle stiffness, probably because of paresis or hypotonia. Then the stretch reflexes are involved, and the amount of the stretch reflex depends, as you know, on the kind of spasticity, duration of spasticity, and so on. This is short-range spasticity. We are not interested in saying anything about the cross-bridges, rather we are interested in muscle stiffness during holding. Later, after the 30 ms, the dynamic reflexes play an additional role, of course, and have a modifying influence on muscle stiffness; as you know, they can modify what is going on in your limb. This can be measured quantitatively, but for differential diagnosis, it's obviously much better to do this clinically.

Dr. Struppler: I do not have very many measurements for dystonia behavior. It depends on when you measure; after 10 or 20 ms they develop stiffness. For this kind of measurement, when you say you have hypotonia, you have to exclude the concomitant triceps antagonistic muscle. We measure the amount of triceps activity as a routine. When you do this motor task, you do not usually have any considerable activity in your triceps antagonistic muscle, but it should be done because many people say that you have a cocontraction. The cocontraction has to be excluded even during flexion holding.

Instrumental Assessment of Rigidity

W. Greulich, K. Zeppenfeld, and W. Gehlen

Introduction

The valid and general clinical method of testing muscle tone, applied up to this date, is the assessment of muscular resistance to passive stretch [5]. As early as 1937, Schaltenbrand [10] rightly pointed out that classifying the resistance to passive motion of patient's limbs by hand is a subjective method and that therefore an objective method of measuring tone is necessary.

Ever since muscle tone began to be measured by mechanic devices, mechanomyographic methods have been in the fore front. Mosso [7] and Rieger [8] were the first to perform myographic tests on human beings. They stretched the flexors and extensors of the knee joint by means of exerted weights, from which they obtained curves which showed the relation between tension and muscle length.

In 1929, Schaltenbrand first used a spring dynamometer and from 1958 onward he used strain gauges to measure force required to produce a definite degree of flexion of any relaxed limb over a certain distance [9,11]. Later Watts et al. [14] used a different way of measuring force: a torque motor for measuring the tone. It consisted of assessing the rigidity at the elbow represented by the slope of a curve when torque is plotted against angular displacement.

In the 1960s it was electromyographically possible to show that in rigid muscle at rest, a steady discharge of single motor units appears and while maintaining the stretch continuous tonic activity occurs in the stretched muscle [12]. On the other hand, under conditions that decrease the load on a rigid muscle, a burst of electromyogram (EMG) activity appeared. This shortening reaction with an increase of EMG activity when a rigid muscle is passively shortened is, according to Denny Brown [2], of diagnostic significance with regard to latent rigidity.

From the pathophysiological point of view, reflex tests and F wave analyses have added further importance to rigidity [1]. Figure 1 gives a general view of the various methods of mechanical assessment of rigidity.

Above all the rigidity in patients with Parkinson's disease is a matter of raised muscle activity in passive stretching [6]. It was our aim to create a method which would take account of this aspect. Furthermore, as far as the usual clinical assessment of rigidity is concerned, a statement about agonists and antagonists of the elbow joint should be made. We therefore chose the myointegration method,

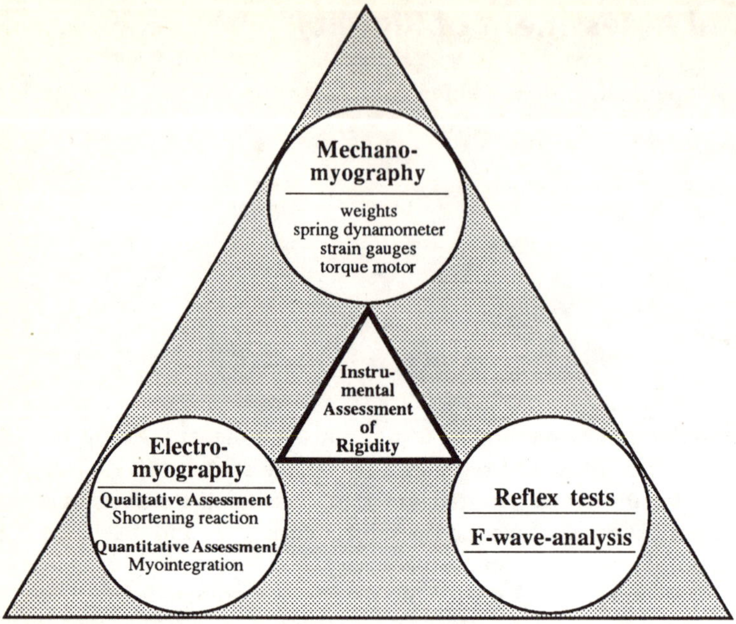

Fig. 1. Methods for instrumental assessment of rigidity

which has turned out well in assessing the effectiveness of L-dopa [3,4]. We also improved the method shown by Gehlen and Eisenlohr [4] using passive arm movements with the help of an electrical device with variable velocity.

Methods

The upper arm is placed horizontally on a semicircular acryl support (Fig. 2, *1*), while the forearm is strapped to an acryl pan (*3*), which is mounted on the lever arm (*2*) of a motor (*5*) and which swings in vertical direction. By means of a crank disc (*4*) and a crank rod (*6*), it is possible to transform the circulation of an electric motor (*5*) into a vertical angle movement with changeable angle size.

As measurement for the rigidity, EMG activity is simultaneously deducted over the M. biceps brachii and M. triceps brachii (Fig. 3). EMG activity now comes via an amplifier to a rectifier circuit. The integrator generally contains a condenser; the condenser's function is to sum up the tension during a 1-min period of measurement.

Afterwards, the analog value proportional to the EMG activity was changed to digital value by an analog–digital (AD) converter and appeared on a counter. A computer connected to the circuit provided the online data capture. Alternating current and tremor artifacts that might falsify the results were detected in time with the aid of an EMG monitor. For rest and passive movement, we determined

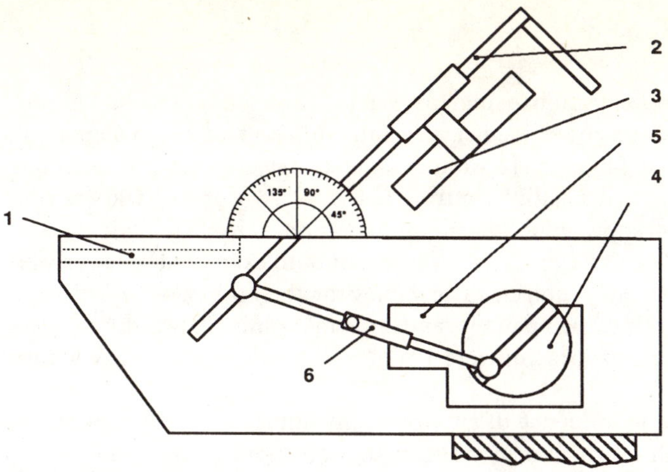

Fig. 2. Vertical myotonograph. See text for details

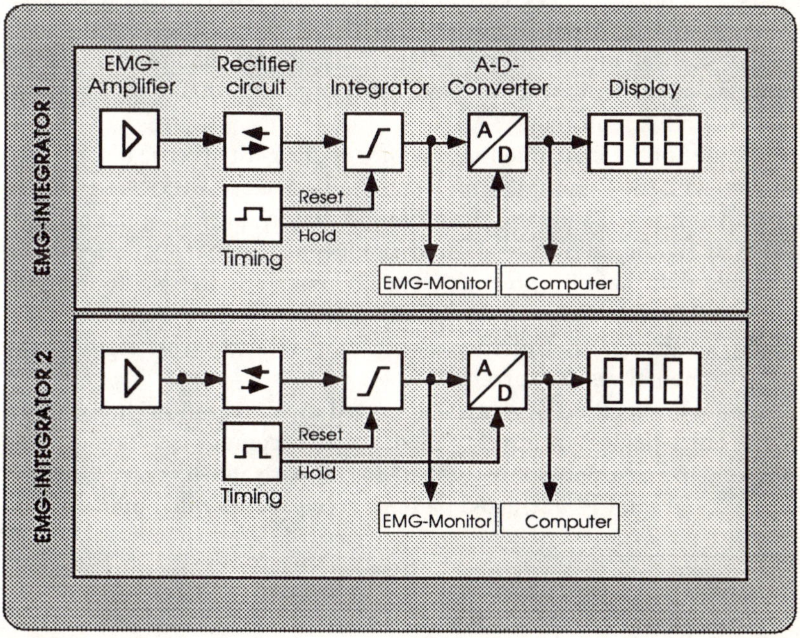

Fig. 3. Quantitative assessment of rigidity by means of myointegration. *EMG*, electromyogram; *A–D*, analog–digital

the myointegration values for the M. biceps brachii and M. triceps brachii. Before each movement, phase 3 rest values were determined for the agonist and the antagonist. Then the passive movement of the arm starts with 30 flexures and extensions per min, in which the elbow angle reached 70°. This phase of movement lasts 8 min. Analog to the start, the assessment ends with a 3-min rest period.

Results

Motor-supported myointegration using the vertical myotonograph at rest and during passive arm movement yielded significantly different values in 65 patients with Parkinson's disease (49 men, 16 women; median age, 64.4 ± 9.5 years) compared with 50 age-matched healthy controls (24 men, 26 women) with normal muscle tone. Figure 4 shows that the myointegration values of patients with Parkinson's disease at rest and during movement of both examined muscles were higher than those of normal subjects. The values for the M. biceps brachii were 119.12 mV × min in parkinsonian patients and 32.24 mV × min, in healthy subjects, the values for the M. triceps brachii were 121.60 mV × min and 62.90 mV × min, respectively.

In order to judge the influence of gravity on myointegration, we constructed another myotonograph in which arm movements were carried out with help of a 450-W alternate current motor in a horizontal direction (Fig. 5). As Fig. 6 shows, the values were 20% higher on average during vertical arm movement than horizontal movement. The differences, however, were not significant. Furthermore, Fig. 6 shows that vertical and horizontal values increased for the first 3 min. After the third minute, values tended to stabilize. This indicated that a minimum of 4–5 min of test period is required.

The significance of the instrumental assessment of rigidity (vertical myotonograph) compared with the Columbia University Rating Scale (CURS) was tested in 550 patients with Parkinson's disease. It was found that the parkinsonian patients with no degree of rigidity clinically showed significantly higher myointegration movement values than healthy normals (Fig. 7). Furthermore, we found that electromyographically there was no difference between degree 0 (absent) and degree 1 (slight) of the CURS. In patients with moderate to severe rigidity, the clinical and instrumental results correlate.

To what extent the method of motor-supported myointegration can be taken as proof of the efficiency of antirigidity medication becomes clear through the example of biperiden and amantadine sulphate in comparison with corresponding values of the CURS. A total 17 untreated patients received biperiden in increasing

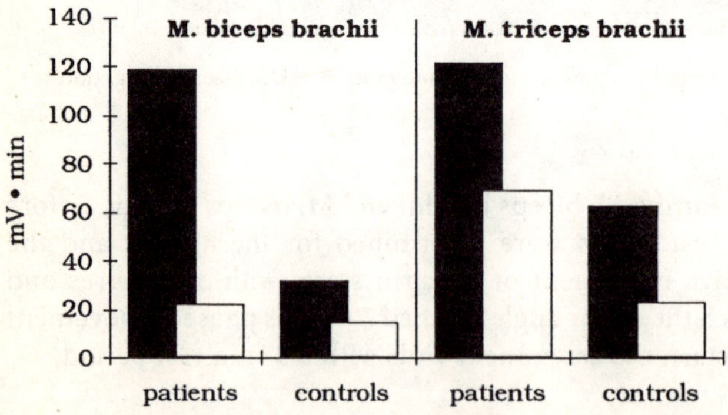

Fig. 4. Myointegration in 65 patients with Parkinson's disease and 50 healthy subjects using a vertical myotonograh. *Black bars*, movement; *white bars*, rest

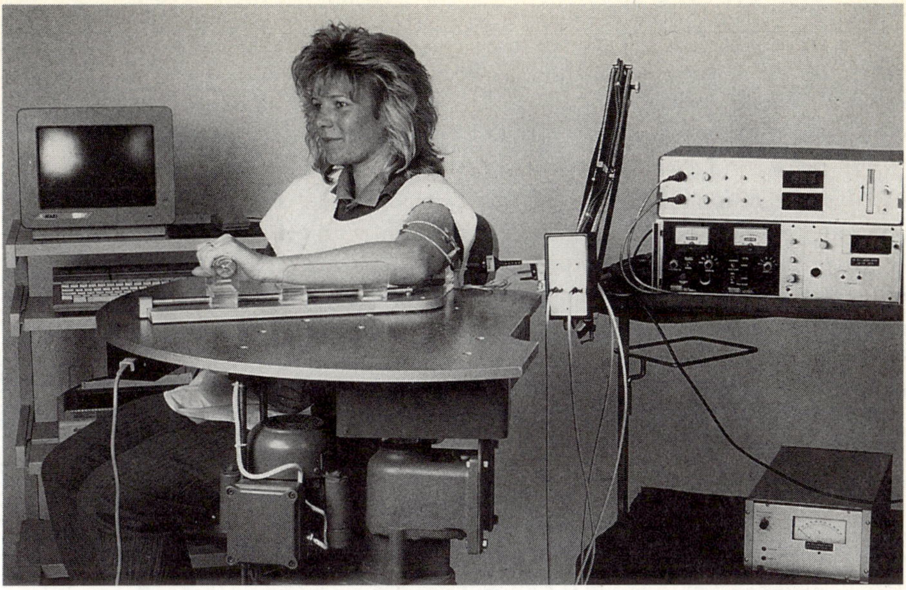

Fig. 5. Horizontal myotonograph

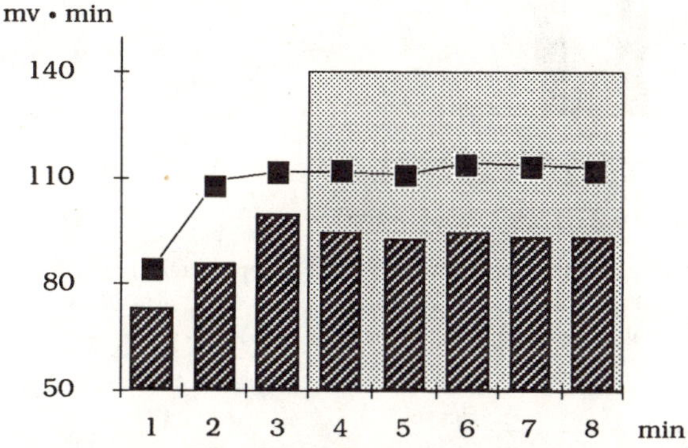

Fig. 6. The effect of gravity on quantitative assessment of rigidity (M. biceps brachii) by means of different myotonographs. *Black boxes*, vertical movement; *shaded boxes*, horizontal movement

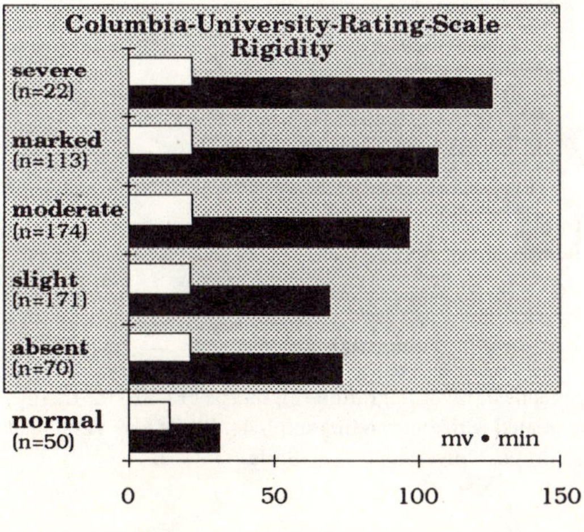

Fig. 7. Quantitative assessment of rigidity by means of myointegration (M. biceps brachii) based on the clinical score of the Columbia University Rating Scale. *White bars*, rest; *black bars*, movememt

doses. In the course of 42 days of tests, the myointegration values (vertical myotonograph) showed a significant decrease, particularly during the period of movement (Fig. 8).

In the second case, 26 untreated patients received amantadine sulphate (Fig. 9). Myointegration measurement was carried out regularly during a period of 6 months, accompanied by clinical examination with the CURS.

In the steady state (168th day) with an average dose of 332 mg amantadine, the integration values during movement showed a significant decrease (vertical myotonograph). At rest, the mean values showed a decreasing tendency with no significance. At the end of the sixth month, amantadine sulphate was withdrawn for a period of 6 days, followed by treatment at the dosage mentioned above. The

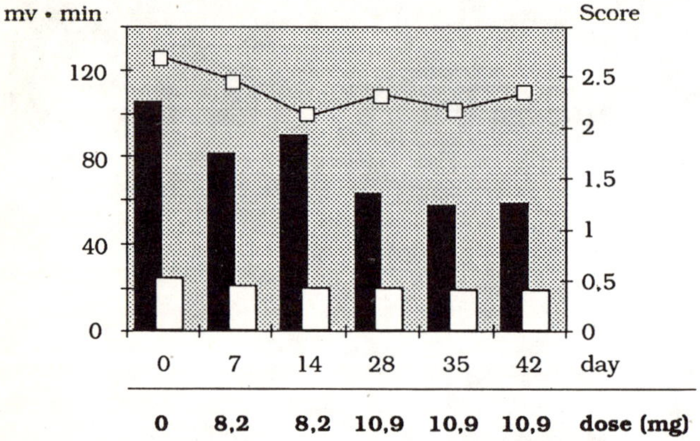

Fig. 8. Quantitative assessment of rigidity by means of myointegration (M. biceps brachii) for therapy control in 17 patients with Parkinson's disease treated with biperiden. *White bars*, rest; *black bars*, movement; *white squares*, rigidity on Columbia University Rating Scale (CURS)

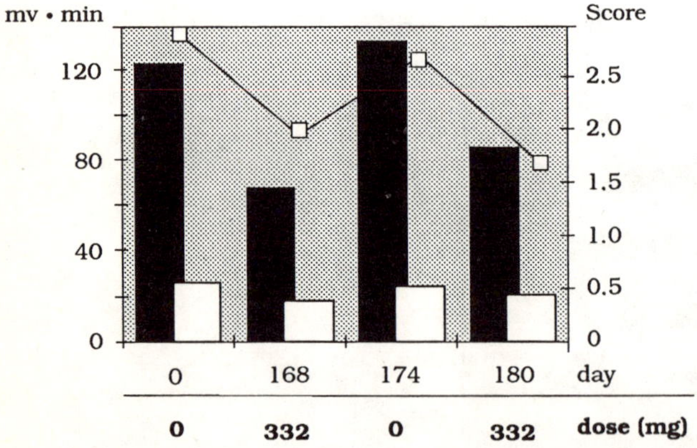

Fig. 9. Quantitative assessment of rigidity by means of myointegration (M. biceps brachii) for therapy control in 26 patients with Parkinson's disease treated with amantadine sulphate. *White bars*, rest; *black bars*, movement; *white squares*, rigidity on Columbia University Rating Scale

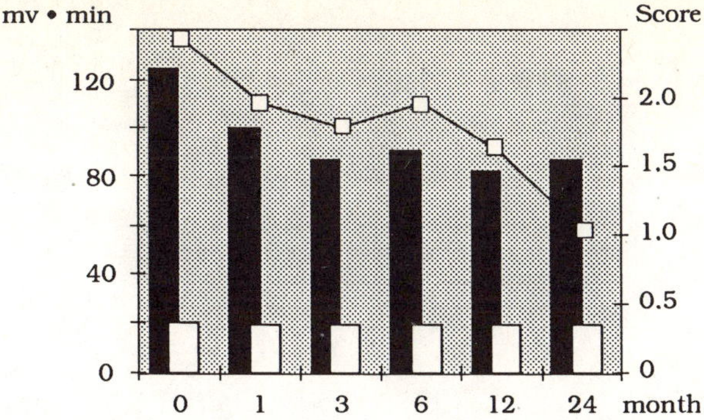

Fig. 10. Quantitative assessment of rigidity by means of myointegration (M. biceps brachii) for long-term therapy control in 25 patients with Parkinson's disease. *White bars*, rest; *black bars* movement; *white boxes*, rigidity on Columbia University Rating Scale (CURS)

drug discontinuance caused a significant increase in the myointegration values, while resumption of treatment decreased the values significantly.

The instrumental assessment of rigidity does not only indicate the effect of a particular drug, but is also a method for long-term therapy control. Figure 10 summarizes the results of 25 parkinsonian patients over 2 years; their medication is listed in Table 1.

Discussion

The necessity of judging Parkinson symptoms dates back more than 30 years [13]. Today there are two test categories: the subjective, qualitative examination of Parkinson symptoms and dysfunctions by means of rating scales and the objective, quantitative method of measurement by means of instrumental techniques. Both methods convert clinical symptoms into numerical data in order to be able to arrive at a statistical calculation, but only instrumental assessments enable measurements to be made over a longer period of time independent of an observer.

We developed the procedure of motor-supported myointegration, which has proved to be good in many respects. Thus, objective proof of the efficiency of biperiden and amantadine sulphate was obtained. The rigidity-reducing effect of biperiden after 42 days treatment with 10.9 mg per day (mean) amounted to 46% and for amantadine sulphate (332 mg per day) in steady state 47%. Compared with the instrumental assessment of rigidity, clinical measurement showed only an average reduction of 14% by using biperiden, which was not significant. By using amantadine, the results of both methods were equal.

This means that for biperiden our technique was more sensitive than clinical measurement; for amantadine sulphate, it gave almost the same results. The value of motor-supported myointegration was also seen in assessments of parkinsonian

Table 1. Two-year course of medication (dose and number of patients) of a total of 25 patients with Parkinson's disease

Month	Amantadine sulphate[a] (mg)	number of patients	Madopar 125[b] (mg)	number of patients	Nacom 100[c] (mg)	number of patients	Selegiline[d] (mg)	number of patients	Bromocriptine[e] (mg)	number of patients	Lisuride[f] (mg)	number of patients
0	300	[8]	390	[12]	316	[3]	9	[9]	10	[8]	–	–
1	323	[11]	417	[12]	340	[5]	10	[11]	13	[8]	–	–
3	363	[12]	423	[13]	400	[4]	10	[12]	14	[8]	–	–
6	390	[10]	411	[12]	400	[4]	9	[12]	15	[9]	–	–
12	373	[11]	414	[13]	329	[7]	10	[16]	14	[9]	0.6	[1]
24	336	[7]	426	[16]	325	[6]	9	[17]	13	[9]	1.6	[3]

[a] PK-Merz (Merz).
[b] 100 mg levodopa and 25 mg benserazide (Roche).
[c] 100 mg levodopa and 25 mg carbidopa (DuPont).
[d] Movergan (Asta Medica).
[e] Pravidel (Sandoz).
[f] Dopergin (Schering).

patients over a long period; a reduction of rigidity could be observed over 2 years, independently of the observer. The observation that patients with Parkinson's disease who clinically had no rigidity, but had higher myointegration values during movement compared with healthy persons, is indicative of the sensitivity of motor-supported myointegration.

References

1. Delwaide PJ (1985) Are there modifications in spinal cord functions of parkinsonian patients? In: Delwaide PJ, Agnoli A (eds) Clinical neurophysiology in parkinsonism. Elsevier, Amsterdam, pp 19–32
2. Denny-Brown D (1962) The basal ganglia and their relation to disorders of movement. Oxford University Press, London
3. Eisenlohr J, Gehlen W (1979) Quantitative Messung des Muskeltonus bei Parkinson Kranken vor und während Madopar-Therapie. Fortschr Neurol Psychiatr 47:331–346
4. Gehlen W, Eisenlohr J (1974) Quantitative Rigormessung bei Morbus Parkinson. Nervenarzt 45:22–29
5. Hopf H (1974) Tonusprüfung (Mechanomyographie). In: Hopf HC, Struppler A (eds) Elektromyographie, Lehrbuch und Atlas. Thieme, Stuttgart, pp 201–209
6. Marsden C (1990) Neurophysiology. In: Stern GM (eds) Parkinson's disease. Chapman and Hall Medical, London, pp 456–457
7. Mosso A (1896) Description d'un myotonomètre pour étudier la tonicité des muscles chez l'homme. Arch Ital biol 25:346
8. Rieger R (1926) Untersuchungen über Muskelzustände. Fischer, Stuttgart
9. Schaltenbrand G (1929) Muscle tone in man. Arch Surg 18:1874–1885
10. Schaltenbrand G (1937) Myographische Untersuchungen in der Klinik. Dtsch Z Nervenheilkd 142:1–17
11. Schaltenbrand G, Hampl F (1958) Über einen neuen Myographen. Dtsch Z Nervenheilkd 178:276–288
12. Steinbrecher W (1965) Elektromyographie in Klinik und Praxis. Thieme, Stuttgart
13. Teräväinen H, Calne D (1980) Quantitative assessment of parkinsonian deficits. In: Rinne UK, Klinger M, Stamm G (eds) Parkinson's disease – current progress, problems and management. Elsevier North-Holland, Amsterdam, pp 145–164
14. Watts R, Wiegner A, Young R (1986) Elastic properties of muscle measured at the elbow in man. II. Patients with parkinsonian rigidity. J Neurol Neurosurg Psychiatry 49:1177-1781

Discussion

Dr. Watts: How long does it take you to do your test on a given person.

Dr. Zeppenfeld: I remember the effect of gravity on myointegration. After the third minute, in general values tend to stabilize, so if you only want to choose one value, a period of 5 min would be enough. Including placing the electrodes, I guess it takes about 15 min altogether.

Dr. Muenter: Every once in a while you run into patients that simply cannot relax and contract in a kind of a semivoluntary fashion. Does that pose a problem with your technique in terms of contaminating the results?

Dr. Zeppenfeld: In patients who are not able to relax completely or who show a tendency to resist or assist the movements which could be detected by EMG monitoring, the test was interrupted or the values of this test period were excluded. But patients usually get accustomed after a few minutes of test period, and therefore over a test period of 15–20 min, it wasn't a problem in the end.

Tremor Assessment in Clinical Trials

P.G. Bain and L.J. Findley

Introduction

During the last two decades there has been an increasing number of clinical trials evaluating the effect of drugs on tremor severity. Trial organisers have appreciated that "open" studies may produce misleading results and consequently have utilised randomised double-blind protocols for definitive studies, in order to minimise bias. In practice, these trials have relied heavily on accelerometry as the objective method of measurement and clinical rating scales and patient self-assessments as the subjective methods.

As the purpose of a clinical trial is to determine whether or not a particular therapy helps patients, it is vital that the outcome measures relate to disability. Otherwise, the outcome measures become abstractions and of no practical importance. The validity of a trial depends upon the method used for assessing tremor severity relating, in a meaningful way, to changes in the patients' daily lives.

The reliability of the methods used in a trial to assess tremor should be known prior to the start of the study, because this information will influence the number of patients required to show a specific size of therapeutic effect. It might also suggest to the trial organisers that specific raters are replaced or rating systems changed to more reliable ones.

Reliability can be measured by statistical methods, for example Cohen's kappa coefficients [1], to provide numerical values for the interrater and intrarater reliability of raters using a specific rating scale. The use of weighted kappa coefficients has been widely acknowledged as suitable for assessing reliability because they are distribution free, allow credit for partial agreement between raters, and correct for agreement due to chance. They also make use of individual items in the rating scale and correct for differences in the raters' mean scores [2,3]. Kappa scores are conventionally interpreted as shown in Table 1.

The reliability of the various subjective rating scales used to assess tremor in the clinical trials published up to now has never been assessed. This oversight must cast some doubt on the results of these trials. Furthermore, the question of whether or not accelerometry provides a valid index of tremor-induced disability has never been formally examined.

Table 1. Interpretation of kappa scores

Kappa coefficient	Strength of agreement
<0	Poor
0.00 – 0.20	Slight
0.21 – 0.40	Fair
0.41 – 0.60	Moderate
0.61 – 0.80	Substantial
0.81 – 1.00	Almost perfect

Methods of Assessing Tremor Severity

Subjective Assessments

Patient Disability Self-Questionnaires

Studies have shown that, in general, patients give an accurate account of their own physical disability, providing that no concurrent mental illness is present [4]. The principle problem is to provide patients with a questionnaire that is readily understood and which can be transcribed into numerical values for statistical analysis. An example of an activity of daily living questionnaire is shown in the Appendix. The patients were asked when using this questionnaire to circle a number (next to each item) which described most accurately how easy or difficult it was for them to perform the relevant activity. The sum of the scores for each item was then converted into percentages, with zero implying no disability and the higher the percentage, the more disabled the patient.

Comparison of the various questionnaires available concerning activities of daily living reveals the principle problem inherent in this method of assessment, namely what items should be included within the questionnaire?

In particular, is any specific item a good indicator of patients' overall disability (e.g., dominant hand function) or are several items required to assess this? Is utilisation of all the item (elemental) scores and their addition to give a "total" score appropriate (because in individual patients, the scores for specific items may well be correlated and are, therefore, not independent variables)? Does the utilisation of a scale having several interrelated items increase the reliability of the overall score? What proportion of the questionnaire should reflect dominant hand function, bimanual function, toiletting or mobility?

The composition of tremor self-questionnaires deserves further study, because improvement in the patients' activities of daily living is the principal objective of symptomatic treatment. Furthermore, patients' views on changes in their own disability are likely to be highly influential on whether or not they comply with therapy.

Tremor Rating Scales

Tremor rating scales have been widely employed for documenting changes in tremor severity during clinical trials. The composition of these scales has differed considerably from trial to trial, although there has been very little discussion about the relative merits of each design [5–12].

We would suggest that several aspects of rating scale design can be improved upon by:

1. Relating the severity of tremor to the parts of the body that are affected.
2. Keeping the scores for each anatomical site separate and not amalgamating them or producing an average (as this does not make sense and causes useful information to be lost).
3. Avoiding the inclusion of measurements of disability or handicap within an impairment scale.
4. Optimising the number of gradations (steps) within the scale. Too few steps will produce an insensitive scale, but increasing the number amplifies the difficulty of consistent judgement. However, increasing the number of steps also decreases the significance of a "unit" error, so that true score variance is altered advantageously for reliability [13–14].

A tremor rating scale, which we designed with these specifications in mind, is shown in Appendix B. This scale was chosen after experimenting with various alternatives because raters found it easy to use. The scores obtained by raters employing this scale correlated well with the results – root mean square (rms) acceleration – of accelerometry and patients' self-assessments of their own disability. The raters' scores were also assessed for their inter- and intrarater reliability using Cohen's kappa coefficients and were found to be in the moderate to almost perfect range for postural tremor of the upper limbs and head tremors. The assessments were performed from videotapes of 20 patients with essential tremor or the tremor associated with dystonia (P.G. Bain and L.J. Findley, unpublished observation).

No other tremor rating scale has been assessed in this way or been shown to correlate with disability.

Spiralography and Handwriting Impairment

It is routine clinical practice to obtain specimens of handwriting and spirals from tremulous patients. However, can the tremor apparent in a spiral or piece of handwriting be scored reliably and does the score correlate with disability?

We assessed the inter- and intrarater reliability of four raters' scores for the tremor visible in 20 spirals and handwriting specimens. A 0–10 subjective scoring system was used and the results analysed using kappa coefficients. The raters produced scores that had inter- and intrarater reliabilities in the fair to almost perfect ranges. The results also showed good correlations with those obtained using the clinical rating scale shown in Fig. 1, upper limb rms acceleration, and patients' self-assessments of disability (P.G. Bain and L.J. Findley, unpublished observation).

Improvements in the reliability of this method could be obtained by having a collection of previously graded spirals and writing specimens to refer to whilst scoring.

The simplicity of this technique could allow assessments to be carried out by postal survey; providing the way in which a spiral is to be drawn has been stand-

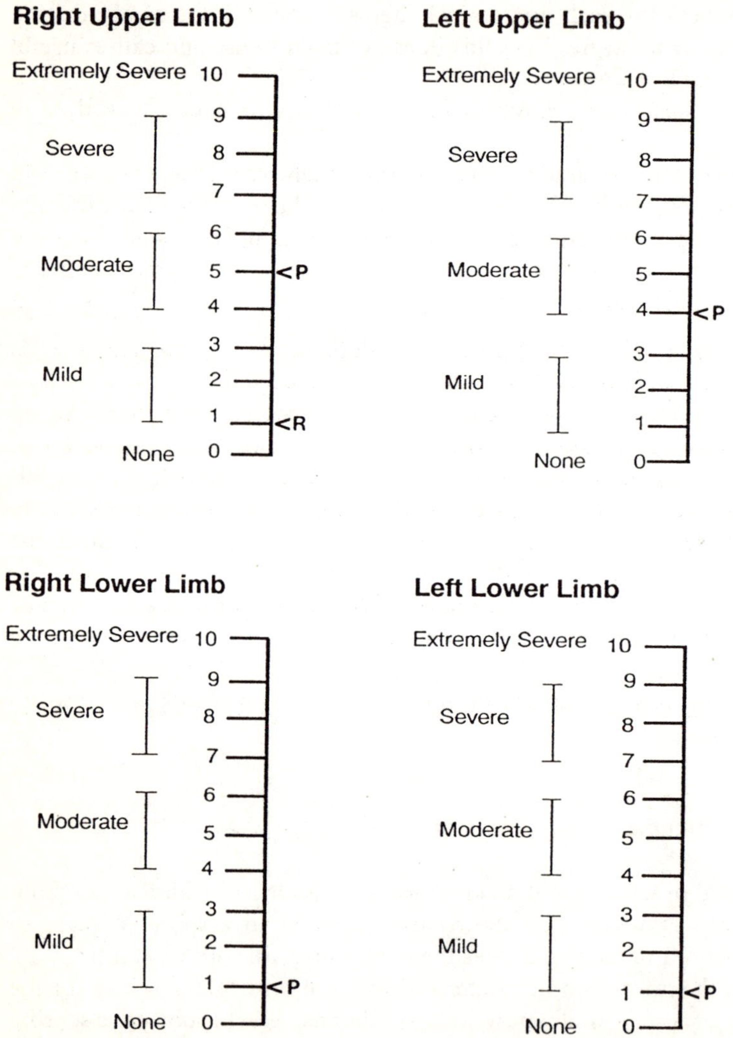

Fig. 1. The rating scale: an example is shown of a patient with grade 5 right and grade 4 left upper limb postural tremor (*P*), grade 1 right upper limb rest tremor (*R*) and grade 1 lower limb P. A similar system can be used for grading head tremor

ardised beforehand. A further advantage with this technique is that, because patients will have learnt to write and draw in childhood and will have practised subsequently, there is unlikely to be a significant training effect caused by serial assessments. This is not the case with accelerometry or more complex hospital-based techniques.

There is one drawback to spiralography, which is that it is rather over-sensitive to fine tremors. This lack of selectivity can be minimised by asking the patients to hold the pen in a normal way and not at the top.

Objective Assessments

Accelerometry

Piezo-resistive linear accelerometry has been widely adopted as the most suitable objective method of quantifying tremor. The accelerometer signals can be amplified and analysed on line to produce averaged spectra which display the rms magnitude of the frequency components as a function of frequency.

There are several difficulties with this technique: Firstly, most studies have used uniaxial accelerometers, which only record tremor in one dimension. Second, accelerometers can only reflect tremor activity at their site of attachment (usually the dorsum of the hand for the upper limb). Third, low-frequency, high-displacement tremor components (intermittent "jumps") produce little effect on the dominant peak of an averaged spectra, but are the events most likely to disrupt a piece of work. Fourth, hospital-based accelerometric assessments have been shown to produce a significant trend towards lower tremor amplitudes at successive evaluation of untreated patients [15]. This introduces a training effect or bias that would have to be accounted for during a clinical trial. Finally, recent studies have shown that the magnitude of acceleration of the dominant spectral peak did not correlate with the disability of patients with postural tremor (P.G. Bain and L.J. Findley, unpublished observation). This observation must put the validity of using standard accelerometric techniques during clinical trials in question. Perhaps accelerometry could provide more meaningful results if recordings were obtained during specific tasks; for example, drawing a spiral rather than a maintained posture. However, this remains to be seen. In the meantime, overemphasis on accelerometry should be avoided in clinical trials.

Volume of Water Spilt From a Cup

The volume of water spilt from a cup, held at arm's length by the patient for 1 min, has been used to provide a simple objective measurement of tremor severity [16]. The method is cheap and could be used by patients to make serial, home-based self-assessments. Our studies have shown that the volume of water spilt correlated well with the degree of tremor documented in spirals and with the peak amplitude of tremor, obtained by accelerometry whilst holding the cup. However, this method is relatively insensitive to fine-amplitude tremors (P.G. Bain and L.J. Findley, unpublished observation).

Conclusion

Tremors are highly complex phenomena that vary continuously with the state of activity of the patients. The parameters of tremor alter from beat to beat and from minute to minute, making assessment of severity extremely difficult. However, some method of quantifying tremor severity is necessary if the natural histories of tremors are to be understood and the influence of drugs comprehended. There are advantages and disadvantages to each of the techniques commonly employed.

Patient disability self-questionnaires provide the most meaningful results in terms of deciding whether or not a particular treatment has actually helped patients with their activities of daily living. However, further research is required to produce optimal questionnaires.

Tremor rating scales must be carefully designed and evaluated for intra- and interrater reliability prior to use in a clinical trial. This would allow, if necessary, trial organisers to switch scales or drop particularly unreliable raters. It would also provide some indication of the number of patients required to show a specific size of therapeutic effect. Without this information, the results of a clinical trial relying upon a tremor rating system are questionable.

Spiralography provides another simple, subjective method of assessing tremor severity which correlates well with disability. It can be sufficiently reliable for the purposes of a therapeutic trial and provides a permanent, objective record of patients' tremors. It has the additional potential advantage of allowing data to be collected by post.

Accelerometry, which is the most frequently used objective method of measuring tremor severity, provides an accurate record of two tremor indices: (1) the magnitude of the rms acceleration and (2) the frequency of the principal peak in a spectrum. However, our studies have shown that neither of these measures correlate with the tremor-induced disabilities of patients with postural tremor. Furthermore, the results of trials relying upon accelerometry should be interpreted with caution, because serial hospital-based recordings produce a systematic bias that will tend to over-estimate the beneficial effects of two drugs involved in a comparison study and the size of a placebo effect. Perhaps the results of accelerometry could be improved upon by recording during specific tasks rather than standard postures, but this remains to be seen.

Finally, the volume of water spilt from a cup provides a potentially attractive method of recording tremor severity in an objective way. However, it is insensitive to low-amplitude tremors and the test–retest reliability of the technique is unknown.

Acknowledgments. We would like to thank the Wellcome Trust for funding this research and Michael Gresty, Marie Vidailhet, Madhuri Behari, Paul Atchison, and Judit Mally for their help with various parts of this study.

Appendix. Activities of Daily Living Self-questionnaire

For each item, circle the number which describes how easy or difficult it is for you to perform the activity:

1. Cut food with a knife and fork	1	2	3	4
2. Use a spoon to drink soup	1	2	3	4
3. Hold a cup of tea	1	2	3	4
4. Pour milk from a bottle or carton	1	2	3	4
5. Wash and dry dishes	1	2	3	4
6. Brush your teeth	1	2	3	4
7. Use a handkerchief to blow your nose	1	2	3	4
8. Use a bath	1	2	3	4
9. Use the lavatory	1	2	3	4
10. Wash your face and hands	1	2	3	4
11. Tie up your shoelaces	1	2	3	4
12. Do up buttons	1	2	3	4
13. Do up a zip	1	2	3	4
14. Write a letter	1	2	3	4
15. Put a letter in an envelope	1	2	3	4
16. Hold and read a newspaper	1	2	3	4
17. Dial a telephone number	1	2	3	4
18. Make yourself understood on the telephone	1	2	3	4
19. Watch television	1	2	3	4
20. Pick up your change in a shop	1	2	3	4
21. Insert an electric plug into a socket	1	2	3	4
22. Unlock your front door with the key	1	2	3	4
23. Walk up and down stairs	1	2	3	4
24. Get up out of an armchair	1	2	3	4
25. Carry a full shopping bag	1	2	3	4

Key: 1 Able to do the activity without difficulty
2 Able to do the activity with a little effort
3 Able to do the activity with a lot of effort
4 Cannot do the activity by yourself

References

1. Francis DA, Bain PG, Swan AV, Hughes RAC (1991) An assessment of disability rating scales used in multiple sclerosis. Arch Neurol 48:299–301

2. Landis JR, Koch GG (1977) The measurement of observer agreement for categorical data. Biometrics 3:159–173
3. Hall JN (1974) Inter-rater reliability of ward rating scales. Br J Psychiatry 125:248–255
4. Brown RG, MacCarthy B, Jahanshahi M, Marsden CD (1989) Accuracy of self-reported disability in patients with parkinsonism. Arch Neurol 46:955–959
5. Webster DD (1968) Critical analysis of the disability in Parkinson's disease. Mod Treatment 5:257–282
6. Duvoisin RC (1970) The evaluation of extrapyramidal disease. In: de Ajuriaguerra J, Gauthier G (eds) Monoamines, noyaux gris centraux et syndrom de Parkinson. Masson, Paris, pp 313–325
7. Lieberman A, Dziatolowski M, Gopinanthan G et al. (1980) Evaluation of Parkinson's disease. In: Goldstein M, Calne DB, Lieberman A, Thorner MO (eds) Ergot components and brain function: neuroendocrine and neuropsychiatric aspects. Raven, New York, pp 277–286
8. Fahn S, Elton RL, members of UPDRS committee (1987) Unified Parkinson's disease rating scale. In: Fahn S, Marsden CD, Goldstein M, Calne DM (eds) Recent developments in Parkinson's disease, vol 2. Macmillan, New York, 153–163, appendices I, II
9. Koller WC (1986) Dose response relationship of propranolol in the treatment of essential tremor. Arch Neurol 43:42–43
10. Cleeves L, Findley LJ (1988) Propranolol and propranolol LA in essential tremor: a double-blind comparative study. J Neurol Neurosurg Psychiatry 51:379–384
11. Muenter MD, Danbe JR, Miller PM (1991) Treatment of essential tremor with methazolamide. Mayo Clin Proc 66:991–997
12. Findley LJ, Cleeves L, Calzetti S (1985) Primidone in essential tremor of the hands and head: a double-blind controlled clinical study. J Neurol Neurosurg Psychiatry 48:911–915
13. Landy FJ, Farr JL (1980) Performance rating. Psychol Bull 87:72–107
14. Nunnally JC (1978) Psychometric theory. McGraw-Hill, New York, chap 15
15. Cleeves L, Findley LJ (1987) Variability in amplitude of untreated essential tremor. J Neurol Neurosurg Psychiatry 50:704–708
16. Mally J (1989) Aminophylline and essential tremor. Lancet 2:278–279

Discussion

Dr. Hallett: Could you perhaps say one or two words more as to what you mean by the difference between kinetic tremor and intention tremor?

Dr. Findley: The talk was not about that, it was about what came out of this study. We thought the assessors understood kinetic tremor as the tremor of movement and intention tremor as the exacerbation tremor as the limb approached the target. We thought that was very clear, but when we actually looked at their figures, in fact the individual observers had great difficulty in separating these, so we had to get around that. If we wanted to look at movement tremor, we would get around it by asking them to look at the tremor of midmovement.

Dr. Klotz: How do you evaluate the spirals?

Dr. Findley: When the assessors were looking at the videos, they assessed the spirals which had been taken at the time the patient came to the laboratory. They were asked to order the spirals in order of best to worst and then they gave a numerical 0–10 grading on the spiral.

Dr. Klotz: Taking into consideration the test–retest reliability, how big do differences in the individual patient have to be for you to be able to say whether he got better?

Dr. Findley: I can't answer that from the data, but it is a very important question.

Dr. Watts: If you had a 24-h measure of tremor, if somebody could wear a device and you could get the dominant frequency, then that kind of application of accelerometry might be much more beneficial than a measurement at one time.

Dr. Findley: I'm not sure that would tell us anything more than this method. The technology is not easy, as you know, and it's limited to a few people. What we need are practical, reliable, reproducible, validated ways of measuring tremor, and I think this method or something like this method would give us that.

Dr. Watts: I think you're right as far as what's available right now, but I think that technology will become available such that if you have a simple, easy measurement that everybody can have and everybody can use, then you can quantify during a period of waking how often and for how long a person has a 7-Hz tremor.

Dr. Fahn: It was interesting to hear how you rated the spirography – that the sheets of paper were sorted by the assessor and by comparison of the severity – but you might get better results on your Kappa because they did it that way and then they can give a ranking which is a 9, which is an 8, and so forth. But if you had a single sheet of paper with somebody's tremors or spirals and you had to ask this person to give it a number, it may not come out as a high Kappa.

Dr. Findley: I agree with that, but the purpose of this was for clinical trials when the system we applied could have been carried out.

Dr. Fahn: I suggest that if you take your sheets of paper and you photograph them together on a single sheet of paper – this is a 10 score, this is a 9 score, and this is what the assessors eventually gave ratings to. Then you have a standard, a gold standard to look at and when a new patient comes along and draws a spiral, you can compare that spiral with your sheet of paper and all your standards and say this is a 5 score. I'd like to see that assessed – the individual against the standard that you've made – and see what the Kappa is. If it looks good, then that could be used as a reliable trial.

Dr. Findley: I agree with that.

Dr. Muenter: You alluded to the fact that you excluded head and voice tremor. Would you mind describing to us what you would consider to be the best methodology to grade those two types of tremor?

Dr. Findley: Head tremor grading certainly works just as well using the same techniques. Voice tremor is a disaster using this technique, and the reason it's a disaster is that the assessors have very great difficulty in recognizing what is voice tremor and what isn't. One of the factors was the presence of head tremor with voice tremor; some assessors interpreted the voice tremor as head tremor interfering with voice and others interpreted it as voice tremor. So it's a question of definitions and semantics. I haven't got a good way of assessing voice tremor, but for head tremor you can use the same rating technique.

Frequency, Amplitude, and Waveform Characteristics of Physiologic and Pathologic Tremors

G. Deuschl, J. Timmer, H. Genger, C. Gantert, C.H. Lücking, and J. Honerkamp

Introduction

Tremor is defined as a rhythmic, not necessarily sinusoidal periodic oscillation of one or more body parts. Tremor occurs in normal man as well as in patients with pathologic conditions and is one of the most distressing symptoms of various extrapyramidal movement disorders. There are differences between various forms of tremor, which can be distinguished by clinical investigation alone. Physiologic tremor has a low amplitude and can not usually be seen with the naked eye. Pathologic tremors occur in a variety of diseases, of which essential tremor (ET) and Parkinson's disease (PD) are the most frequent ones. In ET, the tremor is usually present during posture and action, whereas it is present during resting conditions in PD. Moreover, ET is a mono-symptomatic disease, but PD is characterized by additional symptoms (bradykinesia and rigidity). However, these differences are not seen in every case and it has been estimated that in the early stage of the disease, 20% of patients with ET are misdiagnosed as having PD and vice versa (L. Findley, personal communication). This is due to the fact that there is considerable overlap of tremor characteristics, especially in the early phase of the disease. The tremors of PD may present with atypical characteristics and if additional symptoms of PD are lacking or are only mild, a differential diagnosis may be difficult [4]. Hence, the development of additional criteria based on objective measurement would be helpful for differential diagnosis.

The present paper summarizes our recent attempts to analyze tremor curves of normal subjects and patients with quantitative statistical and mathematical methods. We are limiting the present report to postural tremors seen in normal subjects and patients with ET or tremor in PD. The data have been analyzed with emphasis on the differential diagnostic aspects of these mathematical tests.

Patients and Methods

A total of 64 patients with idiopathic PD and 29 patients with ET were investigated. The diagnosis was based on clinical criteria in the patients [3, 5], and 85 normal subjects served as controls.

All the subjects and patients underwent standardized tremor recording [2]. They were seated in a special comfortable chair with the forearms fixed in a horizontal position. The hands could move freely and the fingers were fixed together with elastic tape. Recordings were obtained in all of the patients and normal subjects with outstretched hands. The accelerometers were fixed 9 cm distal to the ulnar styloid process over the middle phalanx. The weight of the accelerometers was 8 g and their frequency response was linear between 0.3 and 100 Hz. The wrist extensor and flexor muscles were recorded, but are not included in the present analysis. Accelerometer data (bandpass, 0.5–100 Hz) were converted at a rate of 300 Hz per channel and stored on a personal computer.

Each record covered a 34-s tremor period and was subsequently analyzed by Fast-Fourier analysis [3]. From the power spectrum of the accelerometer data, the maximum amplitude (peak amplitude) and the corresponding peak frequency, defined as the tremor frequency at the peak amplitude, were determined. In addition, the total power defined as the integral of the spectrum between 1 and 20 Hz was calculated.

Part of our data was analyzed using two further mathematical tests. The tremor curves obtained unilaterally at the right hand of 85 normal subjects, 24 patients with PD, and 15 patients with ET were included. For this purpose, all the accelerometer data were normalized so as to have a mean value of zero and a standard deviation of one. Therefore, no amplitude information was included for the mathematical calculations in these two tests.

The first test was a calculation of the third momentum defined as

$$m = 1/(n-1)\ \Sigma\ \mathrm{x}(t)^3$$

which gives a measure for the skewness of a distribution if the data are normalized. In other words, this test shows if the third power of the positive and the negative values of the tremor amplitude are skewed to one side.

The second test was to investigate the invariance of the tremor curve to time inversion. The mathematical formula of this test are complicated and the interested reader is referred to the mathematical literature [6]. The idea behind this test, however, is simple. A purely linear gaussian stochastic process or a sinusoidal time series or any function of such a time series is invariant no matter whether it is analyzed forward or backward. It is also well known that nonlinear oscillations do not show such a time reversal invariance. Our tremor curves of normals are regarded as such linear gaussian stochastic time series [7]. If the waveform of a time series is significantly asymmetric, it is intuitively clear that the curve differs from its inversion. As a measure for the strength of noninvariance, the difference between conditional expectations in forward and backward direction are analyzed. The measure (D) is an estimate of:

$$D := \max_{\tau}\left(\int (E\{x(t-\tau)\,|\,x(t)=y\} - E\{y(t+\tau)\,|\,x(t)=y\})^2\,dy\right)$$

where E is conditional expectation and τ is time lag.

The conditional expectations are estimated via kernel regression estimators [7].

Results

The hand tremor frequency of postural tremor in normal subjects varies between 6.5 and about 10 Hz (see Fig. 1). The percentage plot shown in Fig. 1 displays the cumulative number of patients at their appropriate tremor frequency in a normalized form. For each frequency value, it can be determined how many of the patients have lower or higher frequencies (percentile). Hence, it is possible to determine the

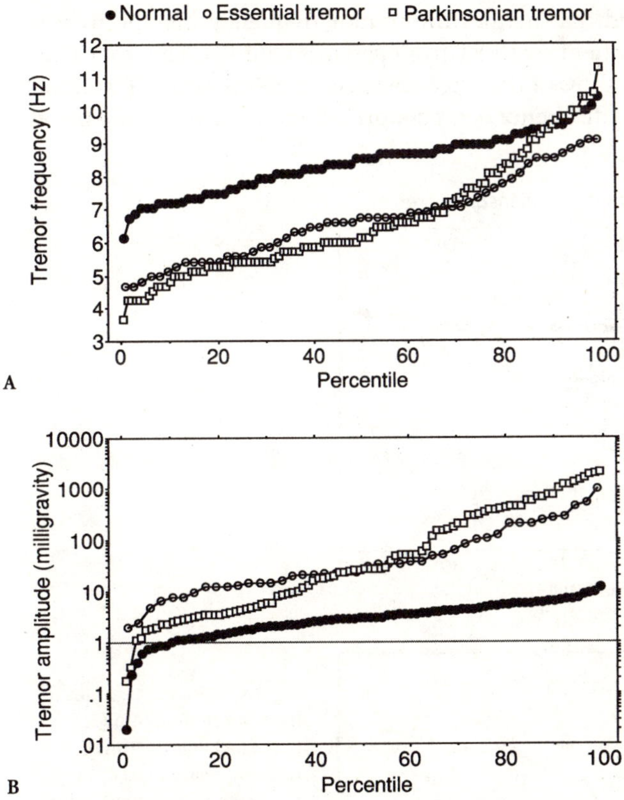

Fig. 1A,B. Tremor frequency (A) and amplitude (B) of 85 normal subjects, 64 patients with Parkinson's disease (PD), and 29 patients with essential tremor (ET) are arranged in order of magnitude in a percentage plot. Each symbol represents the value of one hand. With this kind of display the efficacy of a criterion in distinguishing between the different populations can be seen. By drawing a horizontal line in A at the level of 6.5 Hz, it is evident that 40% of the patients with ET and 55% of the patients with PD can be separated from the normals on the basis of this criterion alone. Even higher values can be obtained on the basis of the criterion of amplitude (B). It is evident that a quite good distinction between normals and patients is possible, but not between the different diseases quality of separation between the different conditions (normal, ET, PD) by drawing a horizontal line. In the case of the tremor frequency, it is evident that 40% of the patients with ET and 55% of the patients with PD have lower frequencies than the normal subjects. However, the remaining patients could be thought to be normal subjects if only this criterion is taken into consideration.

Figure 1B shows the amplitudes of all the normal subjects and patients in a percentage plot. By definition, the tremor amplitudes are a major criterion to separate normal and pathologic tremors. It can be seen from this display that the tremor amplitudes of normal subjects are always below 10 milligravities (1/1000 of gravitation). About 30% of the patients with PD and about 15% of the patients with ET have tremor amplitudes below these values. This is mainly due to the fact that patients were included who had unilateral pathologic tremors and hence, the test does not show abnormalities in their normal hand.

It should be emphasized that neither the tremor frequency nor the tremor amplitude can distinguish patients with ET from patients with PD. The test calculating the third momentum shows differences between patients with ET and patients with PD (Fig. 2A). This difference is even more pronounced when looking at

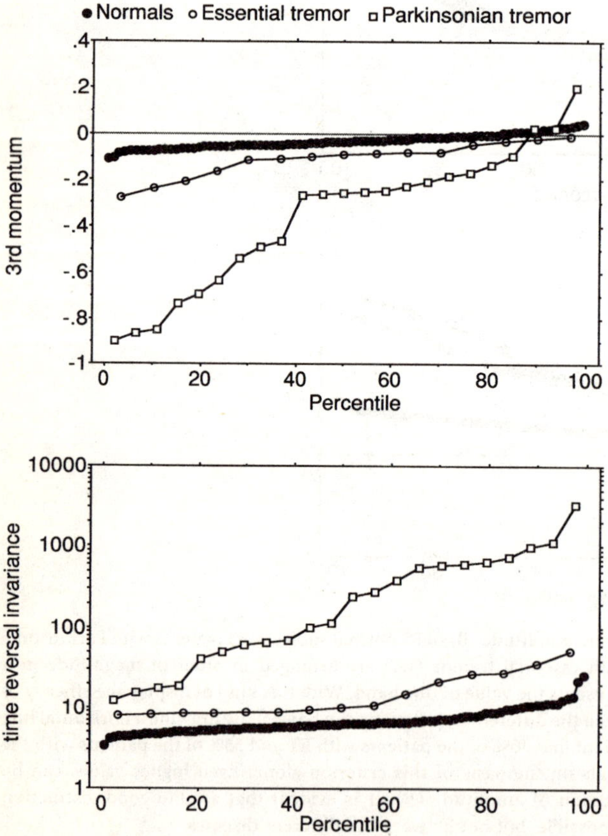

A

B

Fig. 2A,B. Percentage plot of the third momentum (3rd power; A) and the time reversal invariance (B) of 85 normals, 15 patients with essential tremor (ET), and 24 patients with Parkinson's disease (PD). These criteria provide quite a good distinction between patients with ET and PD, but that between normals and ET is only poor the invariance to time reversal of the tremor curves (Fig. 2B). More than 70% of the patients with PD can be distinguished from the ET patients on the basis of this criterion. On the other hand, distinguishing between normals and patients with ET is almost impossible.

Discussion

The present tests provide a rational basis for distinguishing between normal and pathologic tremors on the basis of quantitative tremor measurements alone. It should be emphasized that the distinctions that we have shown here rely only on the information of a 34-s tremor recording during postural conditions. It is evident that the tremor amplitude is quite a good means of distinguishing between normal and pathologic tremors, as the definition of pathologic tremors is based on this difference. The tremor frequency is already known to be a poor criterion to distinguish between normal and pathologic tremors. The present data demonstrate that neither amplitude nor frequency can be used to distinguish between different tremor forms of pathologic tremors such as ET and tremor in PD.

The data show that the calculation of the third momentum and the time reversal invariance seem to be promising mathematical methods to separate different forms of pathologic tremors. In about 70% of the patients with pathologic tremors, tremors of PD and ET can be separated on the basis of this criterion alone. In contrast, the distinction between normals and patients with ET is only poor. Such a high selectivity of a mathematical method must be due to a difference in the physiologic properties of ET and tremor in PD. This difference is shown in Fig. 3, where examples of physiologic tremor and pathologic tremors are displayed. Even by looking at these tremor curves, it is evident that physiologic tremor and ET are nearly sinusoidal, whereas the tremor of PD is nonsinusoidal, thereby providing the basis for differences of the quantitative values of the third power and the time reversal invariance. If we are aware of this particular feature of these tremors, we can even see it upon clinical observation. In clinical terms, the differences obtained in these two tests correspond to the pill-rolling quality of the tremor waveform seen in PD, but not usually in ET.

The present tests show that further work seems to be justified to identify mathematical methods which could distinguish between different forms of tremor. Future work on larger groups of patients has to concentrate on the question of whether these tests are selective and sensitive for a rational differential diagnosis. When combining different types of mathematical analysis, it is evident that higher percentages of distinctions between the different forms of tremor may be achieved. In any case, the present data provide the basis for a more detailed and sophisticated analysis of simple tremor curves and may help to further understand the physiology underlying different forms of tremors.

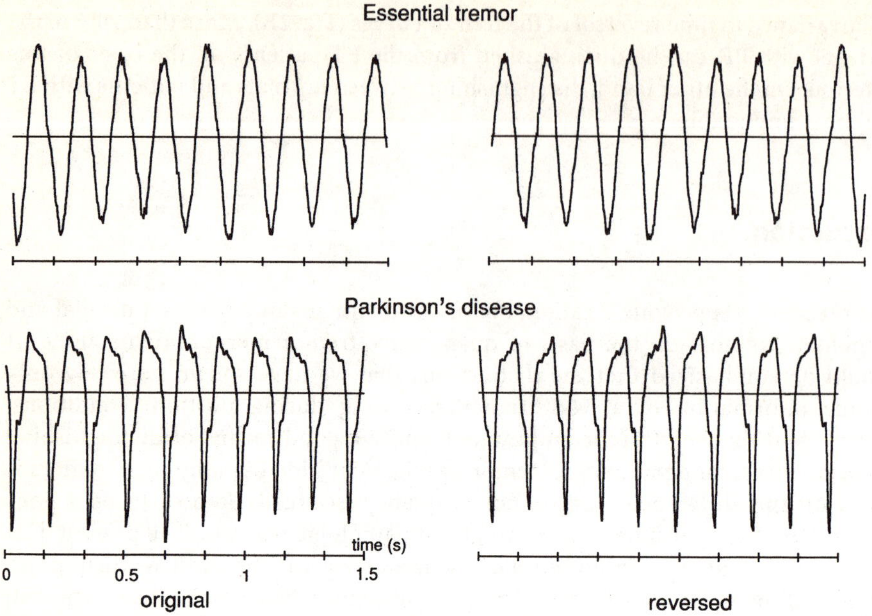

Fig. 3. *Left*, accelerometer curves of the tremor in a patient with essential tremor (ET; top) and a patient with Parkinson's disease (PD; *bottom*). The curves have been normalized. *Right*, the mirror reversed images of these curves are displayed to visualize the difference, which is mathematically picked up with the test of the third momentum and the test for time series invariance to reversal

References

1. Deuschl G (1992) Tremor-Syndrome. In: Hopf H CH, Poeck K, Schliack H (eds) Neurologie in Praxis und Klinik. Thieme, Stuttgart, pp 4.53–4.73
2. Deuschl G, Blumberg H, Lücking CH (1991) Tremor in reflex sympathetic dystrophy. Arch Neurol 48:1247–1252
3. Elble RJ, Koller WC (1990) Tremor. Johns Hopkins University Press, Baltimore
4. Findley LJ, Capildeo R (1984) Movement disorders: tremor. McMillan, London
5. Findley LJ, Koller WC (1987) Essential tremor: a review. Neurology 37:1194–1197
6. Gantert C, Honerkamp J, Timmer J (1992) Analyzing the dynamics of hand tremor time series. Biol Cybern 66:479–484
7. Timmer J, Gantert C, Deuschl G, Honerkamp J (1993) Characteristics of hand tremor time series. Biol Cyber 70:75–80

Discussion

Dr. Findley: Were you're looking at rest tremor, the low frequency tremor?

Dr. Deuschl: We looked at rest tremor, but the idea was with these kinds of tests to have completely the same conditions. We have all these data for rest tremors in these patients, but they were not included in the analysis that I presented here.

Dr. Findley: Because your wave form looks very much like that of rest tremors in Parkinson patients, the lower frequency tremor.

Dr. Deuschl: You will see that type of wave form in most of the patients with Parkinson's disease, also during postural conditions.

Dr. Hallett: Following up that particular question in patients with Parkinson's disease, do you think that there is only one type of tremor that they have or are there in fact multiple types of postural tremor?

Dr. Deuschl: We tried to answer that question in a different study. The final outcome was that – according to a number of different tests that we did with these patients – there are two types of tremor in Parkinson's disease. One is the resting and postural tremor and the other one is the action tremor that you can see in these patients. They can be clearly separated by means of different factor analyses and by different means of tests.

Dr. Hefter: You used the face plane in plots. I predict that everything that you presented with the face plane plots can already be seen in the spectrum and these plots are already available since the harmonics should reflect what you have presented. Did you try to take into account the amount of harmonics or the amplitude of the harmonics in the spectrum to distinguish essential tremor in Parkinson's disease patients?

Dr. Deuschl: It helps in some respects, but it is not as good as these kinds of methods because in some cases it's very difficult to decide whether you already have a harmonic at the appropriate frequency spectrum or not. These kinds of tests seem to be superior, clearly superior to just looking at the frequency analysis.

Dr. Inzelberg: About your patients with essential tremor: some of these patients have agonist - antagonist cocontraction and some of them have alternating agonist - antagonist contraction. Is there any difference between the wave forms of your recordings for these patients?

Dr. Deuschl: We couldn't see any clear differences in the wave form. The only difference was that the ones with alternating contraction had slower frequencies.

Dr. Noth: What was your criterion to separate essential tremor from Parkinson tremor? At the beginning of the disease, it's not so easy, and when where's a clear-cut difference why do you need another criterion to separate them?

Dr. Deuschl: In these kinds of tests you always use either patients with clear Parkinson's disease or clear essential tremor and then you try to look for other measures. The next step can be to look at unselected patients, to see whether it helps you to really separate them. That's the usual procedure that we use.

Interaction Between Voluntary and Involuntary Movements

H. Hefter and H.-J. Freund

Involuntary and voluntary movements share a common final pathway. Therefore, the question arises as to whether they merely superimpose or whether they interact and mutually influence each other. As a simple approach to this problem, we have chosen three types of voluntary movements and have studied the interaction between tremor and these types of voluntary movements. In the presentation here, we mainly concentrate on parkinsonian patients. Analysis of the interaction between voluntary and involuntary movements in other patient groups can be found elsewhere [7–9].

Modifications of Tremor Frequency and Amplitude with Changes of Posture

One of the simplest voluntary motor tasks is a tonic muscle activation. However, even this simple voluntary movement changes amplitude and frequency of tremor considerably. This is illustrated in Fig. 1: tremor was recorded where in four Parkinsonian patients at rest (the hand was semipronated and supported at the ulnar side with the fingers III-V flexed and the index finger relaxed and free to move) and under maintenance of constant horizontal posture (the entire arm, forearm, hand, and fingers were stretched out in the horizontal position in the midsagittal plane with the forearm completely pronated). Tremor was recorded by attaching an accelerometer to the index finger with adhesive tape. The acceleration signal was Fast-Fourier-transformed and the power spectrum density function was calculated. In Fig. 1, it is quite obvious that the change of position from rest (lower part) to continuous activation of muscle groups while holding the position (upper part) may increase or decrease tremor frequency, regardless of whether the parkinsonian patient suffers from the tremulous type (the two examples on the left side) or the akinetorigid type of Parkinson's disease (PD; the two examples on the right side; for the classification of PD patients, see [3, 11]). Usually, tremor amplitude increases with changes of posture from rest to hold. The only exception is the highly synchronized typical tremor at rest in PD, which may become desynchronized, with the power spectrum becoming broader and the tremor amplitude lower. This implies that a careful control of position has to be mentioned when results on tremor frequency and amplitude are presented and that not only

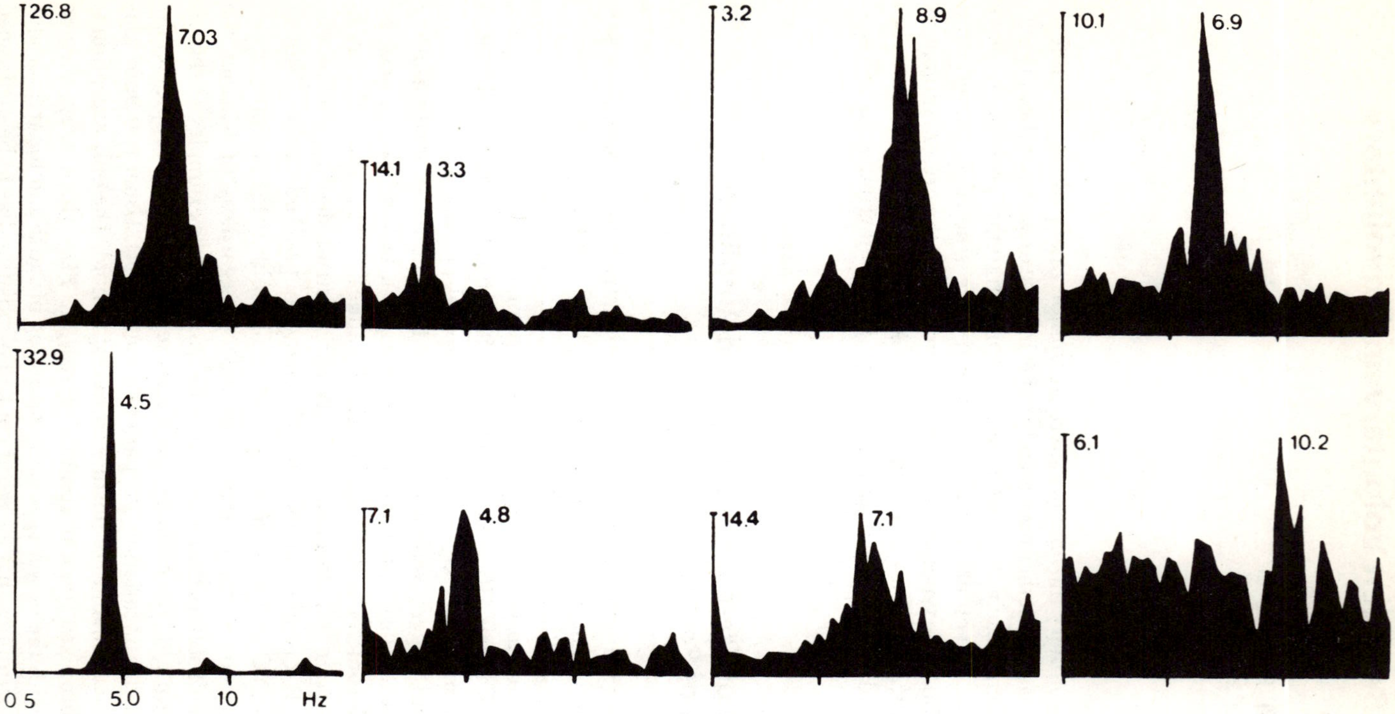

Fig. 1. Comparison of the spectral analysis of finger oscillations in parkinsonian (PD) patients (the *left* four spectra are recorded from two patients with the tremulous type, the right four spectra are recorded from two patients with the akinetorigid type of PD) shows that an increase and a decrease of tremor frequency may occur in both patient subgroups when the hands are stretched out (*top*) starting from a resting condition (*bottom*)

a simple linear summation of voluntary and involuntary activation occurs at the alpha-motoneural level.

Interaction Between Voluntary and Involuntary Alternating Activity

Most rapidly alternating movements form another type of voluntary movements with an alternating electromyographic (EMG) activity pattern similar to that of tremor [12]. During the performance of rapidly alternating movements, the voluntary and involuntary index finger oscillations couple and the tremor works as an attractor (see [4]), implying that the voluntary movements are performed at the same rate as the tremor rate (see Fig. 2). This 1:1 coupling of voluntary and involuntary movements is usually found in patients with a considerable tremor. In patients with a weaker tremor (with tremor peak frequencies larger than 5 Hz), other types of coupling may be found, for example a 1:2 coupling. Even a 2:3 coupling was noticed in a parkinsonian patient with a strong 6.1-Hz tremor who succeeded to perform 4.6-Hz alternating index finger movements over a period of time.

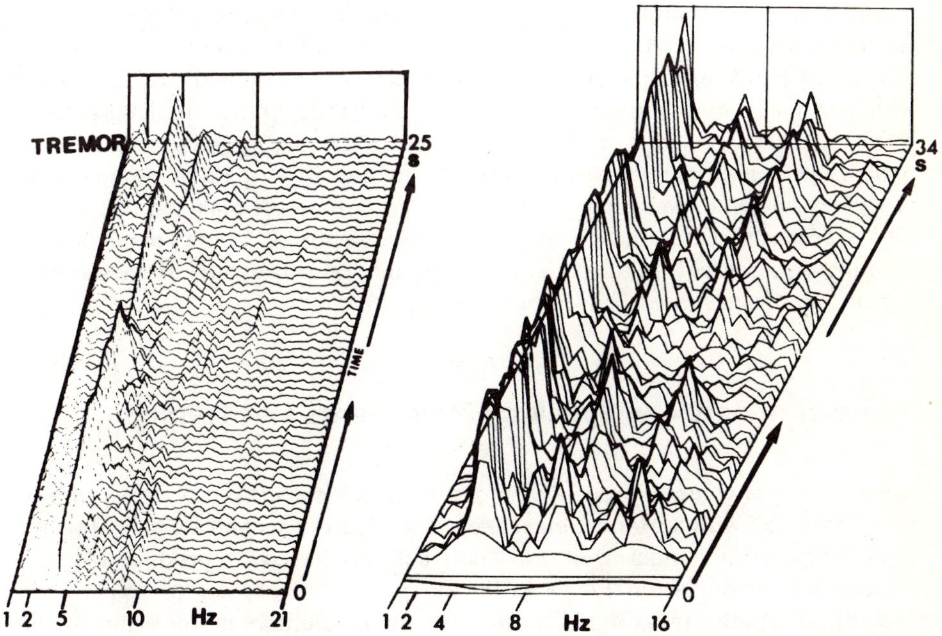

Fig. 2. Voluntary alternating index finger movements were performed with the same frequency as the tremor peak frequency in a parkinsonian patient with typical tremor at rest. Thus, the tremor drives the motor system in tremulous patients

Table 1. Interaction between tremor and voluntary alternating activity

Patient group	Fingers examined (n)	Patients examined (n)	Tremor (mean ± SD)	Alternating movement (Hz; mean ± SD)	t test ($p <$)
Physiological tremor	54	42	8.53 ± 1.91	7.25 ± 1.41	0.002
Essential tremor	39	23	7.83 ± 1.69	5.81 ± 1.49	0.002
Parkinson's disease	89	48	6.93 ± 1.75	5.17 ± 1.40	0.002
Huntington's chorea (HC)	51	33	5.49 ± 1.85	4.63 ± 1.46	0.05
Risk of HC	88	47	7.23 ± 1.75	5.90 ± 1.34	0.002
Cerebellar lesion	23	12	6.67 ± 2.04	4.26 ± 1.47	0.002
Upper motoneuron syndrome	19	12	7.93 ± 1.83	5.10 ± 1.80	0.002
Polyneuropathy	7	5	7.05 ± 2.25	4.16 ± 1.22	0.05
Myopathy	11	7	8.77 ± 1.28	5.12 ± 1.39	0.002
Multiple sclerosis	10	6	8.53 ± 1.86	5.23 ± 1.41	0.002

The 1:1 coupling of tremor and voluntary movement rate has an important implication which was hypothesized by Richard Jung years ago: "Nobody can move faster than he trembles." Thus, a lower tremor rate limits the frequency range of voluntary, alternating movements and is therefore an important factor for the akinesia of tremulous patients. We tested Jung's hypothesis in nine patient groups and it was confirmed in all cases. We analyzed 39 hands in 23 patients with essential tremor, 89 hands in 48 parkinsonian patients, 51 hands in 30 patients with Huntington's chorea, 88 hands in 47 subjects at risk of developing Huntington's disease, 23 hands of 12 patients with a cerebellar lesion, 19 hands of 12 patients with an upper motoneuron syndrome, seven hands of five patients with a polyneuropathy, 11 hands of seven patients with a myopathy, and ten hands of six patients with multiple sclerosis. It turned out that in all patient groups, peak frequency of tremor was highly significantly larger than the maximal rate of rapidly alternating hand movements, with two exceptions: in the patients with Huntington's chorea and the patients with peripheral neuropathy, there was only a weak significance (see Table 1; for details see [5]).

Interaction Between Speaking Movements and Tremor

Another type of voluntary repetitive motor behavior is speaking. Normal subjects prefer to speak with a production rate of about 4–5 per second syllable [14]. We have developed a standardized test where subjects have to reproduce 13 given frequencies ranging from 1.0 to 8.0 Hz by saying the syllable "ta" repetitively [6,9,10]. Also in this test a significant interaction of voluntary motor behavior and tremor can be demonstrated. For example (Fig. 3), in a patient with Wilson's disease, the response frequency did not exceed 3.5 Hz as long as target frequencies did not exceed 5.0 Hz, and 3.5 Hz the approximate tremor peak frequency observed

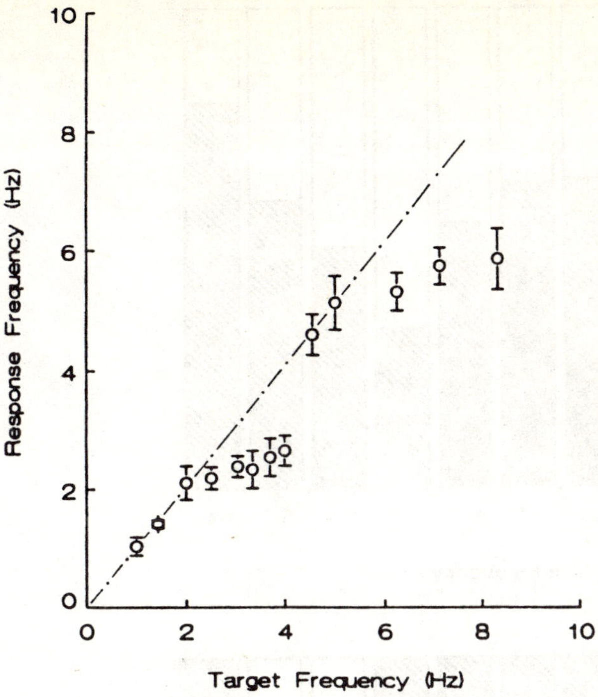

Fig. 3. Considerable hastening at 5.0 Hz in a patient suffering from Wilson's disease with a 3.5- to 4.5 Hz tremor

in this patient. At target frequencies higher than 5.0 Hz, the response frequency suddenly increased to 5.0 Hz and did not change any further. The explanation for this finding is that the response frequency was attracted by the tremor frequency from both sides. However, from a certain frequency on this attraction failed and the responses jumped to another "limit cycle" (see [4]). Thus, hastening is not only found in Parkinson's disease [1,10], but also in patients with Wilson's disease. Therefore, it is not a typical clinical sign of parkinsonian speech as mentioned elsewhere [2,13], but mainly reflects the coupling between voluntary speech movements and involuntary tremor oscillations.

The interesting question is whether hastening of voluntary finger movements occurs at the same frequency as hastening of speech movements does. This was analyzed systematically in 15 parkinsonian patients. It is obvious that speaking and finger movements have to be tested separately, since it is well known that during simultaneous speech and extremity movements both movements are highly coupled. Plotting the percentage of hastened and reduced response frequency for both finger and speech movements in our patient group against target frequency (Fig. 4), it turns out that hastening did indeed occur at the same frequency for both speech and extremity movements.

In summary, these results demonstrate that tremor and voluntary movements interact and do not sum up linearly. Especially during repetitive voluntary motor activity, coupling phenomena occur as predicted by the theory of nonlinear coupled oscillators.

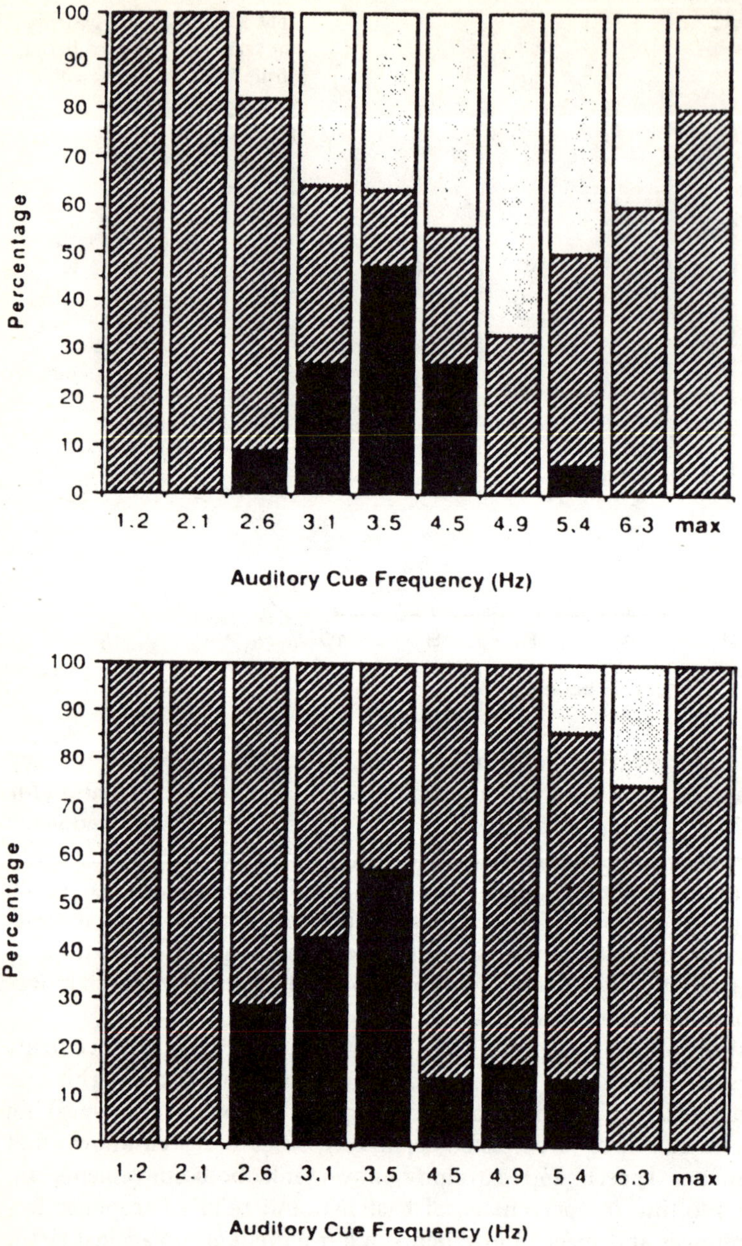

Fig. 4. Comparison of the percentage of hastened responses in 15 parkinsonian patients (voluntary finger movements in the *upper* part; repetitive speech movements in the *lower* part). Hastening occurs at exactly the same frequency for the extremity and the speaking movements. *Shaded bars*, normal; *white bars*, too slow; *black bars*, too fast responses in comparison to target frequency

Acknowledgment. This study was supported by grants from the Deutsche Forschungsgemeinschaft (SFB 194, A5).

References

1. Ackermann H, Ziegler W (1989) Die Dysarthrophonie des Parkinson-Syndromes. Fortsch Neurol Psychiatr 57:149–160
2. Canter GJ (1963) Speech characteristics of patients with Parkinson's disease I. Intensity, pitch and duration. J Speech Hear Res 28:221–229
3. Gerstenbrand F, Poewe W, Klingler D (1983) Therapeutic efficacy of beta-adrenergic blocking agents in parkinsonian tremor. In: Yahr MD (ed) Current concepts of Parkinson disease and related disorders. A symposium by the Extrapyramidal Research Group of the World Federation of Neurology. 23 Sept 1981, Kyoto, Japan. Excerpta Medica, Princeton, pp 112–123
4. Glass L, McMackey (1988) From clocks to chaos. The rhythms of life. Princeton University Press, Princeton, pp 2–25
5. Hefter H (1990) Untersuchungen zur Zeitstruktur willkürlicher Bewegungen von Normalpersonen und Patienten mit motorischen Störungen. Dissertation, University of Düsseldorf
6. Hefter H, Hömberg V, Freund H-J (1988) Quantitive analysis of voluntary and involuntary motor phenomena in Parkinson's disease. In: Przuntek H, Riederer P (eds) Early diagnosis and preventive therapy in Parkinson's disease (Key topics brain research). Springer, Vienna New York, pp 65–73
7. Hefter H, Logigian E, Witte OW, Reiners K, Freund H-J (1992) Oscillatory activity in different motor subsystems in palatal myoclonus. A case report. Acta Neurol Scand 86:176–183
8. Hefter H, Witte OW, Reiners K, Niedermeyer E, Freund H-J (1994) High frequency bursting during rapid finger movements in an unusual case of epilepsia partialis continua. Electromyogr Clin Neurophysiol 34:95–103
9. Hefter H, Arendt G, Stremmel W, Freund H-J (1993) Motor impairment in Wilson's disease II: slowness of speech. Acta Neurol Scand 87:148–160
10. Logigian EL, Hefter H, Reiners K, Freund H-J (1990) Does tremor pace the motor system in Parkinson's disease? Ann Neurol 30:172–179
11. Poewe W, Gerstenbrand F, Ransmayr G (1983) Klinische Manifestationstypen des Parkinson-Syndroms. Neuopsychiatr Clin 2:223–227
12. Sabra AF, Hallett M (1984) Action tremor with alternating activity in antagonist muscles. Neurology (Cleveland) 34:151–156
13. Van Lancker DR, Canter GJ (1981) Temporal organisation in the accelerated speech of a Parkinson's patient. UCLA Work Pap 3:209–237
14. Volkmann J, Hefter H, Freund H-J (1992) Impairment of temporal organization of speech in basal ganglia diseases. Brain Language 43:386–399

Discussion

Dr. Deuschl: You showed us a picture of a resting tremor in a patient who presumably did an extension movement, and this kind of extension movement was still disturbed by resting tremor. Did you find this very often? Because as I understand it, usually before doing a voluntary movement the resting tremor completely stops and then you do the movement. Is that wrong?

Dr. Hefter: We have done a study on what happens to the resting tremor when you perform for example a voluntary action, and what you see is that in some patients the amplitude goes down, while the frequency stays more or less the same. In others, you see a tremendous increase in tremor during the waiting period and there is no silent period. Sometimes, there may be some silent period. We also did a study in normals on the silent period, and we don't usually find one. It may depend on the muscle you're analyzing: the less inertia you have, the less often you find silent periods.

Dr. Deuschl: So the resting tremor is definitely used to voluntary movements?

Dr. Hefter: I would say it disturbs the performance of voluntary movements. One particular woman did not start her voluntary movements in phase with the resting tremor. You have to wait for the right phase of the movement, and patients with bilateral myoclonus did that, but this woman started the voluntary burst between the tremor bursts.

Long-Term Measurement of Tremor

S. Spieker, E. Scholz, M. Bacher, and J. Dichgans

Introduction

The development of new treatment strategies for tremor requires an objective and reproducible method for tremor quantification. Subjective rating, even using standardized scores, very often leads to contradictory results between patients and physicians. Objective methods have so far usually only been performed during short periods and therefore have not taken the high variability of tremor into account.

Our method of long-term electromyogram (EMG) recording provides an objective measure of tremor occurrence (as percentages of time intervals), intensity, frequency, and diurnal variation. The method has already been described previously [1,2]; here it will briefly be reviewed. New data concerning its reproducibility and its use in a preliminary evaluation of therapy with budipine are added.

Methodology

Data Acquisition

Surface EMG activity is recorded from both extensor carpi radialis and flexor carpi ulnaris muscles. EMG signals are amplified and stored on a small Medilog recorder, originally designed for long-term EEG recordings. Patients are free to move around and maintain their normal daily activities as outpatients, and maximum recording time is 24 h. The band width of 0.5–100 Hz is mainly limited by the tape velocity of 2 mm/s. The recorded tape is replayed on an Oxford PMD 12 system, and EMG signals are AD converted and stored on a PC. Sampling rate is 4000 Hz, corresponding to 200 Hz under real time conditions.

Data Analysis

Data analysis is successively performed at intervals of 5.12 s. It consists of four steps:

1. Quality control and artifact elimination
2. Demodulation of the EMG signal
3. Calculation of the power spectrum and detection of tremor
4. Calculation of overall tremor occurrence over the entire recording period from all of these intervals.

These steps will be discussed separately.

Quality Control and Artifact Elimination

Most artifacts in EMG recordings consist of low-frequency changes of the signal baseline (Fig. 1a). Therefore, the percentage of values which exceed a defined range can be used as an indicator of signal quality. Data segments with more than 10% of values outside the normal range are not considered further for analysis. Most voluntary activity is not affected by this process. Strong activity, though, might be counted as artifact, so that patients are asked to refrain from strenuous physical work on the day of recording.

A digital filter with a cutoff frequency of 10 Hz further eliminates low-frequency artifacts. The result of this step is depicted in Fig. 1b.

Demodulation

Extraction of the tremor signal is based on describing EMG activity in terms of amplitude modulated noise:

$$y(t) = c(t)n(t)$$

where $y(t)$ is EMG signal, $n(t)$ is band-limited, gaussian white noise, and $c(t)$ is activity level, which in the case of tremor periodically varies and thus modulates the noise.

By rectifying (in this case squaring) and then low-pass filtering, high-frequency noise is eliminated and the tremor frequency, previously encoded solely in the frequency of the amplitude modulation, can be extracted. The square root is then taken to relinearize the data. Fig. 1c shows the demodulated signal.

Power Spectra and Detection of Tremor

Power spectra are calculated for sequential periods of 5.12 s by a Fast-Fourier Transformation (FFT) algorithm (Fig. 1d). Spectral resolution is 0.2 Hz. Smoothing is achieved by averaging three consecutive spectra, now representing 15-s intervals, and for each interval the main frequency is determined and its intensity calculated.

Intensity is defined as signal to noise ratio (SNR), which is the sum of the three highest spectral values of the dominant peak divided by three times the noise level of the spectrum.

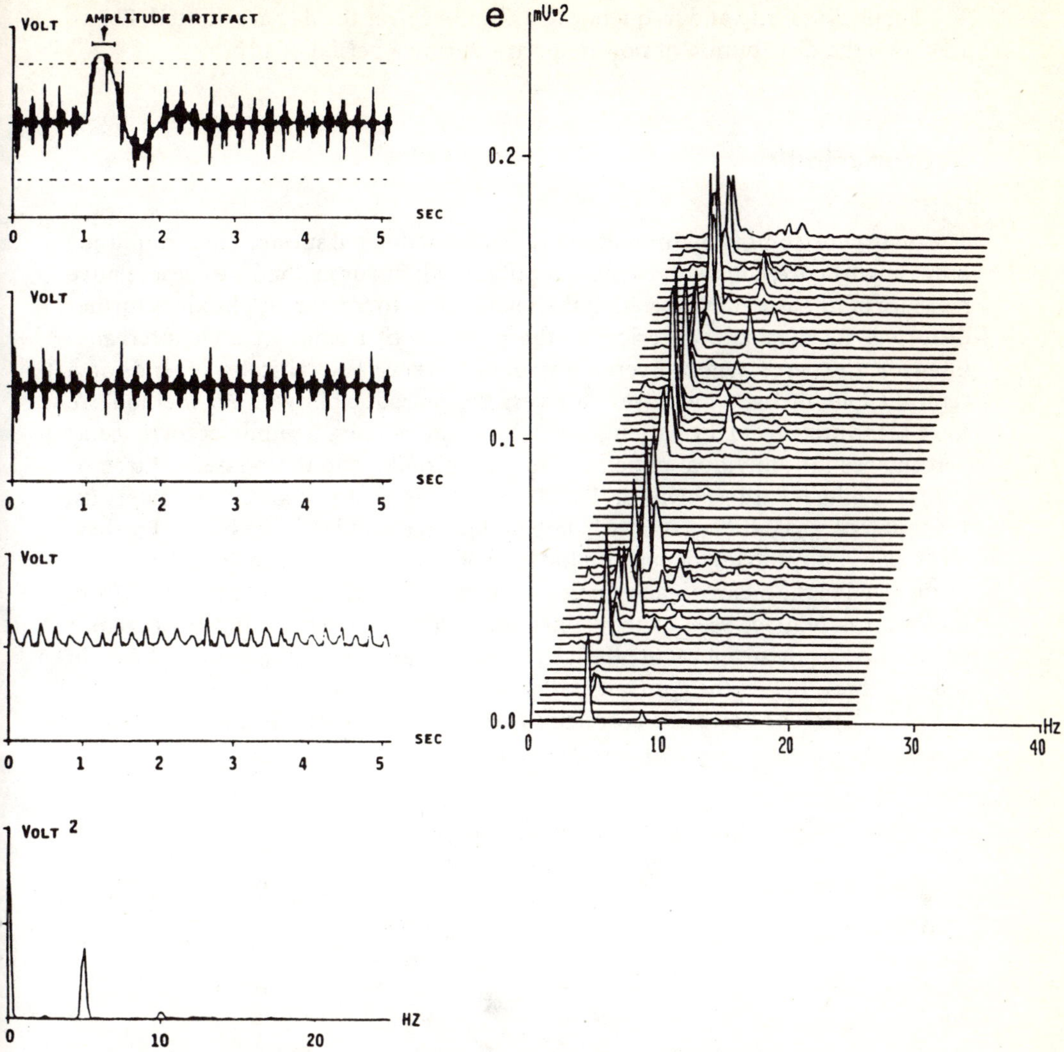

Fig. 1a–e. Results of each step of the analysis procedure. **a** Raw signal. **b** Artifact elimination. **c** Demodulation. **d** Power spectrum. **e** Distribution of power spectra over the day

An interval is defined as containing tremor if the dominant peak is between 3.7 and 10 Hz and the SNR is greater than 4.

Overall Tremor Occurrence

Tremor occurrence during the entire period of interest, which is usually 10 h, is given as a percentage of intervals which fulfill the criteria for tremor.

Finally, intensity and frequency distributions over the day are plotted. Figure 1d shows the distribution of power spectra during a period of 10h.

Reproducibility

The main shortcoming of this method is that demodulated surface EMG amplitude only roughly correlates with tremor amplitude [3]. In our method we use a relative measure of intensity (SNR), so that the relationship to tremor amplitude is further distorted. As the main criterion of the presence of tremor in each interval is intensity, the percentage of overall tremor occurrence also critically depends on a reproducible intensity measure. To assess the reproducibility of our method, we took recordings from 19 patients on 3 consecutive days. Tremor occurrence as percentages for individual patients – 16 parkinsonian and three essential tremor (ET) patients – are shown in Fig. 2. ET patients are marked by asterisks. Intersubject variability was much larger than intrasubject variability. Furthermore, variability did not depend on the level of tremor occurrence. If the values are normalized to the mean of each single patient and the difference of each value from the mean is plotted, 95% of the values are within a range of ±10.5% of tremor occurrence. As these figures are derived from evaluation of a 10-h period (the main waking time), 10% is the equivalent of 1h.

Calculation of Pearson's correlation coefficients between two single days reveals values of 0.93, 0.89, and 0.87, respectively.

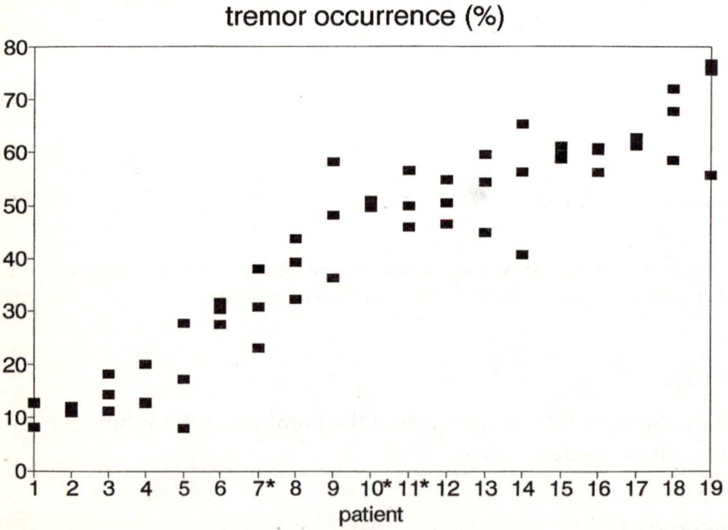

Fig. 2. Reproducibility of long-term measurements. Tremor occurrence as a percentage of time intervals is shown for 16 parkinsonian patients and three essential tremor (*) patients. Patients are aligned according to the mean value of tremor

Strictly speaking, these reproducibility data do not "validate" the method. First, reproducibility also depends on the day to day variability of tremor itself. Secondly, for validation, EMG recordings have to be compared with other methods, e.g., accelerometer recordings. Nevertheless, the good reproducibility suggests that the method is reliable and therefore suitable for therapy studies.

Further Methodological Considerations

The gold standard for quantitative tremor recordings is certainly accelerometry, but for our purposes, EMG has some undeniable advantages. Surface electrodes are totally independent of orientation and position of the arm, whereas accelerometers are critically sensitive to the constant acceleration of gravity and, in addition, to precise placement exactly in the plane of tremor. They are sensitive to mechanical artifacts, which occur preferentially in the tremor frequency range, and they are quite delicate structures that can easily be damaged. Accelerometry is therefore not suitable for long-term recordings under daily life conditions. Technical considerations strongly favor EMG for this purpose.

Therapy Evaluation

The following is an example of the usefulness for therapy evaluation. In an open pilot study, seven tremor-dominant parkinsonian patients were studied before and after treatment with budipine. Budipine is a novel antiparkinson agent, a piperidine derivative, whose exact mechanism of action is not known [4]. It has some anticholinergic effects and it has been shown to be an *N*-methyl-D-aspartate (NMDA) antagonist [5].

Concomitant medication was kept stable during the study. Three patients did not respond, but four showed a remarkable reduction. Overall tremor occurrence decreased by a mean of 21.8 ± 26.7%.

Interestingly, when comparing treatment effects measured by this method with doctors' rating and with patients' self-rating, there is a good correlation with the patients' assessment, whereas doctors' ratings seem to be completely random.

Conclusion

We think that this method is reliable, provides an objective measure for tremor, and is useful for therapy evaluation. However, exact validation by direct comparison of EMG and accelerometry has yet to be done.

References

1. Bacher M, Scholz E, Diener HC (1989) 24 Hour continuous tremor quantification based on EMG recording. Electroencephalogr Clin Neurophysiol 72:176–183
2. Scholz E, Bacher M, Diener HC, Dichgans J (1988) Twenty-four-hour tremor recordings in the evaluation of the treatment of Parkinson's disease. J Neurol 235:475–484
3. Elble RJ and Koller WC (1990) Tremor. John Hopkins University Press, Baltimore
4. Jellinger K, Bliesath H (1987) Adjuvant treatment of Parkinson's disease with budipine: a double-blind trial versus placebo. J Neurol 234:280–282
5. Klockgether T, Jacobsen P, Löschmann P-A, Turski L (1992) The antiparkinsonian agent budipine is an N-methyl-D-aspartate antagonist. J Neural Transm PD-Sect Park Dis Dement Sect 5:101–106

Discussion

Dr. Fahn: Can this method differentiate between when a patient is "off" with tremor versus "on" with dyskinesia. Does this method make a distinction to dyskinesias when you don't see the patient? Is it specific?

Dr. Spieker: It can specifically assess the demodulated tremor signal. For dyskinesias, I think you have to have a concomitant recording of accelerometry.

Dr. Deuschl: If you don't apply the frequency analysis and just integrate the signals and later on subtract both from each other, you could probably use this method to measure dyskinesias.

Dr. Spieker: Could you differentiate between voluntary activity and dyskinesias? I don't think you could.

Dr. Hallett: In how much of your recordings do you have artifacts such that you have to throw the data out? The reason I ask that is that presumably the most likely time when you get a high amount of artifacts is when you have a high amount of tremor with some other movements. So the fact that you throw out some of the activity data may in some way invalidate some of what you are trying to measure.

Dr. Spieker: Most voluntary activity is not affected by this process. Strong activity, however, may be counted as artifact, so patients are asked to refrain from strenuous physical work when we are recording. From these reproducibility measures, the mean artifact was about 8%, but I think it is a problem in patients with strong tremor, where you have to be careful that it is not counted as artifact.

Dr. Hallett: If you bandpass the input differently, would you have less of this artifact from the beginning?

Dr. Spieker: First of all, you cannot bandpass it differently, because of the limitations of the setting, which was actually designed for recording EEG. I do not know what it does to the artifact, but I do know what it does to the tremor.

Dr. Lücking: As you use the EMG, this method is sensitive enough to see subclinical tremor, too. Did you record at night, because it was mentioned that even the Parkinson tremor doesn't stop during sleep and continues, though in a rather subclinical way, only detected by EMG.

Dr. Spieker: We record overnight in our patients and we usually only evaluate the mean waking time. I looked at a couple of night time recordings especially from patients with a very marked and enhanced tremor and I did not find anything. What I will do is go back and change the criteria for detection of tremor and change the signal to noise ratio that is needed for detection and see whether, with a little more sensitivity, I could find something. Up to now I have not found anything.

Dr. Findley: If your signal to noise ratio is less than 4, is the signal rejected?

Dr. Spieker: It is defined as being "not tremor."

Dr. Findley: Conceptually, this must be the right way to look at tremor, recording over periods of time. But you're measuring a mean; how does that correlate with disability?

Dr. Spieker: In parallel, we asked patients, let's say before and after treatment, whether they also found a reduction according to our measures; in general, it correlated very well, much better than the doctors' rating from just a few minutes in the office. It's astonishing that in this budipine study, the three patients who did not respond reported a reduction of tremor, but we will do a double-blind study for this. In general, it correlates very well with the patients' evaluation.

Kinematics of Standing Posture Associated with Aging and Parkinson's Disease

M. Hallett, V. Panzer, and T. Zeffiro

Introduction

Falling is a serious problem in both aging and Parkinson's disease. An increased incidence of falls is a major source of neurological disability in the elderly [9, 10, 21], and a survey of 100 patients with Parkinson's disease showed that 38% had a history of falling, and 13% fell more than once a week [12]. Falling was associated with "postural instability" and was not much influenced by dopaminergic therapy. Falling was also associated with increasing age of the patients. It is also well known that Parkinson's disease has an increased incidence with age. It is clearly important to understand the causes of falling in both aging and Parkinson's disease. Aging itself is likely to be at least one of the causes of falling in Parkinson's disease, but there may also be independent causes.

Posture can be defined as the particular position of parts of the body. Standing posture is the orientation of the parts of the body to each other and to the base of support while standing. Balance is the ability to maintain standing posture and, in particular, not to fall. Falling is avoided by maintaining the center of gravity (COG) of the body over the base of support. Theoretically, it would seem that balance should be assessed by measuring the deviations from a fixed posture. However, normal people are not rigid objects, but have some oscillation about a mean position. Some movement might even have beneficial effects, such as to maintain a steady flow of sensory input, avoiding adaptation of sensory receptors. Thus, it is necessary to differentiate normal and pathological deviations from a mean posture.

For methodological reasons, largely related to the availability of equipment, balance has been measured in a variety of ways. Mechanical devices have been used to measure the motion of the body, which is usually referred to as sway. Movement of the trunk or hip has been measured to approximate motion of the COG, which is located near the hip when the body is standing. Recently, many studies have utilized a force plate to measure the center of pressure (COP). A force plate consists of a rigid surface with force sensors underneath. The position of the COP in the plane of the force plate is calculated from the force sensors.

A force plate measures all the of the forces acting on it, and a dominant force comes from gravity acting on the COG of the body. If there were no forces other than gravity, the COP would lie immediately below the COG and could be a measure of its position in the anterior–posterior (A-P) and medial–lateral (M-L) directions. The COP can have no measure of the distance of the COG from the base of support. However, outside forces acting on the body and movements of individual body parts are also measured by the force plate and will lead to dissociation between the position of the COP and the COG. If these forces are weak, the differences will be small. Traditionally, in the study of posture, it has been assumed that these forces are small in quiet standing. Therefore, the COP has been used as a measure of the COG, but this method has not been well validated, particularly in patients or the elderly. Measures of the COP, in one or two dimensions, can include the mean position with respect to base of support, total path length, maximum deviation of sway, and frequency analysis.

Given that deviations of body parts and of the COG will give rise to movements of the COP, the "sway" of the COP has often been used as a measure of balance. It has generally been assumed that more sway means more instability. Indeed, this has been used successfully in the assessment of patients with cerebellar dysfunction [4]. Given that some sway is normal, the amount of sway, taken by itself, must be interpreted carefully. The real measure of balance is the ability to maintain the COG over the base of support. Thus, for example, a few large movements that bring the COG near the edge of the base of support might demonstrate poor balance, whereas frequent smaller movements that generate more motion, but are "well controlled" might indicate better balance.

We have studied quiet standing in the elderly and in patients with Parkinson's disease by measuring the COG and positions of body segments, as well as the COP. We will summarize our findings and compare them with those of previous studies.

Methodology in Our Laboratory

Two-dimensional position (or kinematic) data were sampled at 50 Hz with a modified video-based infrared marker detection system (VICON, Oxford Metrics, Inc.). Four cameras recorded the position of reflective markers (25-mm foam spheres) attached at eight bony landmarks on the right side of the body (i.e., in front of the ear, the shoulder, the lateral epicondyle of the elbow, the radial styloid at the wrist, the anterior superior iliac spine, the head of the fibula at the knee, the lateral malleolus of the ankle, and the base of the fifth metatarsal of the foot). COP data were obtained at 200 Hz from a force platform (AMTI type OR6-3A, Advanced Mechanical Technology, Inc.).

The subjects were asked to stand upright with a freely chosen foot position for 30-s trials with the eyes open (vision corrected by glasses, if necessary) and closed. Each trial yielded one stabilogram. The position and COP data were transferred to a VAX 11/750 computer for reduction and analysis.

Three-dimensional coordinates for each body marker were calculated from the individual camera views using software specifically designed for this system (AMASS, Adtech Co.) The COG was calculated from the actual position of each body segment measured in three-dimensional coordinates using segment mass and inertial characteristics from Dempster [3]. A six-segment model (lower arm, upper arm, trunk and head, upper leg, lower leg, and foot segments) was analyzed for each video frame.

As a measure of the total sway path, we calculated the total extent of displacement (TEX) of all segment and whole body coordinates in the vertical and A-P planes of motion and of whole body measures only (COG and COP) in the M-L plane of motion. This yielded 13 measures (head vertical, head A-P, shoulder vertical, shoulder A-P, hip vertical, hip A-P, knee vertical, knee A-P, COG vertical, COG A-P, COG M-L, COP A-P, and COP M-L), representing the total path of the coordinate during the last 20 s of the stabilogram.

In addition, we evaluated the variability (VAR) about the path of each coordinate, which yielded 13 additional measures. This was done by calculating the standard deviation about the quadratic fit to the same 20-s period to remove any linear or quadratic trend in the data. When no trend was evident, the higher-order terms dropped out and yielded a value equivalent to the standard deviation about the mean. This parameter represents the standard deviation value of the departures from a central position, which can be defined as the average magnitude of an individual segment or whole body postural adjustment. For further explanation of this procedure, see Panzer and Hallett [14].

Comparison of the COP and the COG

In all of our studies, the COP was a close measure of the A-P and M-L position of the COG, but it clearly was not the same. In particular, it contained many more high-frequency components apparently representing accelerations of body parts that do not alter the COG. These additional movements of the COP do not necessarily represent instability. The extreme example is the balance beam performer, whose complex body segment motions help maintain the COG over the very small base of support [16]. Comparison of the COP and the COG may indicate the nature of the strategy used to maintain posture. The measures differ, and the results of studies using these two measures also differ, as summarized below.

Aging

Many studies have assessed sway in aging. Sheldon [19] was the first to suggest that increased sway might contribute to falling. He studied oscillations of the shoulders while subjects stood with their eyes closed or while they tried to minimize their motion while watching a pencil drawing their movements. He found an increase in sway in both tests in subjects older than age 50. Overstall et al. [13] assessed hip movement in the A-P direction and found that it increased with age. Brocklehurst et al. [1] found the same, but indicated that their population was "frail" and that the increased sway was associated with loss of vibration sense. In studies of sway using the speed of pelvic displacement measured with a lightly tensioned self-recoiling wire, Fernie and Holliday [6] suggested that sway increased with age, but later Fernie et al. [7] found no association between sway and age or between sway and falling.

Era and Heikkinen [5] studied the COP with aging in the setting of eyes open, eyes closed, and standing on one foot. In all three tests, they found an increase in COP motion with aging. The increase was only slight with the eyes open and much more prominent when standing on one foot. They also found a correlation with vibration sensation, grip strength, and level of fitness. Wollacott et al. [22] measured COP motion and found no statistical increase with aging with the eyes open or closed. They also studied standing on a surface that was servorotated in the ankle axis in equal proportion to the A-P sway of the COP. The servorotation eliminated, or at least confused, the proprioceptive input. This task was clearly more difficult and brought out differences with aging. Horak et al. [11] also measured COP motion and likewise found no significant changes with aging on a fixed surface, but did observe differences with a servorotated surface. In a comprehensive study of age-related changes in postural control. Peterka and Black [17] measured sway with a rod attached to the base of support and the subject's hip. They found no increase in sway with age in quiet standing on a stable platform with the eyes open or closed. However, when the platform or visual surround were servoed, there were increases in sway with aging.

In our study of quiet standing in aging [16], we studied 24 subjects (13 men and 11 women), aged 21–78 years. We used a regression analysis to test for the effects of age, sex, and vision. As an effect of age, there was a decrease of the TEX of the head A-P and an increase of the VAR of the head vertical, hip vertical, and COG vertical. The only effect of closing the eyes was an increase of the COP A-P. (Women had larger values than men of the TEX of the head vertical, COG M-L, and COP M-L and of the VAR of the hip vertical, knee vertical, and COG M-L.)

We found no changes of the COP with aging with the eyes either open or closed. The increase in the vertical VAR of the head, hip, and COG without an increase in the TEX of these same parameters indicates an increase in large movements with a concomitant decrease in small movements. As noted earlier, an increase in large movements might suggest decreasing stability, but because these movements are in the vertical direction, these changes are unlikely to be related to stability. Note that these changes in vertical motion could not have been detected with a COP measure.

Also of interest was our finding of an increase in the TEX of the COP A-P with the eyes closed but no concomitant increase in the COG A-P. Thus, in this normal population, the increase in sway noted with the eyes closed was not associated with a decrease in stability.

Some studies have shown an increase in body or COP motion with normal aging in quiet standing, but the most recent ones, including ours, have not, indicating that if there is any increase in sway, it is small. Additionally, increases in sway, when seen, might be due to confounding factors that are difficult to eliminate. Aging is clearly associated with problems such as cognitive impairments, sedative use, sensory loss, muscular weakness, lack of fitness, and poor vision [20]. These problems may have affected some studies more than others.

Parkinson's Disease

There have been only a few studies of quiet standing in Parkinson's disease. Gregoric and Lavric [8] studied the COP in normal subjects and patients standing in the Romberg position with the eyes open. On average, they found somewhat more sway in the patients, but the results were highly variable, and many patients swayed less than normal. They did a frequency analysis of the sway and found decreased frequencies of 0.5–1 Hz. They also assessed the mean position of the COP and found it, on average, to be displaced backward in the patients, but some patients were displaced more forward than normal. Dichgans et al. [4] and Bronstein et al. [2] found no difference in COP motion between the eyes open condition or the eyes closed condition. In the latter study, however, an abnormality was detected in patients tested in a situation where vision was misleading. Schieppati and Nardone [18] also found no difference in COP motion between the eyes open or the eyes closed. They did find, however, an abnormality of the mean position of the COP that correlated with the severity of the disease. In mild disease, the mean COP was backward, and with increasing severity it moved forward, so that with severe disease it was forward of the normal position. Thus, the mean COP position was in the normal range for patients with disease of intermediate severity.

We have repeatedly studied a patient with Parkinson's disease in order to assess the sensitivity of these measures to changes in the parkinsonian state [14]. The patient had marked "on–off" fluctuations; in the off state, he had poor balance and was bradykinetic and rigid, but in the on state he had good balance and was mobile with dyskinesia. The two states were best discriminated with the TEX of the head, shoulder, and knee vertical and of the shoulder and the COP A-P and with the VAR of the COG vertical and of the head, shoulder, and hip A-P. In the off state, motion decreased in the A-P direction and increased in the vertical direction. Decreased motion in the A-P direction during the off state was most apparent clinically. This suggests that in Parkinson's disease decreased sway could possibly be a correlate of poor balance.

We report here our study of a larger group of patients with Parkinson's disease. A preliminary note has already been published [15]. We studied ten patients with Parkinson's disease (nine men and one woman), aged 30–75 years, with Hoehn and Yahr stages from I to V. The results were compared with those of ten normal subjects (nine men and one woman), aged 38–78 years, who were individually age- and sex-matched with the patients. The patients were studied when optimally medicated.

Table 1. Values of TEX[a] parameters

Parameter	Normal (mean ± SD; mm)	Patient (mean ± SD; mm)	P[b]
Head			
Vertical	285.9 ± 76.6	354.0 ± 75.7	NS
A-P	451.6 ± 103.7	554.1 ± 101.3	0.003
Shoulder			
Vertical	262.9 ± 39.2	359.2 ± 160.3	NS
A-P	421.4 ± 60.6	538.2 ± 127.2	0.001
Hip			
Vertical	241.3 ± 62.2	373.4 ± 157.0	0.001
A-P	542.8 ± 179.0	688.6 ± 468.2	NS
Knee			
Vertical	266.3 ± 179.8	442.9 ± 224.0	NS
A-P	420.7 ± 110.1	588.3 ± 209.1	0.003
COG			
Vertical	143.6 ± 36.1	207.44 ± 80.1	0.002
A-P	254.1 ± 58.8	338.2 ± 204.2	NS
M-L	166.3 ± 57.5	252.4 ± 153.7	NS
COP			
A-P	241.3 ± 100.7	380.6 ± 199.0	NS
M-L	230.7 ± 53.5	354.9 ± 287.2	NS

A-P, anterior–posterior direction; M-L, medial–lateral direction; COG, center of gravity; COP, center of pressure; NS, not significant.
[a] Total extent of displacement of body segment and whole body coordinates (see text for details).
[b] Paired *t* test, values corrected for the number of comparisons.

A three way analysis of variance was carried out for the TEX and the VAR separately, utilizing the patients and normal subjects, the eyes open and closed, and the 13 parameters of posture as the repeated measure. The results are shown in Tables 1 and 2. For the TEX, patient values were greater than those of the normal subjects ($p = 0.0026$). There was no significant difference of vision. The repeated measures were significantly different ($p < 0.0001$). Post hoc paired *t* tests were assessed for the differences between patients and normal subjects, using $p < 0.004$ as the level of significance ($p < 0.05$ corrected for the 13 comparisons). The measures that showed significant differences were vertical movements of the COG and the hip and A-P movements of the head, shoulder, and knee (Figs. 1, 2).

For the VAR, patient values were generally larger than those of the normal subjects, but the difference did not reach significance ($p = 0.0687$). The repeated measures differed ($p < 0.0001$). The interaction of patients and normal subjects and the repeated measures was also significant ($p = 0.0009$), indicating differences between patients and normal subjects on some of the measures, but not all, and not always in the same direction. Again, vision was not significant. None of the measures differed between patients and normal subjects on the corrected, post hoc, paired *t* test.

Table 2. Values of VAR[a] parameters

Parameter	Normal (mean ± SD; mm)	Patient (mean ± SD; mm)	P[b]
Head			
Vertical	0.699 ± 0.203	0.766 ± 0.204	NS
A-P	4.536 ± 1.455	6.411 ± 3.402	NS
Shoulder			
Vertical	0.777 ± 0.204	0.845 ± 0.312	NS
A-P	4.043 ± 1.330	5.687 ± 3.093	NS
Hip			
Vertical	0.701 ± 0.185	0.795 ± 0.310	NS
A-P	2.969 ± 1.132	4.128 ± 2.334	NS
Knee			
Vertical	0.481 ± 0.118	0.687 ± 0.366	NS
A-P	1.427 ± 1.066	1.985 ± 1.127	NS
COG			
Vertical	0.504 ± 0.282	0.503 ± 0.210	NS
A-P	2.892 ± 1.890	3.422 ± 1.970	NS
M-L	1.710 ± 1.253	1.990 ± 1.458	NS
COP			
A-P	3.666 ± 1.916	4.811 ± 2.426	NS
CM-L	2.308 ± 1.283	2.935 ± 1.884	NS

A-P, anterior–posterior direction; M-L, medial–lateral direction; COG, center of gravity; COP, center of pressure; NS, not significant.
[a] Variability about the path of each coordinate (see text for details).
[b] Paired *t* test, values corrected for the number of comparisons.

The abnormalities that we have found for Parkinson's disease are clearly different than those identified for aging. In Parkinson's disease, the amount of movement (TEX) is increased, but, in general, the oscillations about the mean position (VAR) are not significantly increased. In some patients, this pattern of abnormality was explicable by a tendency for slouching and continuous or intermittent flexion of the posture during the test. Interestingly, however, such movement does not give rise to significant net displacement of the COG or COP and, therefore, does not indicate a loss of stability.

For the patients, a correlation analysis was done between the Hoehn and Yahr stages and the different measures. Significant values were found for the TEX of the hip vertical ($p = 0.018$) and knee A-P ($p = 0.003$) and for the VAR of the COP A-P ($p = 0.023$). The first two parameters were also found to be significantly different between normal subjects and patients.

Our results agree with those of most earlier studies that failed to find a significant increase in COP motion in patients with Parkinson's disease. On the other hand, our more complete observations showed that these patients have a significant increase in the movement of some parts of the body and that these movements may become more marked with increased severity of the disease. Although balance clearly worsens with the severity of Parkinson's disease, our study failed to

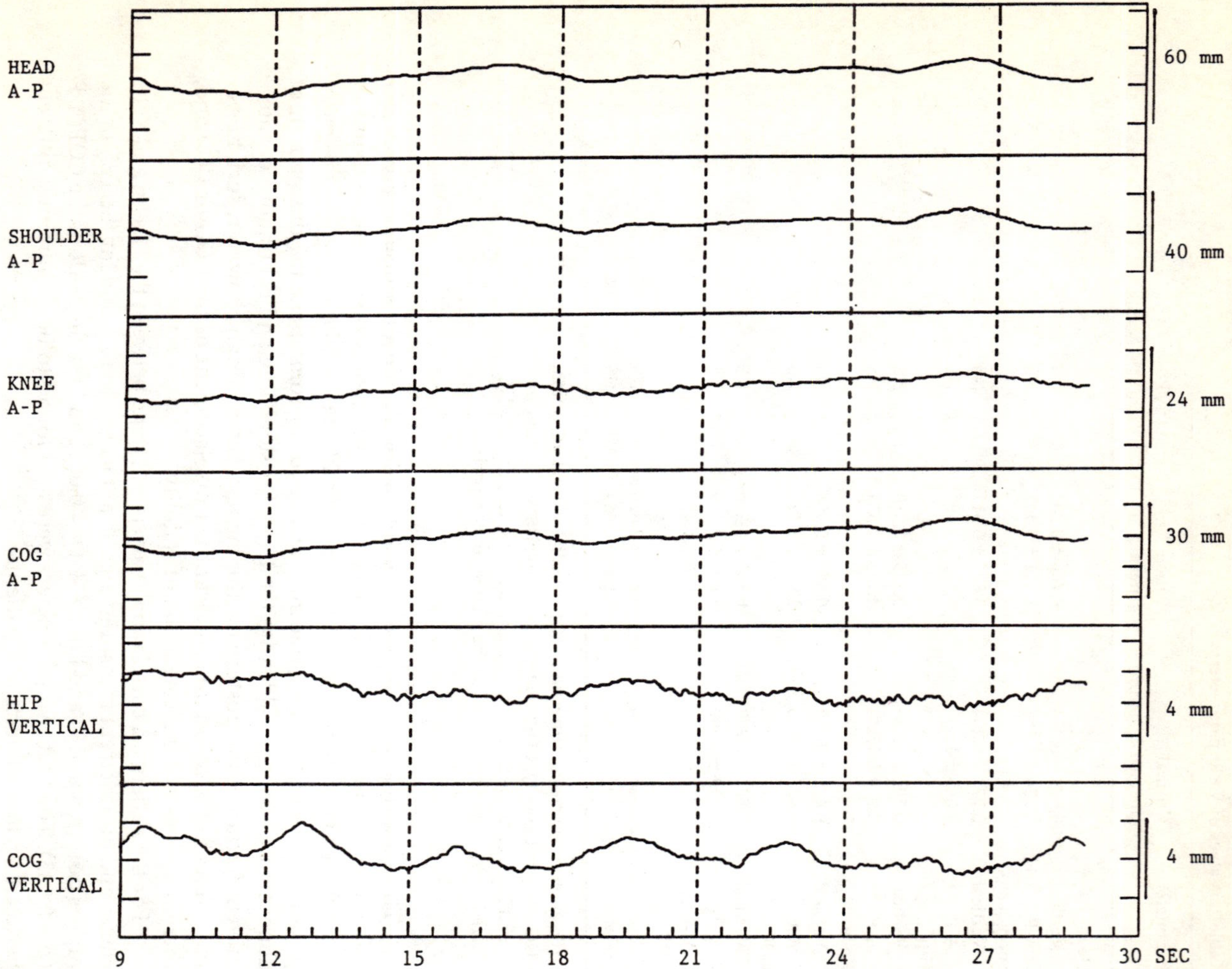

Fig. 1. Selected parameters of standing posture in a 38-year-old normal man age- and sex-matched to the patient illustrated in Fig. 2. *A-P*, anterior–posterior; *COG*, center of gravity

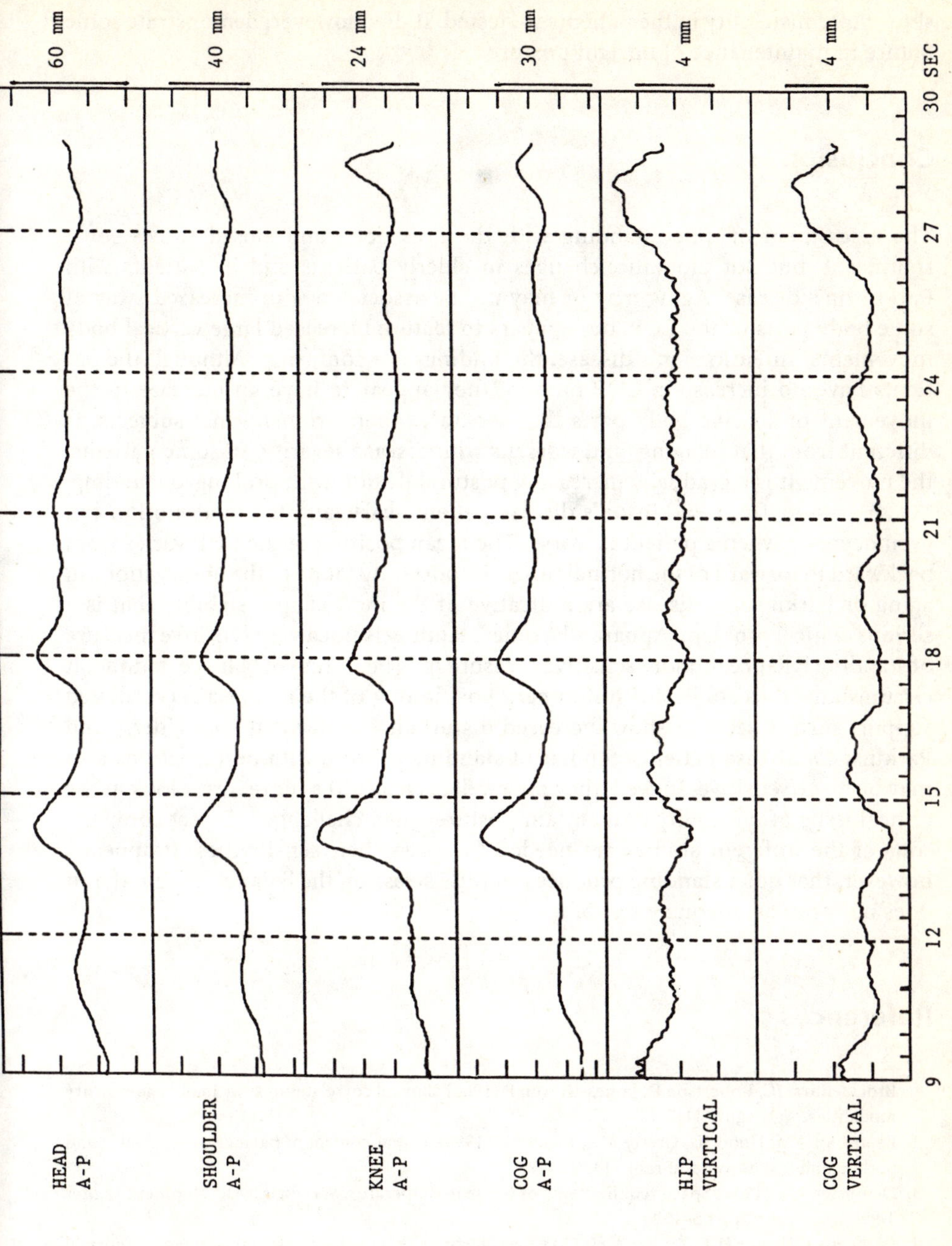

Fig. 2. Selected parameters of standing posture in a 37-year-old man with Parkinson's disease. Note the irregularly appearing brief flexion movements. *A-P*, anterior–posterior; *COG*, center of gravity

show more instability in the patients we tested. It did, however, demonstrate some failure in maintenance of upright posture.

Conclusion

The assessment of quiet standing with the eyes open and closed shows some significant, but not dramatic, changes in elderly patients and in patients with Parkinson's disease. Aging may or may not be associated with increased sway of some body parts or the COP, but appears to feature increased large vertical body movements. In Parkinson's disease, the findings are confusing. Although the patients have no increase in COP motion, they appear to have an increase in the movement of specific body parts that separates them from normal subjects, is different from that in aging, and worsens with disease severity. In some patients, the movement is a gradually increasing postural flexion with prolonged standing. Yet the results from Parkinson's disease patients vary, and the total motion can even decrease when a patient is worse. The mean position of the COP varies from backward to forward of the normal range. Importantly, none of the observations in aging or Parkinson's disease are indicative of the increasing instability that is a serious clinical problem. Apparently, quiet standing is not a very sensitive measure of standing balance. A more sensitive measure may be testing of balance in difficult circumstances, as studies with Romberg positioning of the feet or a servorotated support surface seem to show increased disturbance of sway in both elderly and Parkinson's disease patients. Studies of standing posture with perturbations also may be more sensitive. Indeed, they may well even afford a more direct look at the critical issue of the ability to maintain posture when challenged. Direct comparisons of the different studies are needed to assess their sensitivities. It appears, however, that quiet standing produces so little stress on the balance system that it does not offer an adequate test of it.

References

1. Brocklehurst JC, Robertson D, James-Groom P (1982) Clinical correlates of sway in old age-sensory modalities. Age Aging 11:1–10
2. Bronstein AM, Hood JD, Gresty MA, Panagi C (1990) Visual control of balance in cerebellar and parkinsonian syndromes. Brain 113:767–779
3. Dempster WT (1956) Space requirements of the seated operator. Wright Air Development Center Technical Report, pp 55–159
4. Dichgans J, Diener H-C, Müller A (1985) Characteristics of increased postural sway and abnormal long loop responses in patients with cerebellar diseases and parkinsonism. In: Struppler A, Weindl A (eds) Electromyography and evoked potentials: theories and applications. Springer, Berlin Heidelberg New York, pp 68–74
5. Era P, Heikkinen E (1985) Postural sway during standing and unexpected disturbance of balance in random samples of men of different ages. J Gerontol 40:287–295

6. Fernie GR, Holliday PJ (1978) Postural sway in amputees and normal subjects. J Bone Joint Surg [Am] 60A:895–898
7. Fernie GR, Gryfe CI, Holliday PJ, Llewellyn A (1982) The relationship of postural sway in standing to the incidence of falls in geriatric subjects. Age Ageing 11:11–16
8. Gregoric M, Lavric A (1977) Statokinesimetric analysis of the postural control in parkinsonism. Agressologie 18A:45–48
9. Gryfe CI, Amies A, Ashley MJ (1977) A longitudinal study of falls in an elderly population. I. Incidence and morbidity. Age Ageing 6:201–210
10. Hindmarsh JJ, Estes EH Jr (1989) Falls in older persons. Causes and interventions. Arch Intern Med 149:2217–2222
11. Horak FB, Shupert CL, Mirka A (1989) Components of postural dyscontrol in the elderly: a review. Neurobiol Aging 10:727–738
12. Koller WC, Glatt S, Vetere-Overfield B, Hassanein R (1989) Falls and Parkinson's disease. Clin Neuropharmacol 12:98–105
13. Overstall PW, Exton-Smith AN, Imms FJ, Johnson AL (1977) Falls in the elderly related to postural imbalance. Br Med J 1:261–264
14. Panzer VP, Hallett M (1990) Biomechanical assessment of upright stance in Parkinson's disease: a single-subject study. Clin Biomech 5:73–80
15. Panzer VP, Zeffiro TA, Hallett M (1990) Kinematics of standing posture associated with aging and Parkinson's disease. In: Brandt T, Paulus W, Bles W, Dieterich M, Krafczyk S, Straube A (eds) Disorders of posture and gait 1990. Thieme, Stuttgart, pp 390–393
16. Panzer VP, Bandinelli S, Hallett M (1995) Biomechanical assessment of quiet standing and changes associated with aging Arch Phys Med Rehabil 76:151–157
17. Peterka RJ, Black FO (1990) Age-related changes in human postural control: sensory organization tests. J Vestib Res 1:73–85
18. Schieppati M, Nardone A (1991) Free and supported stance in Parkinson's disease. Brain 114:1227–1244
19. Sheldon HJ (1963) The effect of age on the control of sway. Gerontol Clin 5:129–138
20. Tinetti ME, Speechley M, Ginter SF (1988) Risk factors for falls among elderly persons living in the community. N Engl J Med 319:1701–1707
21. Wolfson LI, Whipple R, Amerman P, Kaplan J, Klienberg A (1985) Gait and balance in the elderly. Two functional capacities that link sensory and motor ability to falls. Clin Geriatr Med 1:649–659
22. Woollacott MH, Shumway-Cook A, Nashner LM (1986) Aging and posture control: changes in sensory organization and muscular coordination. Int J Aging Hum Dev 23:97–114

Discussion

Dr. Paulus: What do you mean by vertical body sway? I am not sure if I understand that correctly.

Dr. Hallett: One of the interesting aspects of being able to look at individual body parts as opposed to the center of pressure is that you can look at movement in the vertical direction. The center of pressure doesn't have any vertical parameter to it of course; it's only forward and backward and side to side. With any particular body part it can go forward and backward, side to side, and also up and down, so that if there is an increased vertical movement of the center of pressure, it can go up and down, but it won't go forward and backward or side to side.

Dr. Paulus: So you do not claim that the body height increases, but just that the pressure varies?

Dr. Hallett: There isn't any change in the center of pressure. The center of gravity can go up and down as the body goes down and up. There are vertical differences as to where the center of gravity is or vertical differences as to where the head is, but the center of pressure can't change its vertical position.

Dr. Allum: How do you distinguish between a vertical change and a displacement of a body part, and a rotation of that body part forward or backward, because then you also have a vertical displacement? In other words, if your measurements included trunk rotation forward and backward, which would cause a vertical displacement of a part and, for example, bending of the knees, which as you just demonstrated causes purely vertical displacement. Are your measurements capable of doing that?

Dr. Hallett: What we did is look at each of these parameters separately. We took, for example, the actual position of the knee marker and looked at its movement forward and backward, side to side, and up and down. Some of the movements may in fact be linked movements; that's what you're talking about, that if there is a particular movement in one direction there may have to be a cojoined vertical movement with it. What we did is look at the individual parameters separately, and these are the results that we came up with. Most of the statistically significant differences were in fact in vertical movements, but without anteroposterior movements.

Dr. Paulus: Just a very short comment about what you claimed about the higher frequency you measure with a platform. I think it's less acceleration of certain body parts and more muscle activity, simply muscle activity acting on the platform, which you can register there but not detect with an optical body motion system.

Dr. Hallett: That's right. Muscle activity creates a force, that's what muscles do, and forces are seen on the platform, because the platform is designed to measure forces. So you are correct that the center of pressure does in fact measure all the individual muscle components, whereas the center of gravity doesn't necessarily see that unless the body is moved from one place to another. That's why the two measurements differ.

Dr. Hocherman: How much of the sway can be explained by breathing?

Dr. Hallett: People have looked at sway with breathing, and there is indeed a certain amount of sway that is synchronous with breathing. In terms of the differences between our normal subjects and the two groups, this doesn't differ, of course. There is a certain amount of normal sway that is due to the breathing motion.

Dr. Fahn: In the case report of a Parkinson's disease patient who had increased sway when the patient was "on," could this be a representation of underlying subclinical possible choreatic movements and, therefore, could this kind of testing be done, let's say as a preclinical test for Huntington's disease or something like that?

Dr. Hallett: The increased sway that patient had when he was "on" was in fact due to dyskinetic movements that the patient had, but the point that I was trying to make was that with increased sway the balance was clearly better. It would also detect movements in Huntington's disease, of course. I'm not sure that it could be used as a test that would be more sensitive than clinical observation.

Dr. Rabey: One of the variables that may affect position in Parkinson's disease patients is the sensory afferent system, not only eyes open or closed. Did you try to change one of the variables, such as being close to a door or to some coloured stripes, to see whether there is a difference in the postural stability of the patients?

Dr. Hallett: We didn't do that in these studies. The only thing that we did here was look at quiet standing with eyes open and eyes closed; if you alter the sensory environment in some way, just as I showed with the aging situation, it might be that Parkinson patients get worse, but that isn't what we looked at here.

Differential Diagnosis of Organic and Psychogenic Vertigo Using Dynamic Posturography

J.H.J. Allum, F. Honegger, and M. Huwiler

Introduction

Dizziness, and with it the risk of losing one's balance, is a common debilitating problem among adults older than 50 years of age. Approximately 10% of all patients visiting a general practitioner complain of being prone to fall [15], due to an unbalanced gait or stance or a sensation of falling or vertigo (an illusion of movement of oneself or the environment). The complexity of the balance system – information from three orientation senses, vestibular, visual, and proprioceptive, is used by the CNS to generate appropriate musculoskeletal responses to regain or maintain equilibrium – places increased diagnostic demands on the examining medical specialist.

Foremost, the specialist needs to be able to distinguish the effects of an organic vestibular disorder on balance corrections and, equally crucially, have an objective indication of whether the patient is simulating or aggravating a balance disorder. Balance tests should, therefore, also provide definitive evidence for a psychogenic vertigo. Estimates of psychogenic vertigo among patients visiting dizziness clinics vary between 10% and 20% [9,14] and have been cited as approximately 2% of patients admitted to the neurology wards of large metropolitan hospitals [12]. Thus, a psychogenic balance disorder may be one of the most frequent types of balance disorders seen by the clinician. Some of these patients expect financial compensation from accident or automobile insurance companies. In order to reduce social and medical costs for the society at large, techniques which provide accurate information on the cause of a balance dysfunction, yet complement conventional clinical testing, offer the best possibility of an objective diagnosis of psychogenic vertigo and ultimately of defining the extent of peripheral or central vestibular deficit.

There are two fundamental reasons why the vestibulospinal reflex (VSR) function should be investigated independently of conventional vestibular test procedures. Conventional clinical testing of the peripheral vestibular system is based mainly on caloric and rotating chair tests, both of which excite the horizontal vestibulo-ocular reflex (VOR). It is possible that the horizontal VOR functions normally, but a pathology exists in the vertical vestibular system (pitch and roll planes) which is overlooked and the patient is incorrectly diagnosed. Given that the horizontal VOR (yaw plane) is not specific for gait or stance instability, this possible oversight has to be carefully considered. Secondly, the VSR and VOR signals reach their target motoneurons via different central neural integration stations and separate peripheral pathways. Central deficits in VOR pathways are based on the interaction between visual and vestibular ocular reflex signals occurring within the brain stem. Optokinetic and pursuit tracking tests appear to be the most sensitive tests for distinguishing central VOR lesions [3].

Often, the Romberg test is used as a screening test of VSR pathology, be it of peripheral or central origin. Modified forms of the Romberg test have also been employed to distinguish abnormalities in visual, vestibular, and proprioceptive contributions to balance control [7,10] and in exceptional cases a psychogenic vertigo [10,13]. However, these tests do not provide objective documentation of a patient's functional disability related either to the extent of his peripheral vestibular deficit or to any muscle activation patterns used to simulate a balance disorder. This is probably because reflex and voluntary muscle activity cannot be separated from one another with the Romberg test. The techniques of dynamic posturography described in this paper specifically fulfill these requirements by examining the relationship between muscle response and biomechanical reactions following a sudden, controlled balance perturbation, usually a translation or rotation of the support surface on which the test subject stands.

Effects of Vestibular Loss on Balance Corrections

A balance perturbation caused by a controlled support surface movement elicits muscle responses in man at several body segments. The amplitude of these responses are dependent on the angular movements of the limbs and include muscle stretch or release and joint rotations, as well as head accelerations [4]. For example, both a rearward translation of the support surface, which, if uncorrected, causes globally forward motion of the body, and a dorsiflexion rotation, which causes a globally rearward falling of the body, may have the same amount of ankle joint rotation but certainly differing knee and hip flexion and head rotations [4]. Hence, the CNS is always faced with the problem of coordinating balance-correcting movements across several body links using a combination of proprioceptive and vestibular information. A vestibular deficit would, therefore, be expected to result in a breakdown of this coordination.

Figure 1 illustrates differences in the responses of normal subjects to those of subjects with a bilateral peripheral vestibular deficit (vestibular loss). The stimuli, dorsiflexion rotations of the support surface, combined with a small amount of rearward translation (0.7 cm), were presented randomly under eyes open conditions. Despite the availability of alternative visual inputs, the responses of the vestibular-loss subjects were consistently smaller than normal in a number of leg and trunk muscles, except for paraspinal (PARAS) muscles and, surprisingly, early stretch reflex responses in soleus (SOL) muscles, which yielded larger than normal responses.

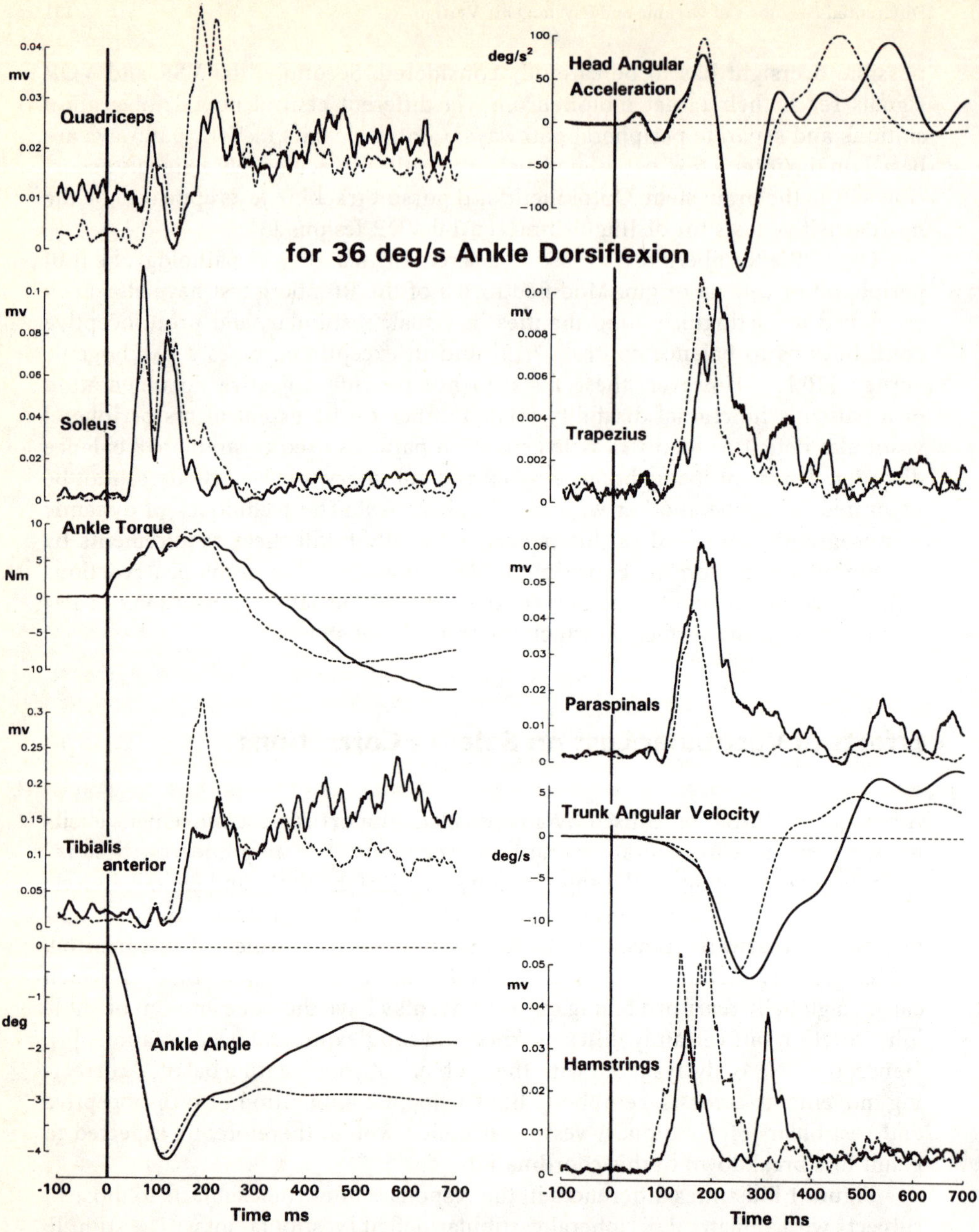

Fig. 1. Muscle activation patterns of normal (---) and vestibular-loss subjects (—) to a support surface movement causing 36°/s ankle dorsiflexion (3.5° dorsiflexion rotation, 0.7 cm rearward translation). All traces are group averages (calculated from the average of nine responses from each of 16 normals and from each of five vestibular-loss subjects). The traces have been aligned in time with the first deflection of ankle angular velocity. Rearward rotations of angles are plotted positively, as is increased plantar flexion torque imposed on the platform. Note the biphasic pulse of head angular acceleration occurring as the stimulus rapidly rotates the foot during the first 100 ms of the stimulus profile (see ankle angle trace). Except for paraspinals and the early soleus responses, muscle responses are weaker in vestibular-loss subjects. (Modified from [5])

The sequence of events causing vestibular-loss subjects to topple over backwards like an inverted pendulum following support surface rotations [1] can be understood by comparing the electromyogram (EMG) and biomechanical traces for normals and vestibular-loss subjects in Fig. 1. The enhanced stretch reflex response in SOL between 50 and 100 ms from the onset of dorsiflexion combined with the decreased tibialis anterior (TA) response after 120 ms provides less stabilizing torque around the ankle joint. The ankle torque trace in Fig. 1 depicts this less rapid change in ankle torque after 150 ms in vestibular-loss subjects. The deficit in ankle joint torque is more pronounced under eyes closed conditions [2]. Normal subjects respond to the toe-up rotation by generating sufficient torque in the lower leg muscles to maintain an upright stance. The rotation of the foot around the ankle joint, which is imposed on the subject by the support surface rotation, is not corrected back to approximately 90°, but remains essentially unchanged. Vestibular-loss subjects, however, begin to topple over backwards when tilted and permit the angle of ankle dorsiflexion to return towards the prestimulus value of approximately 90°. Because the upper and lower legs essentially act as one segment in response to support surface rotations, the upper legs also start toppling over backwards.

The passive movement of the trunk in response to a support surface rotation is first forwards. Coordinated hip-flexing muscle action should then place the trunk in an upright position as quickly as possible, otherwise the continued unchecked forward rotation of the trunk will thrust the hips backward and enhance any toppling effect elicited by weak ankle torques. Precisely how the hip-flexing action of the quadriceps, hamstrings and abdominal and paraspinal muscles is coordinated in normals is not completely understood. It can, however, be surmised from the smaller responses than normal in quadriceps and hamstrings muscles of vestibular-loss subjects, the larger than normal responses in PARAS muscles, and from the trunk angular velocity profiles in Fig. 1 that coordination of this muscle activity is dysfunctional in vestibular-loss subjects and often leads to a fall. The weaker hamstring activity in vestibular-loss subjects first permits the trunk weight to act as a toppling force acting outside the area of foot support behind the ankle joint, then the enhanced paraspinal activity pitches the trunk far too rapidly backwards. At 700 ms, the trunk of vestibular-loss subjects is almost colinear with the legs, and a fall can only be avoided by supplementary TA activity after 300 ms. Such enhancement of TA activity occurs when visual feedback is present (Fig. 1), but is absent with eyes closed [1]. The vestibular-loss patient standing with eyes closed must be supported if a fall is to be avoided following a rapid support surface rotation.

The foregoing description of the effects of a vestibular loss on balance corrections emphasises the importance of TA EMG activity over the 120- to 200-ms period after onset of a jolt to quiet standing in generating stabilizing ankle torque. The optimal period to measure the resulting ankle torque should be delayed some 25 ms to account for electromechanical coupling delays in ankle muscles [2].

Figure 2 shows how the average amplitude of these two variables will change the extent of the clinically defined peripheral vestibular deficit. The bar graphs in

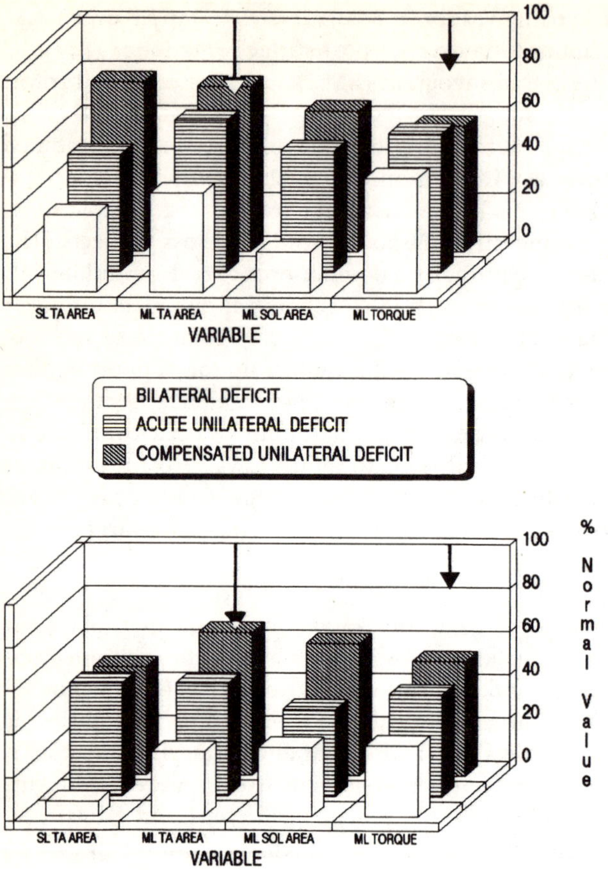

Fig. 2. Percentage decrement in lower leg muscle response and stabilizing ankle torques in three groups (bilateral; acute, unilateral; compensated, i.e. 3 months postacute, unilateral) of peripheral vestibular-deficit subjects. The percentage decrement is with respect to normal values obtained in response to a 36°/s support surface dorsiflexion rotation. Response variables, ordered from left to right in each bar diagram are short latency (*SL*) tibialis anterior (*TA*) electromyogram (*EMG*) area (measured between 80 and 120 ms after onset of platform rotation), medium latency (*ML*) soleus (*SOL*) and TA area (120–200 ms), and ML torque (145–225 ms). Eyes open trials in the *upper* bar graph, eyes closed in the *lower* graph. The *vertical arrows* above ML TA area and ML ankle torque bars indicate one standard deviation of the normal responses. The average response amplitude for the patient groups decreases with increasing severity of the clinically defined deficit (Modified from [2])

Fig. 2 represent the average response amplitudes of three populations of peripheral vestibular-deficit subjects. The data points for each subject in these populations were computed as the average responses for the last seven of ten presentations of a 36°/s toe-up support surface rotation. That is, the first three responses were not included in the averaging process in order to remove the effect of response adaptation from the population measures [11]. Compared to normal responses, which are equally vigorous under eyes open and eyes closed conditions (see Fig. 3), Fig. 2 illustrates that the responses of vestibular-deficit subjects are even smaller than normal under eyes closed conditions. The stepwise decrease in the area under TA activity between 120 and 200 ms (called ML, medium latency, in Fig. 2) and ML (145–225 ms) torque as the extent of the peripheral vestibular deficit (defined on the basis of caloric and rotating chair VOR tests) increases is particularly evident in the lower bar graph of Fig. 2. A bilateral deficit is the most profound deficit, and a compensated unilateral peripheral deficit, the most marginal deficit.

In summary, an organic peripheral vestibular deficit can be characterized by weak VSR following support surface rotation. Responses are decreased over 120–240 ms in TA muscles, and a corresponding weak ankle torque response is elicited over approximately the same time period. Both these responses are even weaker than normal under eyes closed conditions. Repeating the rotations under eyes closed conditions has no effect on normal responses. In addition, responses in PARAS muscles are larger than normal in vestibular deficit subjects. Together, the uncoordinated TA and PARAS activity causes the body to fall backwards as if it were an inverted pendulum rotating about the joints. Normals correct for a support surface rotation by using a combination of hip and ankle rotations [1,4].

Patterns of Balance Corrections Elicited When a Balance Deficit Is Simulated

The pattern of muscle activity generated when a normal subject mimics a balance disorder is, presumably, different from that of a subject with an organic balance disorder. A similar reasoning would suggest that the coordination of link movements (or joint torques) would also be different. In an attempt to determine how the pattern of muscle activity and resulting biomechanical responses might be altered when a balance disorder is simulated by normal subjects, we requested normal subjects to respond to a series of 11 consecutive support surface dorsiflexion rotations of 4° amplitude as if they had a balance deficit. The results are illustrated in Fig. 3. Two sets of traces show completely normal responses. That is, the subjects were asked to return to upright as rapidly as possible without mimicking a balance disorder. One series was presented under eyes open conditions and the other under eyes closed conditions. As expected from previous publications [11], no significant effect of vision was observed (compare dashed and solid lines in Fig. 3).

Three patterns of postural responses emerged when the same group of normal subjects were asked to mimic a balance disorder. All of these patterns appear in the traces labeled "voluntary" in Fig. 3 because these were averaged together (dash-dot lines). The predominant pattern consisted of increased PARAS activity after 150 ms and increased SOL activity after 240 ms, which appeared to rotate the trunk backwards excessively about the hips. This extra activity is marked by stars in Fig. 3. Concomitantly, trapezius is activated, presumably to assist the rearward rotation of the trunk with head rearward pitching. A second pattern was also distinguished by increased SOL activity after 240 ms. Biomechanically, though, a forward flexion of the trunk was developed as the legs pitched backwards (see upper leg

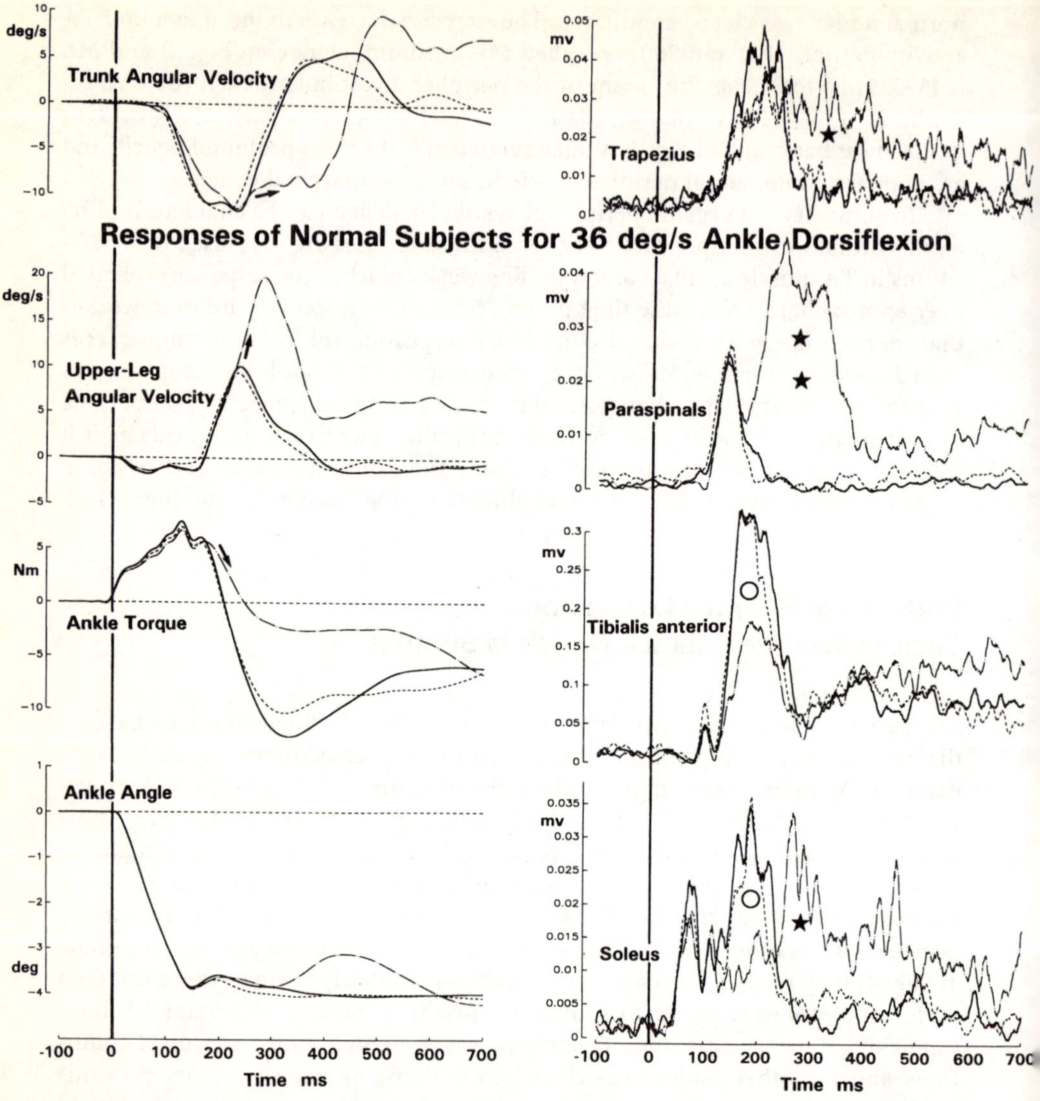

Fig. 3. Comparison of average eyes open (EO) (—), eyes closed (EC) (---), and simulated balance dificit responses, "voluntary" (—•—), from a group of eight normal subjects. The stimulus was a 4°, 36°/s ankle dorsiflexion repeated 11 times for each condition and averaged over the last eight responses. The subjects were asked to respond to the simulated responses labeled "voluntary" as if they had a balance disorder. Otherwise, i.e., for the eyes open and closed responses, the subjects were asked to regain upright stance as quickly as possible. Note the identical response patterns for EO and EC conditions. Increases in electromyogram (EMG) activity for the simulated conditions with respect to EO and EC conditions are marked with *stars*, decreases with *open circles*. Divergences of the biomechanical traces from normal EO or EC conditions are marked with an *arrowhead*. For details of the biomechanical traces, see Fig. 1 and text. Because the subjects respond differently when asked to simulate a balance disorder, the figure is a composite of response types. (Previously unpublished observations from [6])

angular velocity trace in Fig. 3). Finally, the least common pattern involved suppressing TA and SOL activity between 160 and 240 ms (see circles indicating these decreased EMG responses in Fig. 3), so that the body fell backwards like an inverted pendulum.

The biomechanical traces in Fig. 3 provide a composite picture of the aforementioned simulation patterns. Arrows on these traces mark the time point at which a significant divergence from the normal movement strategy occurs. Consistent with the increased activity in PARAS and SOL muscles, the upper leg and trunk angular velocity traces diverge from nonsimulated (normal) responses after 220 ms. Similarly, the decreased activity in SOL and TA muscles after 120 ms causes a divergence of the simulated response torque traces at 170 ms. The general picture emerging from a balance disorder simulation is always for the ankle torque traces to diverge from the sharp decrease in plantar flexion torque observed for normal responses. However, the profile of ankle torque is very different from the shallow decrease in torque seen for vestibular-loss patients (compare ankle torque traces in Figs. 1 and 3), as it starts sharply, then rapidly flattens out or increases. The divergence of upper leg and trunk angular velocity is always in the direction of increased velocity.

In summary, a psychogenic balance disorder can be characterised by strong bursts of muscle activity in SOL and PARAS muscles after 240 ms. Particularly for the PARAS muscles, the amplitude of this activity is greater than the reflex response normally occurring in normal or vestibular-loss subjects between 100 and 160 ms. Anticompensatory movement of the trunk has a much higher velocity than normal after 220 ms and appears to simulate either a rearward or forward falling. Such action is also indicative of a psychogenic balance disorder. A divergence of the ankle torque profile at 170 ms in the direction of increased rather than decreased plantar flexion torque would be consistent with the observation on trunk angular velocity profiles. Finally, greater balance instability under eyes closed conditions compared to full visual feedback is to be expected for subjects with an organic balance disorder. Greater instability associated with the above cited changes in muscle response patterns under eyes open conditions would not be recorded unless the subject was simulating a balance disorder. It should be noted that although the stimuli were presented randomly, they were a series of consecutive dorsiflexion displacements of the same amplitude. Some subjects can suppress TA and SOL response amplitudes (see Fig. 3) prior to activation of PARAS and SOL at voluntary response latencies. Such suppression of TA and SOL activity *without* accompanying activity after 220 ms in SOL and PARAS muscles is not indicative of a psychogenic balance disorder, because TA and SOL EMG activity is also reduced between 120 ms and 200 ms for subjects with organic balance deficits. The following case study demonstrates the application of these criteria.

Case Study of Psychogenic Vertigo

A female patient, born in 1947, had a right cerebellar pontine angle tumor (9 mm in diameter) removed some 6 months prior to our examination. Pre- and postop-

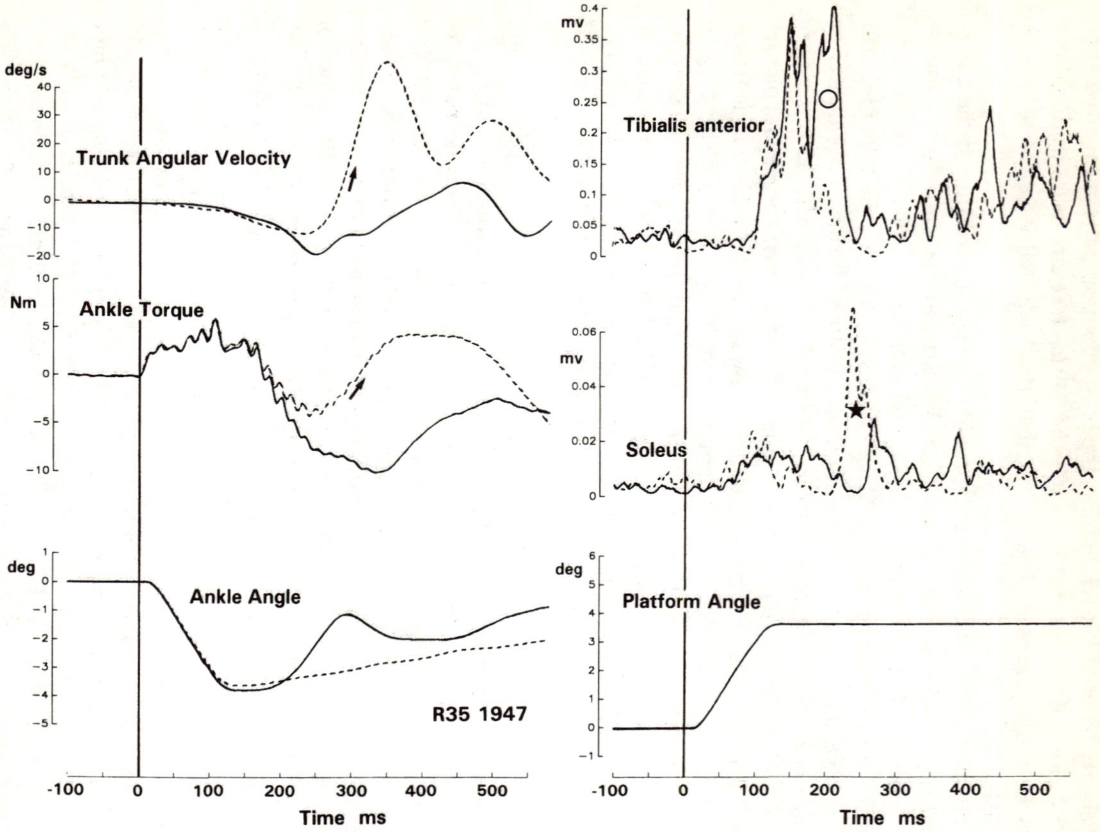

Fig. 4. Case study of suspected psychogenic vertigo. For eyes closed (---) conditions, the subject is voluntarily activating the soleus muscle (SOL) after 200 ms and suppressing tibialis anterior (TA) activity after 170 ms in response to the 3.6° support surface rotation. Trunk muscles are also probably activated voluntarily after 200 ms because the trunk tips back much more rapidly than normal. Note the normal responses for eyes open conditions (—)

erative visual oculomotor tests were normal. Although a canal paresis of 100% right was present postoperatively, a symmetrical response of normal amplitude was observed for the rotating chair tests of horizontal VOR function. The patient complained of increasing loss of balance 5 months postoperatively and a hearing loss on the left (nonoperated) side. A test of otoacoustic emissions and stapedius reflexes indicated normal hearing on the left side. The dynamic posturography results are illustrated in Fig. 4. The responses under eyes open conditions are normal. In contrast, a number of observations from the responses under eyes closed conditions suggest the presence of psychogenic vertigo. Clearly, both the ankle torque and trunk angular velocity traces indicate that the patient was voluntarily tilting the trunk backwards in response to the balance perturbation (see arrows in Fig. 4). The presence of SOL activity at 220 ms (marked with a start) and suppression of TA activity just prior to this time point (marked with a circle) support this conclusion. The patient was advised to seek psychiatric assistance, which positively influenced both her hearing and balance deficits.

Conclusions

Dynamic posturography is unique compared to other conventional clinical vestibular or neurological tests, because the balance task elicited by displacement of the support surface on which the test subject stands is very similar to more natural balance tasks encountered by the elderly. For example, the body displacements occurring when a bus stops suddenly or goes sharply around a curve bear a distinct resemblance to the rotation or translation of the support surface used during dynamic posturography. For both the natural and laboratory test balance perturbations, a number of motor tasks are encountered. Firstly, the center of body mass must be stably positioned within the area of foot support; secondly, movement of the body links should be corrected into an upright stance; and finally, throughout these movements, the head must be steadied so that gaze is stable. The purpose of this brief review has been to describe the types of muscle responses underlying the first two motor tasks and elucidate how these responses are dependent on peripheral vestibular inputs. With this knowledge it is possible to understand how balance movements are affected by an organic balance disorder. This knowledge also enables the examining physician to differentiate between normal and organically pathological VSR function. Because only the amplitudes and not latencies of muscle response are affected by a peripheral vestibular disorder [5], prolonged latencies are strong indications of a CNS or spinal cord lesion [8]. Specific tests of central vestibulospinal deficits using dynamic posturography have yet to be devised.

Another purpose of this review was to identify changes in muscle responses occurring when subjects simulate a balance disorder. These changes in the form of additional bursts of PARAS and SOL activity after 220 ms and characteristic alterations to ankle torque and trunk velocity profiles are relatively easy to pinpoint. This invaluable aspect of dynamic posturography provides a very useful complement to standard clinical tests when assessing cases of psychogenic vertigo.

Acknowledgment. This research was supported by grant 31-30863.91 from the Swiss National Research Fund.

References

1. Allum JHJ, Honegger F (1992) A postural model of balance-correcting movement strategies. J Vestib Res 2:323–347
2. Allum JHJ, Keshner EA, Honegger F, Pfaltz CR (1988) Indicators of the influence a peripheral vestibular deficit has on vestibulospinal reflex responses controlling postural stability. Acta Otolaryngol (Stockh) 106:252–263
3. Allum JHJ, Ura M, Honegger F, Pfaltz CR (1991) Classification of peripheral and central (pontine infarction) vestibular deficits: selection of a neurootological test battery using discriminant analysis. Acta Otolaryngol (Stockh) 111:16–26
4. Allum JHJ, Honegger F, Schiecks H (1993) Vestibular and proprioceptive modulation of postural synergies in normal subjects. J Vestib Res 3:59–85
5. Allum JHJ, Honegger F, Schicks H (1994) The influence of a bilateral peripheral vestibular deficit on postural synergies. J Vestib Res 4:49–70
6. Allum JHJ, Honegger F, Huwiler M (1995) The influence of a simulated balance disorder on dynamic posturography: implications for the diagnosis of psychogenic vertigo (in preparation)
7. Black FO, Shupert CL, Horak FB, Nashner LM (1988) Abnormal postural control associated with peripheral vestibular disorders. Prog Brain Res 76:263–275
8. Diener HC, Ackermann H, Dichgans J, Guschlbauer B (1985) Medium and long-latency responses to displacements of the ankle joint in patients with spinal and central lesions. Electroencephalogr Clin Neurophysiol 60:407–416
9. Drachman DA, Hart CA (1972) An approach to the dizzy patient. Neurology 22:323–334
10. Kantner RM, Rubin AM, Armstrong CW, Cummings V (1991) Stabiliometry in balance: assessment of dizzy and normal subjects. Am J Otolaryngol 12:196–204
11. Keshner EA, Allum JHJ, Pfaltz CR (1987) Postural coactivation and adaptation in the sway stabilizing responses of normals and patients with bilateral vestibular deficit. Exp Brain Res 69:77–92
12. Lempert T, Dieterich M, Huppert D, Brandt T (1990) Psychogenic disorders in neurology: frequency and clinical spectrum. Acta Neurol Scand 82:335–340
13. Nashner LM, Peters JF (1990) Dynamic posturography in the diagnosis and management of dizziness and balance disorders. Neurol Clin 8:331–344
14. Nedzelski JM, Barber HO, McIlmoyl L (1986) Diagnoses in a dizziness unit. J Otolaryngol 15:101–104
15. Sloane PD, Baloh RW, Honrubia V (1989) The vestibular system in the elderly: clinical implications. Am J Otolaryngol 10:422–429

Discussion

Dr. Findley: You showed the vestibularly deficit patients and showed the difference between normals. Peripheral vestibular deficits are adapted in most people. In most people there is adaptation symptomatically for the clinician anyway. Does that cause a change in your findings?

Dr. Allum: No. That sounds as if it were contradictory. It is true that patients with peripheral vestibular deficits adapt and it is also true – as we have shown in earlier work – that those with unilateral vestibular deficits have torque responses in a compensated state which are much greater than those in the acute stage. These patients with bilateral vestibular deficits were tested in the compensated state. I should have stated that, but this I think answers your question.

Dr. Findley: You would expect to see a more dramatic result if you had tested them in the acute stage.

Dr. Allum: Yes, but it's very difficult to find an acute bilateral vestibular deficit. Most of the time it starts off on one side and then it develops on the other side. Sometimes by the time we see the patients, they've already compensated.

Dr. Deuschl: In one of your slides there was a big difference in the quadriceps concerning the baseline. What does this mean? The baseline EMG is much higher here in the patient group. Do they have a preventive strategy?

Dr. Allum: If you look at a vestibularly deficit patient and in particular at his neck muscles, you notice that they are very taut. In fact, such patients often complain of stiff neck muscles, and this is because they use a stiffening strategy. However, when we measured responses, we controlled naturally for the baseline activity, and all areas which I showed you as being statistically significant were with respect to the baseline. You have to make this compensation, otherwise you cannot compare the areas. But yes, you're right. They do increase their background muscle activity. The difference is not statistically significant. In other words, we haven't been able to find a statistical significance.

Dr. Hocherman: Do you see any adaptation or learning changes in response strategy for repeated stimulation?

Dr. Allum: We published an earlier work showing that both vestibularly deficit patients and normals adapt their response size when you present them with stimulus serially – the same stimulus. However, these stimuli were not the same stimulus presented serially; the stimuli were presented randomly and there is some adaptation. We didn't look at that question in detail; what we did was just throw out the first response from all our averages, because we knew they were always large.

Relevance of Posturographic Parameters in the Differential Diagnosis of Parkinsonism

C. Trenkwalder, W. Paulus, S. Krafzcyk, M. Hawken, W.H. Oertel, and T. Brandt

Introduction

In idiopathic parkinsonism, a gait disorder with reduced postural adjustments occurs almost invariably in the advanced stages of the disease [7,11]. The gait disturbance in nonidiopathic parkinsonian syndromes is difficult to differentiate from that in Parkinson's disease (PD). Clinical classification of these gait disorders remains equivocal and we have selected the term "lower body parkinsonism" (LBP; [4]) for our nonidiopathic Parkinson patients suffering from gait disorder, step hesitation, and akinesia of the "lower half." In order to obtain posturographic parameters helpful for differential diagnosis, we compared different methods and evaluations of static postural performance in both groups of patients.

Two results emerged out of this study:

1. Two different parameters for measuring body sway are necessary for differentiation of sway due to slow body shifts and due to parkinsonian tremor.
2. Only with provocative methods is a clear-cut differentiation between different parkinsonian syndromes possible.

Patients and Methods

The patients in both groups suffered from a moderate to severe gait disorder with step hesitation as predominant symptom and reported a history of frequent falls within the last few months. LBP or PD were classified by clinical findings, pharmacological testing with oral L-dopa and apomorphine, and CCT/MRI findings.

LBP Group

The mean age of the 11 LBP patients (eight males, three females) was 70.9 years (range, 61–85 years). Six patients suffered from moderate and five from severe gait disorder with predominant step hesitation and showed negative response to apomorphine and L-dopa.

PD Group

The diagnosis of PD was determined only if patients showed typical symptoms, such as unilateral or bilateral rigidity and/or rest tremor and akinesia, and if oral L-dopa clearly improved motor symptoms. The mean age of the ten patients with PD (seven men, three women) was 64.8 years (range, 51–78 years), and they were classified as Hoehn and Yahr stage III and IV (off period). None of the patients were wheelchair bound. Four patients suffered from severe and six from moderate gait initiation failure. At time of assessment, all patients were treated with L-dopa (200–1000 mg per day), and eight patients with an additional dopamine agonist.

Experimental Procedure

Postural sway during stance was tested with a force-measuring platform (Kistler). The patients were asked to stand as still as possible. As soon as the patient had adopted the position, the data were digitized at a sampling rate of 40 Hz with an analysis time of 25.6 s for each trial. The averaged results of two separate trials were used for the statistics. The patients stood 70 cm in front of a highly structured visual background either with eyes open or with eyes closed and either on a firm foot support or on a wooden footplate placed upon a 10-cm foam slab (further details in [8]). The torque forces were registered by the platform using 12 force transducers.

Data Analysis

These data were converted to reflect the center of foot pressure (CFP). When tracing the change of CFP over time, we calculated the following data:

1. Root mean square values of lateral body sway (RMSx values)
2. Root mean square values of anterior–posterior (A-P) body sway (RMSy values)
3. Sway path (SP) of CFP in the lateral direction
4. Sway path of the CFP in the anterior-posterior direction
5. Total sway path (vector SP) of the CFP during each trial

Items 1 and 2 were obtained by squaring each CFP value, summing up all values, and then taking the square root. In order to obtain SP values, the spatial difference between each CFP value was summed up and divided by the recording time.

Results of Posturography

Differences and Artifacts in Evaluating Root Mean Square and Sway Path Values

Figure 1 demonstrates the results of two extreme possibilities. First (Fig. 1, y1), the subject oscillates on a platform in the A-P direction in order to simulate

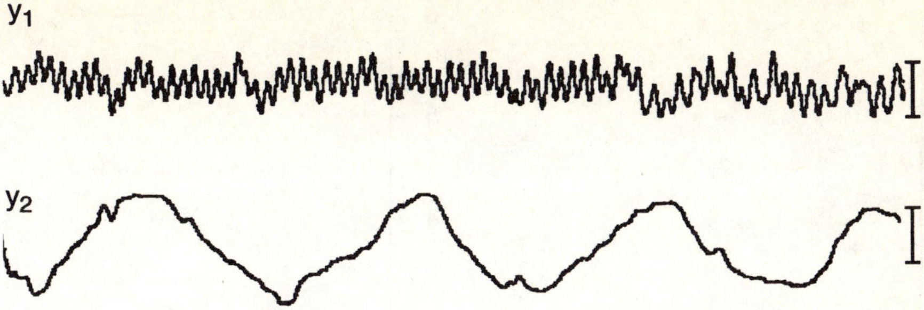

Fig. 1. Kistler y_1: high-frequency movements simulating 3- to 5-Hz tremor in anterior-posterior direction. Sway path anterior-posterior, 10.2 m/min; root mean square (RMS) sway anterior-posterior, 12.5 mm. Kistler y_2: Low-frequency movements (0.1 Hz) simulating slow body shifts in anterior/posterior direction. Sway path anterior-posterior, 1.7 m/min; RMS sway anterior-posterior, 29.3 mm. RMS y values are increased during slow dorsal–caudal (D-C) shifts, whereas sway path A-P rises at higher frequencies comparable with tremor. *Black vertical bar* indicates 0.05 m

parkinsonian tremor. The resulting SP is high (due to the increased distance across which the CFP has traveled over time), while RMS is comparatively low. Second, the subject exhibits a slowly moving CFP (Fig. 1, y2) with a concomitantly low sway path, but a higher RMS sway. The higher RMS sway is caused by the unusually large deviations of the CFP from the baseline, since each digitized data value is calculated from the baseline. Thus, RMS is more sensitive for large, slow oscillations while SP depicts small, high-frequency oscillations.

Comparison of Posturographic Data of LBP and PD Patients and Controls

In order to demonstrate the evidence of methodological differences, we selected the following two conditions:

Standing with Eyes Closed on Firm Foot Support (Fig. 2)

During stance with eyes closed on firm foot support, A-P sway was always higher than lateral sway both in normals and PD patients, but less marked in LBP patients. Medians of A-P and lateral SP values of PD and LBP were also within the normal range of controls ($p > 0.05$, Mann-Whitney test). One parkinsonian patient of the PD group showed moderate rest tremor during the trial, which is reflected as one high SP value in the PD group (see Fig. 2).

Standing with Eyes Closed on Foam

Standing with eyes closed on foam showed higher RMSx and RMSy values of LBP patients when compared with controls ($p < 0.0006$) and with PD patients ($p < 0.05$).

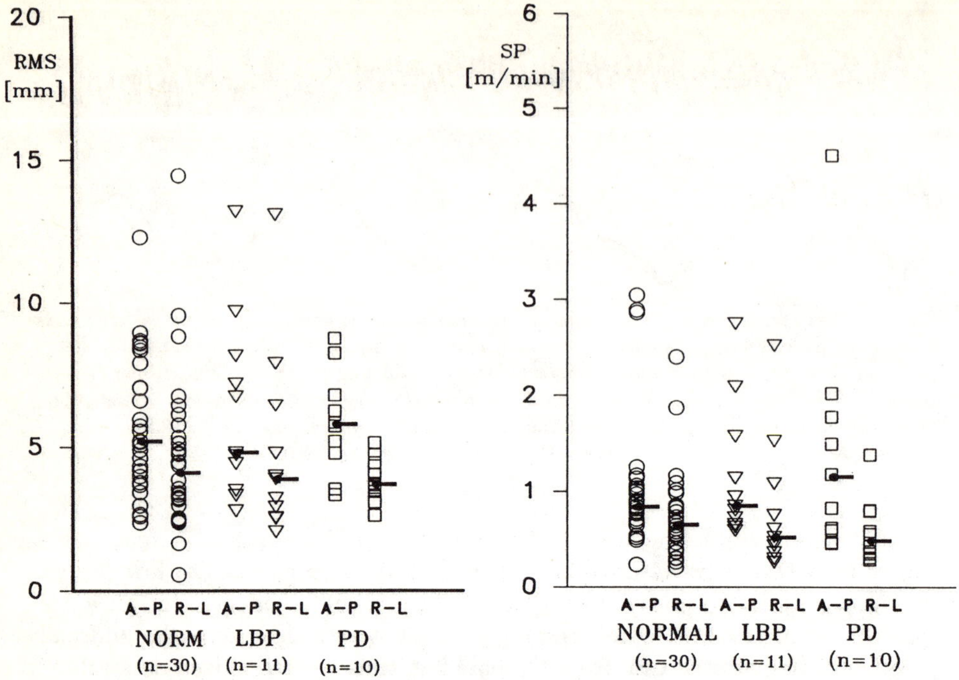

Fig. 2. Anterior–posterior (*A-P*) and lateral (*R-L*) root mean square (*RMS*; *left*) and sway path (*SP*; *right*) values of normals, lower body parkinsonism (*LBP*), and Parkinson's disease (*PD*) patients standing with eyes closed on firm foot support. Medians of RMS and SP values of normals, LBP, and PD patients showed no significant difference ($p > 0.05$, Mann-Whitney test), although SP A-P of PD patients is increased due to one patient presenting with parkinsonian tremor during the trial (A-P SP value, 4.5 m/min). RMS values do not reflect the patient's tremor during the trial

Six of 11 LBP patients were not able to perform the 25-s trial standing and fell. This was the only condition in which PD patients performed significantly worse, with increased RMSx and y values than normals ($p < 0.05$). Lateral and vector SP values were within normal range of controls, and only A-P SP was significantly increased in LBP patients compared with controls ($p < 0.05$). Thus, we conclude that only with provocative methods does posturography turn out to be a sensitive tool for differentiation of parkinsonian syndromes.

Discussion

Posturography is one of the best standardized methods for quantifying ataxia. Calculation of the CFP unequivocally reflects the center of gravity in each subject. The methods of further calculation, however, differ. One possible way is to calculate SP. As a rule of thumb, mean SP values will be approximately 1 m/min in normals when standing with eyes closed on firm foot support. Two independent studies have confirmed this value [5,10]. A different approach is the calculation of RMS values. As demonstrated in Fig. 1, RMS does not simply reflect SP, but rather supplies different information on large, slow body shifts. Both sets of information together may differentiate between parkinsonian patients with and without tremor. Thus, if information on the slow body shifts in parkinsonian patients is required irrespectively of superimposed tremor, measuring RMS values is the appropriate method. If the tremor component is of particular interest, SP will be the better choice.

On posturographic evaluation during stance with eyes open and eyes closed on firm foot support, body sway of PD and LBP patients stayed within the range of normals and all patients maintained balance when standing with eyes closed on firm foot support. These results were obtained in all static methods measuring lateral and A-P SP as well as RMSx and y values. In our investigation, neither PD nor LBP patients could be differentiated from normals when standing with eyes open and eyes closed on the Kistler platform, regardless of the methods applied. This is very well compatible with the normal clinical Romberg test in these patients.

With the reduction of somatosensory information caused by placing the patients on a slab of foam, LBP patients were not able to compensate this artificial instability with visual or vestibular information and presented with significantly higher RMS values than controls and PD patients; two patients lost balance completely. With a lack of visual information, this difference between LBP and PD patients markedly increased, and six of 11 LBP patients could not maintain their balance. Our findings, as well as previous reports [1,3,6,9], show essentially normal static posturographic behavior in PD patients. Particularly patients in early stages of PD maintain stance like normals with no specific SP [1,2,9]. The mechanism of visual stabilization and the reason for its importance for PD patients is still unclear. Bronstein and coworkers [1] supposed that vision also predominates when visual input conflicts with other sensory cues. In their investigations, PD patients were abnormally unstable when the room moved. Thus, provocative methods such as an unstable foot support are an additional requirement for obtaining good quantitation results in PD patients.

In our investigation, static posturographic methods were applied for etiologically different groups of parkinsonian patients. RMS measurements seemed to be more appropriate than SP values in the differentiation of parkinsonian syndromes, because high frequencies of tremor artifacts influence SP values more than RMS values.

Acknowledgment. This work was supported by the BMFT "M. Parkinson und andere Basalganglienerkrankungen."

References

1. Bronstein AM, Hood JD, Gresty MA, Panagi C (1990) Visual control of balance in cerebellar and parkinsonian syndromes. Brain 113:767–779

2. Dichgans J, Diener HC, Müller A (1985) Characteristics of increased postural sway and abnormal long loop responses in patients with cerebellar disease and parkinsonism. In: Struppler A, Weindl A (eds) Electromyography and evoked potentials: theories and applications. Springer, Berlin Heidelberg New York, pp 68–74
3. Dick JPR, Rothwell JC, Berardelli A, Thompson PD, Gioux M, Benecke R, Day BL, Marsden CD (1986) Associated postural adjustments in Parkinson's disease. J Neurol Neurosurg Psychiatry 49:1378–1385
4. FitzGerald PM, Jankovic J (1989) Lower body parkinsonism: evidence for vascular etiology. Mov Disord 4:249–260
5. Hufschmidt A, Dichgans J, Mauritz KH, Hufschmidt M (1980) Some methods and parameters of body sway quantification and their neurological application. Arch Psychiatr Nervenkr 228:135–150
6. Martin JP (1967) The basal ganglia and posture. Pitman Medical, London
7. Nutt JG, Nashner LM, Horak FB (1983) Why do parkinsonian patients fall? Ann Neurol 14:136
8. Paulus W, Straube A, Krafczyk S, Brandt T (1989) Differential effects of retinal target displacement, changing size and changing disparity in the control of anterior/posterior and lateral body sway. Exp Brain Res 78:243–252
9. Schieppati M, Nardone A (1991) Free and supported stance in Parkinson's disease. Brain 114:1227–1244
10. Straube A, Bötzel K, Hawken M, Paulus W, Brandt T (1988) Postural control in the elderly: differential effects of visual, vestibular and somatosensory input. In: Amblard B, Berthoz A, Clarc F (eds) Posture and gait: development, adaptation and modulation. Elsevier, Amsterdam, pp 105–114
11. Traub MM, Rothwell JC, Marsden CD (1980) Anticipatory postural reflexes in Parkinson's disease and other akinetic-rigid syndromes and in cerebellar ataxia. Brain 103:393–412

Discussion

Dr. Allum: Are you saying that the result that Diener had with parkinsonian patients, where he showed an increase in the soleus response to toes-up rotation in those patients between 80 and 120 ms after platform rotation, that you haven't observed the same result?

Dr. Paulus: We saw a tendency, but we did not even reach statistical significance. For us, this was quite a disappointing result.

Dr. Rabey: When you tried to differentiate between idiopathic Parkinson's disease and lower body PD I found that some features that you considered classical for lower body PD are still shared by the patients with idiopathic PD, for example freezing episodes or starting hesitation. My question is this: if you take the group of idiopathic PD, in which some show these features when they don't have any change in the CT or MRI, what happens when you apply your methodology to idiopathic PD with and without those features?

Dr. Paulus: Of course there is an overlap and you really have difficulties to differentiate on a clinical basis between these two groups. We even still have problems in separating the upper half of the patients. So we are not yet happy with the results we have so far. We are still looking for a more sensitive test.

Quantification of Dopaminomimetic Effects on Parkinsonian Symptoms Using Automatic and Voluntary Postural Responses

V. Panzer-Decius, L.M. Nashner, D.J. Beckley, and T.N. Chase

Introduction

Postural abnormalities associated with Parkinson's disease (PD) have been elegantly illustrated by Purdon-Martin [11]. While tremor, rigidity, and bradykinesia can be readily evaluated by the trained clinician, even semiquantitative assessments of the postural deficits associated with this disorder have proven more challenging. The appearance of postural instability is an important marker for progression in PD and symptoms associated with postural deficits are significant targets for pharmacological intervention. The development of appropriate quantitative measures to evaluate posture has thus become an important issue.

One approach to the assessment of postural mechanisms in PD has been to study quiet standing, Results from these studies have demonstrated changes in overall body position [12] and in the position and motion of individual body segments which could in a single patient statistically discriminate levodopa effects [8]. Observed changes appear to reflect modifications in the principal position of the center of gravity (COG). Nevertheless, quiet standing appears to represent an insufficient challenge for studies of postural instability in PD (see Hallett, Panzer and Zeffiro, this volume).

Various perturbations to quiet standing have also been employed to evaluate postural responses. Inappropriate postural response modulation has been postulated as a fundamental deficit, but results from perturbation studies have been controversial. Reactive scaling of postural responses to perturbation has been observed to be normal, whereas predictive responses were scaled inadequately [7]. Lower leg surface electromyographic (EMG) medium- and long-latency responses to postural perturbations were found to be enhanced and delayed (respectively) in PD [13]. After correction for background EMG, Beckley and colleagues [1] found that only patients with evident postural abnormalities (Hoehn and Yahr stage IV) exhibited EMG disturbances. Therefore, it is not clear whether the observed postural response abnormalities to perturbations are characteristic of the disease. Perhaps these abnormalities represent adaptation to the physiological changes of PD or nonspecific neurological deficits.

Significant abnormalities were demonstrated in early-stage PD patients performing a weight-shifting movement during a controlled tracking task [6]. Clinically, it is well known that while patients may be unable to perform a voluntary movement, an external sensory stimulus can enable the initiation of the movement. Perhaps the important distinction lies in the ability to perform predictive voluntary movements.

The goal of these studies was to identify posturographic methods which can be used to quantify symptoms associated with postural deficit. The measures must clearly differentiate between normal and PD and reflect pharmacological effects on the principal symptoms.

Methods

Ten PD patients (mean age, 61; SD, 7.1; range, 51–78) were tested 1.5–2 h after receiving their usual antiparkinsonian medication, and five of these were also tested after withdrawal of all dopaminomimetics for at least 12 h. Ten age-matched (mean age, 61; SD, 6.8; range, 52–79), neurologically intact volunteers served as normal controls.

Quiet standing was evaluated with a standard EquiTest procedure (NeuroCom International) including three 20-s trials in each of six different conditions (eyes open, eyes closed, sway-referenced vision, sway-referenced surface, eyes closed sway-referenced surface, and sway-referenced vision and surface). Postural responses to perturbation were assessed with forward and backward platform translations (series of three translations of small, medium, and large amplitude, representing a continuum from superthreshold to subsaturation stimulus) and toes-up and toes-down platform rotations (series of five in each direction of subsaturation magnitude). Voluntary postural movements were tested with a continuous weight-shifting task: patients made lateral (R-L) and anterior–posterior (A-P) movements at slow, medium, and fast speeds while standing on the force platform. The task and the patient's COG position were displayed on a computer monitor during each trial. One elderly patient (73 years old) did not participate in the voluntary weight-shifting task and his normal control was removed from the data set.

For each condition of quiet standing, equilibrium scores were calculated for all trials. Equilibrium scores are based on the maximum excursion of the COG expressed as a percentage of the height-adjusted theoretical limits of stability (LOS; 100 denotes complete stability and 0 means they have reached the limit or fallen). Equilibrium scores for each condition were averaged for three trials. Average latency of mechanical postural response was calculated for each set of three translations and was measured as the time from onset of force plate translation to initiation of mechanical response. An adaptation score based on the subject's ability to suppress the automatic postural response triggered by the platform rotation was assigned to each of five platform rotations. This score was calculated from integrated force or sway energy in each trial measured after the perturbation.

Movement time and movement amplitude were evaluated separately for voluntary weight-shifting movements. Slow, medium, and fast (3, 2, and 1 s) lateral weight shifts set at 50% of the patient's height-adjusted LOS were shown on the monitor. We measured the amplitude and the time to complete each individual weight-shifting movement (transition). A-P postural movement deficits were evaluated using the same protocol used to test lateral voluntary movements. Patients practiced until comfortable with each task and with each pace. Six complete, continuous transitions were recorded at each pace and the entire series was repeated three times for R-L and A-P movements. Movement time and distance were measured for each transition and results for each direction of movement R-L and A-P at each speed (3 ,2, and 1 s paces) were averaged across three trials.

Student's *t* tests were used to compare patients to normal controls. In addition, the results measured for patients who were tested off medication were compared to those obtained from the same patients on medication.

Results

During quiet standing, equilibrium scores of PD patients were not abnormal and performances were not significantly affected by medication (Table 1). Patients' responses to perturbation were not significantly different from normal or significantly affected by medication. Sway energy measurements after platform rotations did not indicate an abnormal response; however, these values did tend to increase with medication (Table 1). Elderly patients were characterized by age-related deficits observed during quiet standing when the platform was sway referenced and during platform rotations (Fig. 1). Postural response latency to forward and backward platform translations were not significantly delayed.

Significant differences between PD patients and normal subjects were observed for movement amplitude during voluntary weight-shifting movements for R-L transitions at all speeds (Fig. 2) and A-P transitions at medium and fast speeds (A-P 2 s and A-P 1 s; Table 2). Patients were able to match the prescribed movement time, and these values were not significantly different from normal (Table 2). No significant differences were observed in patients tested both on and off dopaminomimetics. However, medication appeared to increase the movement amplitude for A-P medium and fast movements (A-P 2 s and A-P 1 s; Table 2), and when medicated, patients movement times more nearly approximated the prescribed task (Table 2).

Discussion

We chose to evaluate all of the clinical assessment protocols available, including quiet and perturbed standing and predictive voluntary postural movements. Since postural abnormalities associated with age are often confounded with those

Table 1. Mean values ± SD for quiet and perturbed standing

	Normal[d]	Patients[e]	Patients off medication[f]	Patients on medication[g]
Equilibrium[a]				
Eyes open	93 ± 1.9	93 ± 3.4	95 ± 1.9	94 ± 1.8
Eyes closed	90 ± 4.7	89 ± 9.8	92 ± 2.3	92 ± 2.9
Sway-referenced vision	90 ± 4.4	89 ± 6.7	91 ± 2.5	91 ± 3.4
Sway-referenced surface	84 ± 6.1	79 ± 14.5	82 ± 7.7	76 ± 15.6
Eyes closed and sway-referenced surface	67 ± 13.3	70 ± 12.8	66 ± 10.6	69 ± 12.2
Sway-referenced surface and vision	63 ± 12.2	74 ± 14.1	72 ± 10.5	70 ± 15.3
Latency (ms)[b]				
Backward small	149 ± 19.4	146 ± 16.2	149 ± 18.1	141 ± 14.6
Backward medium	131 ± 10.5	146 ± 22.8	130 ± 12.0	131 ± 11.3
Backward large	130 ± 7.7	148 ± 27.7	133 ± 7.6	147 ± 36.8
Forward small	159 ± 11.4	158 ± 17.4	160 ± 16.0	151 ± 12.5
Forward medium	148 ± 10.7	156 ± 20.6	140 ± 10.7	151 ± 18.9
Forward large	136 ± 10.5	143 ± 16.8	134 ± 9.2	139 ± 16.4
Adaptation[c]				
Toes up 1	66 ± 22.3	45 ± 15.7	39 ± 10.5	51 ± 18.1
Toes up 2	56 ± 18.8	48 ± 11.2	48 ± 23.5	53 ± 14.4
Toes up 3	52 ± 16.6	43 ± 22.9	42 ± 10.7	53 ± 32.3
Toes up 4	49 ± 16.0	39 ± 11.1	37 ± 6.8	44 ± 14.7
Toes up 5	50 ± 14.8	41 ± 14.7	38 ± 5.3	47 ± 19.2
Toes down 1	77 ± 36.3	48 ± 19.8	46 ± 14.0	53 ± 22.8
Toes down 2	53 ± 19.2	46 ± 18.4	39 ± 9.5	49 ± 29.4
Toes down 3	42 ± 14.8	38 ± 14.0	37 ± 9.0	42 ± 21.8
Toes down 4	36 ± 9.0	33 ± 9.0	40 ± 13.2	34 ± 14.1
Toes down 5	39 ± 8.3	36 ± 14.2	35 ± 9.3	43 ± 19.3

[a] Scores given are for three trial averages in each of six conditions of quiet standing. (Eyes open, eyes closed, sway-referenced vision, sway-referenced surface, sway-referenced surface and eyes closed, and sway-referenced surface and vision). A score of 100 represents perfect stability and 0 represents a fall. See text for further explanation.
[b] Scores are in ms for three trial averages of mechanical postural response to small, medium, or large platform translations. Forward and backward platform movements results are presented after averaging latencies across legs.
[c] Scores for each of five trials of toes-up or toes-down platform rotations are given individually. Scores represent the amount of sway energy generated after a perturbation. See text for further explanation.
[d] Ten age-matched, normal control subjects.
[e] Ten patients, 1.5–2 h after usual medication.
[f] Five patients off medication for at least 12 h.
[g] Five patients, 1.5–2 h after usual medication.

of PD [9], we controlled for this problem by comparing PD patients with age-matched normal controls. Our goal was to identify parameters specific to PD and responsive to pharmacological treatment. Postural responses to quiet and perturbed standing were not abnormal in PD patients and did not respond to dopaminomimetics.

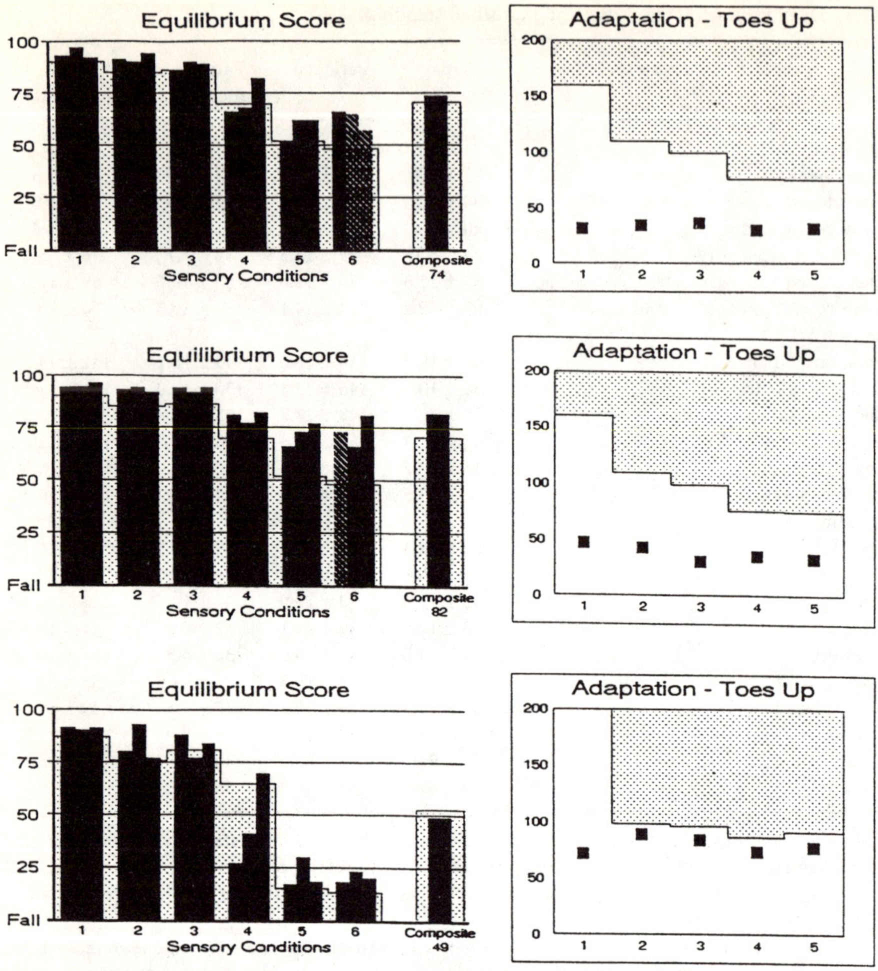

Fig. 1. Quiet and perturbed standing in a 51-year-old patient off (*top*) and on medication (*middle*) and in a 78-year-old patient off medication (*bottom*). Equilibrium scores are *solid bars* on the *left*; scores for three trials for each of six conditions of quiet standing are shown (*1*, eyes open; *2*, eyes closed; *3*, sway-referenced vision; *4*, sway-referenced surface; *5*, eyes closed, sway-referenced surface; *6*, sway-referenced surface and vision). *Striped bars* are trials that were repeated and *bars falling within the dotted background area* represent scores below that of an age-matched normal population. Note the scores for the elderly patient in condition 4, which are abnormal initially and subsequently improve, reaching normal values on the third trial. On the *right* side of the figure, adaptation scores (sway energy) are shown for each of five consecutive toes-up platform perturbations. While no score falls within the age-matched abnormal range (*dotted background area*), the elderly patient has elevated scores that are close to the normal limit

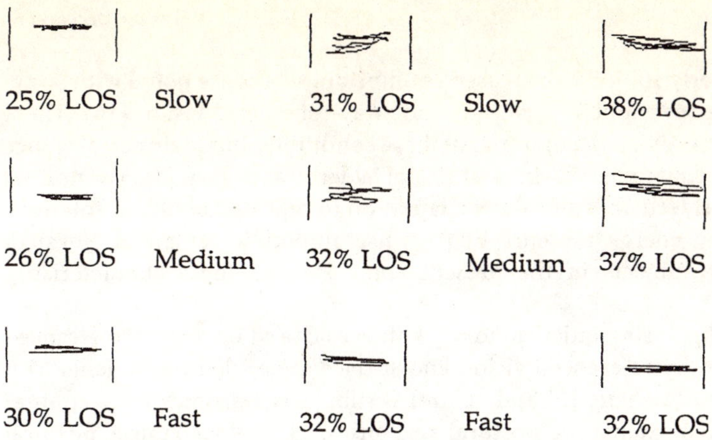

Fig. 2. Lateral (R-L) weight-shifting movements in a 51-year-old patient off (*left*) and on (*middle*) medication and an age-matched (56-year-old) normal volunteer (*right*). The traces shown represent the path of the center of gravity (COG) as the task was performed at slow, medium, and fast speeds (*top to bottom*, R-L 3 s, R-L 2 s, and R-L 1 s). The three individual paths at each speed were averaged to obtain a representative movement amplitude value for each trial. Vertical lines represent 50% of the subjects height-adjusted limits of stability (*LOS*) and numbers shown below each trial represent the average movement amplitude. Note the patient's improvement when medicated and the difference in movement amplitude between the patient and the normal subject

Table 2. Mean values ± SD for voluntary weight shifting

	Normal[c]	Patients[d]	Patients off medication[e]	Patients on medication[f]
Movement amplitude[a]				
A-P 1 s	37 ± 12.8	26 ± 7.6	25 ± 8.3	42 ± 28.4
A-P 2 s	44 ± 13.7	28 ± 11.1	26 ± 6.8	38 ± 17.7
A-P 3 s	39 ± 15.3	30 ± 7.6	32 ± 9.7	30 ± 9.9
R-L 1 s	37 ± 8.1	26 ± 12.2	27 ± 11.3	26 ± 9.8
R-L 2 s	41 ± 8.3	30 ± 7.7	28 ± 4.7	32 ± 5.7
R-L 3 s	36 ± 6.4	29 ± 6.2	28 ± 5.1	30 ± 5.3
Movement time (s)[b]				
A-P 1 s	0.99 ± 0.08	0.96 ± 0.08	0.99 ± 0.10	0.99 ± 0.05
A-P 2 s	1.92 ± 0.12	1.98 ± 0.07	1.83 ± 0.20	1.94 ± 0.11
A-P 3 s	2.91 ± 0.10	2.82 ± 0.16	2.66 ± 0.12	2.95 ± 0.14
R-L 1 s	1.03 ± 0.11	1.05 ± 0.25	1.20 ± 0.43	1.01 ± 0.07
R-L 2 s	2.02 ± 0.09	2.01 ± 0.16	1.96 ± 0.05	1.99 ± 0.13
R-L 3 s	3.00 ± 0.08	2.91 ± 0.22	3.15 ± 0.31	3.00 ± 0.11

[a] Given as percentages of the individuals height-adjusted limits of stability (LOS). Values are averages of three paths and three trials for lateral (R-L) or anterior–posterior (A-P) fast (1 s), medium (2 s), or slow (3 s) voluntary weight-shifting movements. Significant comparisons ($p < 0.05$) between patients and normal controls for Student's *t* tests.
[b] Values are averages of three paths and three trials for R-L or A-P 1-s, 2-s, or 3-s voluntary weight-shifting movements.
[c] Nine age-matched, normal control subjects.
[d] Nine patients, 1.5–2 h after usual medication.
[e] Five patients off medication for at least 12 h.
[f] Five patients, 1.5–2 h after their usual medication.

In normal elderly subjects, decreased equilibrium scores are noted with sway-referenced surface (eyes open or closed) and sway-referenced vision [16]. These subjects did poorly only on the first trial of these conditions, but their performance improved in subsequent trials. In a study of elderly and very elderly normal subjects, the very elderly failed to show adaptation to repeated platform rotations [10], and the sway energy measure of response amplitude remained elevated. Individual elderly subjects in the present study showed these characteristics (Fig. 1).

Specific deficits during quiet standing with eyes closed on a sway-referenced surface and with sway-referenced vision and surface are evident in patients with peripheral vestibular deficits [3] and central vestibular syndromes (in combination with prolonged latency of postural responses; [15]). Mechanical postural response latencies reflect the long-latency EMG response. Patients with central or peripheral pathway lesions such as peripheral neuropathy, multiple sclerosis [5], cerebellar lesions [4], and Huntington's disease [14] are characterized by a generalized increase in sway in all conditions (decreased equilibrium score), in combination with prolonged postural response latencies. Reports of latency response abnormalities in PD have been controversial and are not substantiated in this study.

Whereas measures of quiet standing and of postural responses to perturbation have characteristic patterns in many other patient populations, patients with PD could not be distinguished from an age-matched, normal control group. For patients with PD, these protocols lack the specificity required to be useful as a metric for clinical evaluation and intervention. Apparently, the traditional means of evaluating postural deficit must be expanded to include voluntary postural movements to achieve these goals. It seems clear that the volitional component of movement is fundamental to the parkinsonian deficit.

Predictive voluntary weight-shifting movements are clearly abnormal in PD. We observed an increase in movement amplitude with dopa replacement therapy, but in this small sample of patients, the increase was not significant (Fig. 2). Recently, Beckley and colleagues [2] studied voluntary weight-shifting and automatic postural response latencies in ten patients off dopaminomimetics for at least 12 h and approximately 1 h after their usual dosage and compared them to ten normal control subjects. Their results replicated and extended those reported here. Postural response latencies were not abnormal and did not respond to dopa replacement. Movement amplitude was significantly reduced in PD patients, while movement time was normal. In their sample of ten patients tested on and off medication, movement amplitude significantly improved with dopa replacement, but remained significantly less than that measured in normal subjects. Improvement in these measures were correlated with improvement in Unified Parkinson's Disease Rating Scale (UPDRS) motor subscale ratings for these patients. Increases in A-P movement amplitude were significantly related to ratings of postural instability (retropulsion), while improvement in R-L weight-shifting performance corresponded to changes in ratings of bradykinesia and rigidity, particularly on the patient's dominant side.

In summary, externally paced voluntary movements appear to be the best means of differentiating PD patients from the normal healthy elderly and appear to provide a useful metric for pharmacological intervention. These tests were well tolerated, even in patients with advanced disease. In addition, these test protocols have the advantages of ease of administration, standardization, and commercial availability. Further testing will be needed to resolve their ability to detect PD in the preclinical stages and to monitor disease progression.

Acknowledgment. The authors gratefully acknowledge the technical assistance of Cheryl Manley in making this work possible.

References

1. Beckley DJ, Bloem BR, van Dijk JG, Roos RAC, Remler MP (1991) Electrophysiological correlates of postural instability in Parkinson's disease. EEG Clin Neurophysiol 81:263–268
2. Beckley DJ, Panzer VP, Remler MP, Ilog L (1995) Impairment of paced voluntary postural task in Parkinson's disease (submitted)
3. Black FO, Shupert CL, Horak FB, Nashner LM (1988) Abnormal postural control associated with peripheral vestibular disorders. In: Pompeiano O, Allum JHJ (eds) Progress in brain research, vol 76. Elsevier Science, New York, pp 263–276
4. Dichgans J, Diener HC (1985) Characteristics of increased postural sway and abnormal long loop responses in patients with cerebellar diseases and parkinsonism. In: Struppler A, Weindl A (eds) Electromyography and evoked potentials: theories and applications. Springer, Berlin Heidelberg New York, pp 68–74
5. Diener HC, Dichgans J, Hulser PJ, Buettner UW, Bacher M, Guschlbauer B (1984) The significance of delayed long-loop responses to ankle displacement for the diagnosis of multiple sclerosis. EEG Clin Neurophysiol 57:336–342
6. Krasilovsky G, Gianutsos J (1991) Effect of video feedback on the performance of a weight shifting controlled tracking task in subjects with parkinsonism and neurologically intact individuals. Exp Neurol 113:192–201
7. Nutt J, Horak F, Frank J (1992) Scaling of postural responses in Parkinson's disease. In: Woollacott M, Horak F (eds) Posture and gait: control mechanisms, vol 2. University of Oregon Books, Eugene, pp 4–7
8. Panzer VP, Hallett M (1990) Biomechanical assessment of upright stance in Parkinson's disease: a single-subject study. Clin Biomech 5:73–80
9. Panzer VP, Zeffiro TA, Hallett M (1990) Kinematics of standing posture associated with aging and Parkinson's disease. In: Brandt T, Paulus W, Bles W, Dieterich M, Krafczyk S, Straube A (eds) Disorders of posture and gait 1990. Thieme, Stuttgart, pp 390–393
10. Panzer VP, Kaye J, Edner A, Holme L (1992) Standing postural control in the elderly and very elderly. In: Woollacott M, Horak F (eds) Posture and gait: control mechanisms, vol 2. University of Oregon Books, Eugene, pp 220–223
11. Purdon-Martin J (1967) The basal ganglia and posture. Pittman Medical, London
12. Schieppati M, Nardone A (1991) Free and supported stance in Parkinson's disease. Brain 114:1227–1244
13. Scholz E, Diener HC, Noth J, Friedemann H, Dichgans J, Bacher M (1987) Medium- and long-latency EMG responses in leg muscles: Parkinson's disease. J Neurol Neurosurg Psychiatry 50:66–70
14. Tian J, Herdman SJ, Zee DS, Folstein SE (1992) Postural stability in patients with Huntington's disease. Neurology 42:1232–1238

15. Voorhies RL (1990) Dynamic posturography findings in central nervous system disorders. Otolaryngol Head Neck Surg 103:96–101
16. Wolfson L, Whipple R, Derby C, Amerman P, Murphy T, Tobin JN, Nashner LM (1992) A dynamic posturography study of balance in healthy elderly. Neurology 42:2069–2075

Discussion

Dr. Fahn: In this translational test, I assume that the platform is going backwards, is that what you explained?

Dr. Panzer: Backwards and forwards, sometimes either.

Dr. Fahn: If you just go backwards, there is a slight pulling of the patient forwards instead of backwards.

Dr. Panzer: We also tested with the platform going forwards, and the very surprising thing was that their responses were within normal limits, which suggests that when perturbed by an external stimulus, patients respond.

Dr. Fahn: But the center of gravity isn't really shifted when you do that. When you pull somebody, you're moving the center of gravity backwards.

Dr. Panzer: It is moved significantly in a large translation. I think what happens is there's a voluntary component to the push test that we aren't aware of. When a patient hears a loud sound or sees the stripes on the ground, they can walk, but when they have to walk themselves they often have difficulty. I think the lesson I'd take from this series of studies is that it is really the voluntary component or volitional component that's most effective in these patients. We examined a wide range of patients, and they were all significantly abnormal in their ability to move when they were making the movements, but in a very severely affected, 83-year-old stage IV patient on the platform off medication, the latencies to translation when perturbed were normal. It is very surprising. We were quite shocked when we first did the study. That's what led us to start looking more closely at the volitional components.

Dr. Paulus: I could not show all the data we have, but we also asked the patients to move forward and backward as fast and as far as they could without falling. The Parkinson's disease patients, the idiopathic ones, behaved like the normal subjects. Only the symptomatic lower body patients had a reduced sway of about 20%, they went down to 80%. We didn't find a difference between the idiopathic and the normals in that condition.

Dr. Panzer: When you asked them to make weight shifts forward and backward, were they confused?

Dr. Paulus: The idiopathic Parkinson's disease patients were essentially normal. Only the symptomatic lower body patients had a reduction to about 80% of the amplitude range with an equal frequency.

Dr. Panzer: Did you normalize for the patient's body height in some way?

Dr. Paulus: No, we didn't normalize that. We just compared the 30 normals with the ten and 11 other patients.

Dr. Allum: If I understood it correctly, the parkinsonian patients or the older patients don't have a large initial response and that's the reason why they don't adapt?

Dr. Panzer: They don't need to. It's a flat curve, and they don't have a heightened initial response. It's basically low and flat, which is why I said it is not at all specific for Parkinson's disease.

Posturography in Parkinson's Disease Patients on and off Medication

F. Müller, J. Dichgans, and G.E. Stelmach

Introduction

Problems of postural control in Parkinson's disease (PD) have been considered an essential part of the syndrome since its discoverer's early description of the illness. Patients exhibit a stooped posture with kyphosis and bent knees and arms. This abnormal postural attitude has to be differentiated from insufficient postural stabilization in response to destabilizing body displacements (i.e., when pushed), the tendency to fall from propulsion during initiation of movement or locomotion (kinetic imbalance), and finally the spontaneous loss of balance while standing (static imbalance). Despite modern dopaminergic treatment, unstable posture that results in falling has remained an important medical problem in PD.

In a survey on 100 patients, Koller et al. [11] estimated that 38% of them suffered from falls. While falling was not related to sensory loss, dementia, or other medical conditions, falls correlated with duration of the disease, postural instability, bradykinesia, and rigidity. Surprisingly, frequency of falling correlated only with the severity of postural instability as rated by the clinician. Reliable methods to measure postural instability are thus desirable to identify patients prone to falls and to measure the benefit of possible treatment.

Dynamic Posturography

Dynamic posturography perturbates quiet stance by sudden tilts of a platform to elicit postural reflexes in leg muscles. These are recorded by means of skin electrodes from above the triceps surae (TS) and anterior tibial (TA) muscle. Short (SL)-, medium (ML)-, and long-latency (LL) responses are normal in patients suffering from PD. However, the integrals of ML responses in the stretched TS after a sudden toe-up tilt of the platform have been shown to be significantly increased in PD patients [6,14], when high velocity stimuli (4° at 50°/sec) are applied. Since the reflex activity in TS adds to the backward body movement induced by the perturbation, the increased ML response in PD functionally destabilizes posture. The stabilizing LL responses of TA, however, are normal. LL reflexes are important for stabilization of posture in normals, since they pull the body forward after toe-up tilt of the platform. Modulation of postural reflexes as dependent on functional requirements in normals is significantly impaired in PD patients. This is exemplified by the inability to suppress the ML and LL responses in situations where they are functionally inadequate, e.g., while sitting [7] or standing with support [13].

Static Posturography

Static posturography measures sway behavior when subjects are quietly standing upright on a stable force platform. This method of assessing postural stability has not shown specific impairments - except for tremor - in PD patients [4,5,13]; however, patients were generally tested while on medication.

Effects of Medication

The goal of the present study was to evaluate postural sway in PD patients who are off medication and to compare the results with observed changes after dopaminergic medication has been given. Since visual, vestibular, and somatosensory information have been shown to contribute to control of posture, patients were tested with their eyes open or closed, standing either on a stable support surface or on a layer of thick foam. The latter method minimizes the accuracy of somatosensory feedback both in terms of amplitude and frequency content.

Methods

Subjects

Six patients with idiopathic PD rated to be in stages II and III according to Hoehn and Yahr [8] were tested after their drug treatment had been withdrawn for at least 1 week. When this test session had been completed, patients were given one Sinemet pill (250 mg; levodopa and carbidopa) and the test was repeated 1 hour later. A group of 18 elderly, neurologically normal, adults served as controls.

Apparatus and Procedure

A force platform (AMTI model OR6-5-1) with four load cells was used to measure force and moment components along the x, y, and z axes. Sway behavior in anteroposterior and lateral dimensions was computed and analyzed separately. The experiment consisted of four different conditions: (1) standing on force plate surface with normal vision; (2) standing on force plate surface with eyes closed; (3)

standing on altered surface (a 5-cm layer of foam) with eyes open; and (4) standing on altered surface with eyes closed. For each condition, after an initial adaptation period, subjects were asked to stand with bare feet together without movement on the platform. Signals from the platform were amplified and digitized with a sampling rate of 40 Hz during 160 s in eight distinct periods for each condition. Repeated measure analysis of variance (ANOVA), *t* tests, and Wilcoxon matched pairs signed rank tests were used for statistical comparisons.

Results

In general, patients had no more problems standing on the platform than elderly healthy controls, even when visual and somatosensory information were removed. A typical sway path of a 20-s period is given in Fig. 1 for a PD subject under the four

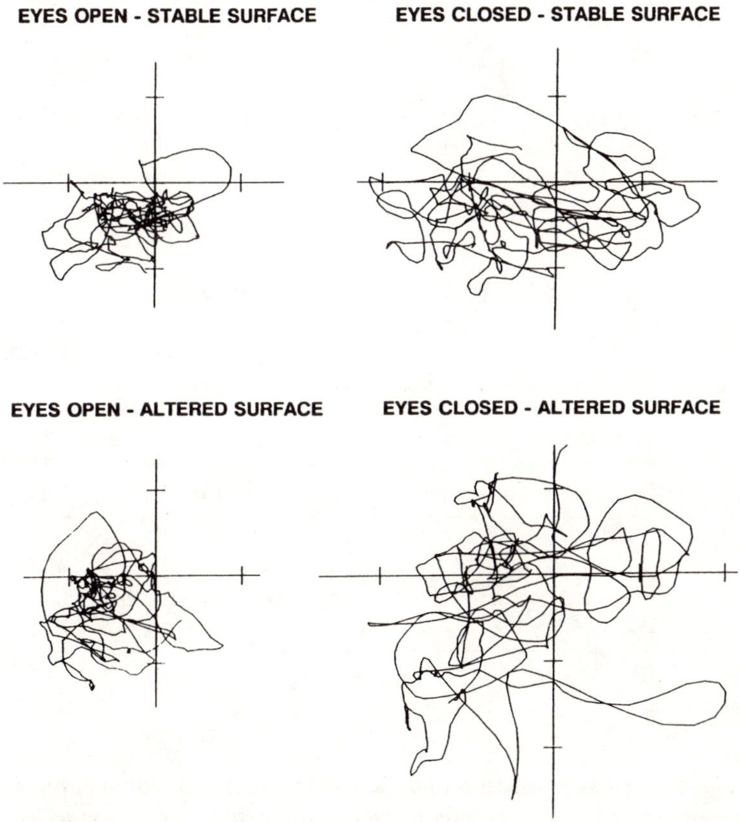

a

Fig. 1a,b. Original recordings of sway path of a patient off (**a**) and on (**b**) medication for each of the four experimental conditions

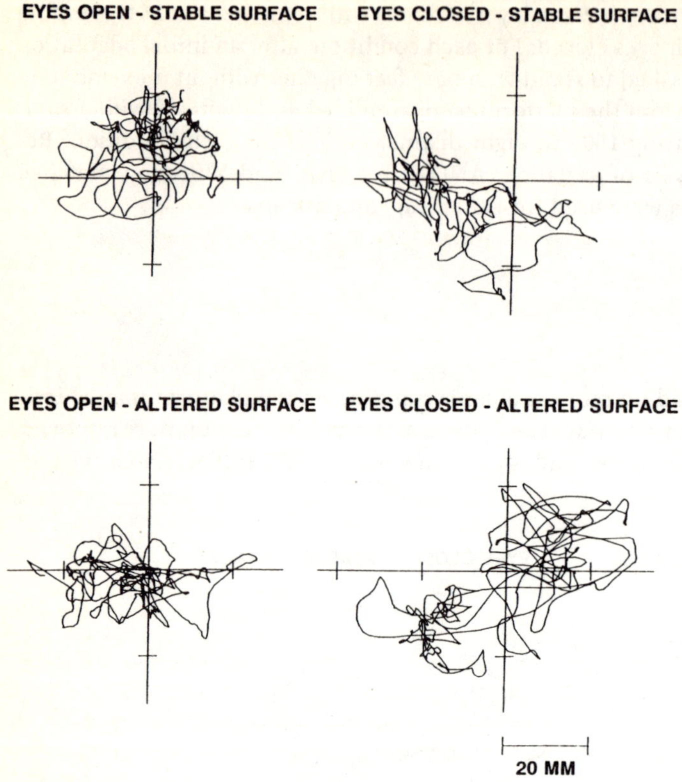

b

Fig. 1b

Table 1. Group means of sway range in the mediolateral (Lat) and anteroposterior (A-P) dimensions and of total sway path for controls and Parkinson's disease patients off and on medication

Conditions	Control			Patient off medication			Patient on medication		
	Lat	A-P	Total	Lat	A-P	Total	Lat	A-P	Total
Vision, normal surface	18.9	16.0	14.3	23.9	20.8	24.6	25.0	21.4	17.6
No vision, normal surface	30.4	26.2	28.2	41.1*	32.4	37.2	30.4**	25.8	23.6**
Vision, altered surface	22.0	21.3	17.6	29.4	26.1	29.6	29.6	26.4	24.8
No vision, altered surface	45.8	38.5	39.8	44.1	41.0	45.0	41.7	41.7	37.6

* $p < 0.05$ for group differences.
** $p < 0.05$ for treatment effect.

different conditions, plotted as a function of on and off medication. For statistical analysis, several indices of sway behavior were calculated: sway range in anteroposterior plane and lateral plane and total sway path. Group mean data are given in Table 1.

Comparison of Group Data

Sway Range

Range of sway behavior gives an indication of how far the center of foot pressure (COP) deviates. Overall, range was not significantly different between patients off treatment and controls, while both groups exhibited a greater sway range along the mediolateral plane than along the anteroposterior plane ($p < 0.001$). Removal of vision affected both groups with a highly significant ($p < 0.001$) increase of 15 mm for all recordings when vision was reduced. The reduction of acuity of somatosensory feedback by alteration of the support surface had a similar, though less pronounced effect in both groups ($p < 0.001$). The removal of vision during stable support affected patients more than controls, which was predominantly caused by an increase in lateral sway range ($p < 0.05$). The combined alteration of vision and proprioceptive information did not cause an additional effect in patients (interaction effect, group by vision by surface condition $p < 0.01$).

Sway Path

Although group means of patients were increased for all conditions, the main effect of group did not reach statistical significance. Only the interaction effect group by vision showed a trend ($p < 0.08$) toward an increased sway path of patients with their eyes closed. While the alteration of visual and somatosensory input considerably increased the sway path ($p < 0.001$), there was no differential effect between patients and healthy controls.

Treatment Effects

Sway Range

Sway range in general was not altered by the administration of Sinemet. However, when patients were tested while off medication and with their eyes closed on a stable surface, an increased sway range in the lateral dimension was observed. After treatment, this increase was reduced in five out of six patients, leading to a mean reduction of 11.7 mm ($p < 0.06$).

Sway Path

After medication, sway path was reduced in five out of six patients in all conditions with eyes closed, i.e., regardless of the type of surface and in the condition with eyes open on a stable support only. Individuals with increased path values without medication showed a larger reduction after the administration of Sinemet. Sway

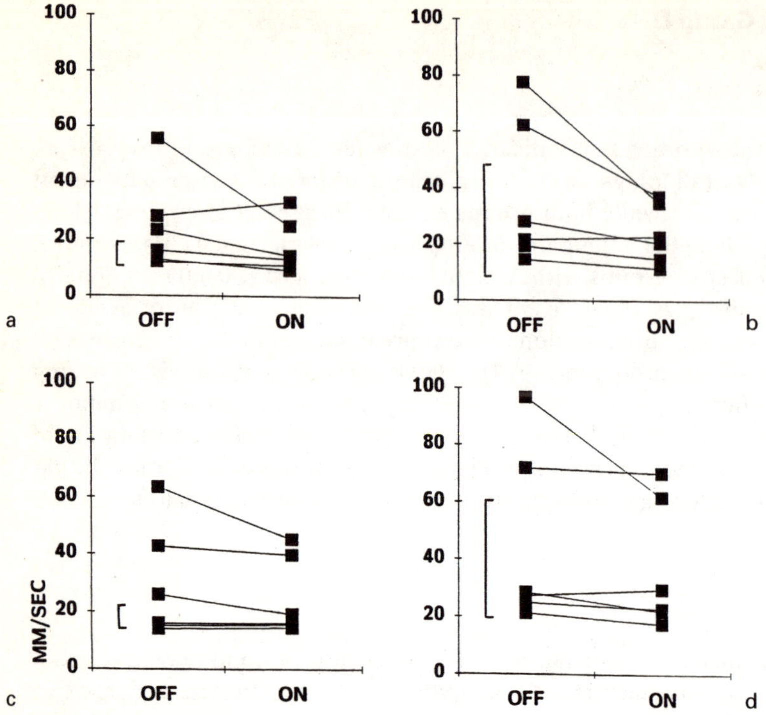

Fig. 2a–d. Mean measures of sway path of each patient ($n = 6$) off and on medication for each of four experimental conditions. **a** Eyes open, stable surface. **b** Eyes closed, stable surface. **c** Eyes open, altered surface. **d** Eyes closed, altered surface. Range (mean ± 1 SD) of control group is indicated by a *bracket*

path measures on and off medication for each individual are given in Fig. 2. The reduction of group means was statistically significant ($p < 0.05$) in the condition with altered vision on normal surface. There was also a statistical trend in the conditions with altered vision and altered surface and with normal vision and normal surface ($p < 0.06$).

Discussion

In general, sway behavior of mildly to moderately affected untreated patients did not show major differences when compared with healthy elderly controls, although there had been a drug wash-out period of more than 1 week. Increased mean values of sway path did not reach statistical significance, which is in accordance with previous studies [13]. In moderately to severely affected patients, a decreased sway range has even been reported [9].

In the present study, sway range measures showed a disproportionate increase when eyes were closed. This finding supports the idea of hyperactive "visuopostural loops" [4] in PD. Interestingly, the alteration of somatosensory information did not induce a comparable instability in patients as alteration of vision. When alterations of visual and somatosensory feedback are combined, balance control depends primarily on vestibular information. Our data do not confirm the postulation that in PD a loss of vestibular function contributes significantly to postural instability [12]. Static posturography did not show a major balance problem in untreated mildly to moderately affected patients. Thus, treatment effects cannot explain the lack of balance impairment found in previous studies using static posturography to test PD patients while on treatment. Rather, postural instability in Parkinson's disease seems to be less a problem of quiet stance, but a phenomenon caused by dynamic conditions such as the initiation of a movement, the movement itself, or need of response to unforeseen environmental obstacles.

In various motor tasks, a single dose of dopamine was able to improve behavioral deficiencies, as was shown, for example, in a complex locomotor task by Johnels et al. [10] and in parkinsonian walking by Blin et al. [2]. In our patients as well, a single dose of dopamine was able to reduce increased sway range and sway path in conditions when visual control was unavailable. Thus, balance control can be improved by dopaminergic treatment and is not exclusively dependent on nondopaminergic mechanisms, as was put forward by Bonnet et al. [3] because of insufficient treatment effects for postural problems in advanced parkinsonism.

In summary, sensitivity of static sway measures in PD is low. It cannot be improved by withdrawing dopaminergic medication, nor by use of an altered support surface to reduce proprioceptive feedback. Dynamic posturography to elicit postural reflexes has a greater potential to detect postural abnormalities in PD patients [7,9,13]. An association between abnormal modulation of postural reflexes and clinically rated balance impairment has recently been established in PD by Beckley et al. [1].

References

1. Beckley DJ, Bloem BR, van Dijk JG, Roos RA, Remler MP (1991) Electrophysiological correlates of postural instability in Parkinson's disease. Electroencephalogr Clin Neurophysiol 81:263–268
2. Blin O, Ferrandez AM, Pailhous J, Serratrice G (1991) Dopa-sensitive and dopa-resistant gait parameters in Parkinson's disease. J Neurol Sci 103:51–54
3. Bonnet AM, Loria Y, Saint-Hilaire MH, Lhermitte F (1987) Does long term aggravation of Parkinson's disease result from nondopaminergic lesions? Neurology 37:1539–1542
4. Bronstein AM, Hood JD, Gresty MA, Panagi C (1990) Visual control of balance in cerebellar and parkinsonian syndromes. Brain 113:767–779
5. Dichgans J, Diener HC, Müller A (1985) Characteristics of increased postural sway and abnormal long loop responses in patients with cerebellar diseases and parkinsonism. In: Struppler A, Weindl A (eds) Electromyography and evoked potentials. Springer, Berlin Heidelberg New York, pp 68–74
6. Diener HC, Dichgans J (1988) Anwendung und Nutzen der statischen und dynamischen Standmessung (Posturographie). Fortschr Neurol Psychiatr 56:249–258
7. Diener C, Scholz E, Guschlbauer B, Dichgans J (1987) Increased shortening reaction in Parkinson's disease reflects a difficulty in modulating long loop reflexes. Mov Disord 2:31–36

8. Hoehn MM, Yahr MD (1967) Parkinsonism: onset, progression, and mortality. Neurology 17:427–442
9. Horak FB, Nutt JG, Nashner LM (1992) Postural inflexibility in parkinsonian subjects. J Neurol Sci 111:46–58
10. Johnels B, Ingvarsson PE, Thorselius M, Valls M, Steg G (1989) Disability profiles and objective quantitative assessment in Parkinson's disease. Acta Neurol Scand 79:227–238
11. Koller WC, Glatt S, Vetere Overfield B, Hassanein R (1989) Falls and Parkinson's disease. Clin Neuropharmacol 12:98–105
12. McDowell FH, Reichert WH, Doolittle K (1981) Vestibular dysfunction in Parkinson's disease. Ann Neurol 10:94
13. Schieppati M, Nardone A (1991) Free and supported stance in Parkinson's disease. The effect of posture and "postural set" on leg muscle. Brain 114:1227–1244
14. Scholz E, Diener HC, Noth J, Friedemann H, Dichgans J, Bacher M (1987) Medium and long latency EMG responses in leg muscles: Parkinson's disease. J Neurol Neurosurg Psychiatry 50:66–70

Discussion

Dr. Paulus: I think it's time to write a paper entitled "Requiem for Dynamic Posturography in Parkinson's Disease." I quote Dr. Scholz, who stated 3 years ago in Bad Kissingen that "We now know that this method is not suited to differentiate between extrapyramidal diseases." Since I have made this personal experience and spent a lot of time on this method, I would like to discourage other people from using this method.

Dr. Müller: I think there are two people here who can comment on that. First of all, I certainly think before doing that we have to repeat some of the studies done comparing postural responses on and off treatment. From Tübingen we cannot report much on this topic. You might be able to answer a little bit more about that, since I understood you tested patients off medication. Most patients in Tübingen were tested on medication. A requiem is too early if there are doubts about whether the patient is really dead, and that's why I think Dr. Nardone is of importance in this auditorium.

Dr. Hallett: Perhaps we can ask Dr. Nardone to comment on this question.

Dr. Nardone: We have recently, for example, presented some important data showing that if you use slower velocities of perturbations, you can better differentiate normals from parkinsonian patients. It might not be the right time for requiems yet.

Dr. Müller: I think there are several more questions to be discussed on this topic, but that was not the main goal of my talk and I don't want to elaborate on that. I wasn't in Portland, but there's another paper by the Portland group in the volume of proceedings, again showing differences between Parkinson's disease patients on and off medication. They analyzed the torque measures that have already been proposed today.

Dr. Allum: I'd like to make a comment if I may about what Dr. Paulus said. The difference that the group of Diener observed was in the so-called medium latency response in the soleus. You did not observe a difference. I would suggest that perhaps one should use a perturbation which is going to enhance this response to such an amplitude that one would be able to measure statistical differences more easily. I don't think the rotation of the support surface is the best way to do that. It may be that for these particular patients, the translation which enhances the soleus response in normals compared to rotation might be a better way of testing the parkinsonian change in this response.

Dr. Panzer: Getting back to your work, which I think is a very interesting study, to what do you attribute patients' decreased ability to use proprioceptive information? Do you have an interpretation of this finding? It's very interesting.

Dr. Müller: We saw no reduction of sway measures by dopamine, but we also saw no difference between patients and controls when testing them with a reduced proprioception. The question is, why do we get no effect of dopamine under these testing conditions? So far we haven't done any studies to test that. It seems as if the proprioceptive information seems less used by Parkinson's disease patients.

Dr. Dobbs: We've been studying maintenance of balance, and the sessions mainly addressed the question of the sway itself and perturbation. There's also the question of the broadening of base. You can obviously compensate the sway by broadening your base, and I wondered whether your dyskinetic patients were doing that. We've actually measured foot separation during walking at free walking speed and we do find it is helpful in differentiating between normals and parkinsonians, and for treatment effect. Maybe one should be looking at this other aspect of the problem.

Dr. Hallett: Are you saying that in your Parkinson's disease patients, they had a broader base than normal while walking? Is that what your conclusion was?

Dr. Dobbs: No, they have a narrower base. On the other hand, patients who are dyskinetic have a broader base.

Dr. Hallett: In the studies that were done at the National Institutes of Health, the base was the same in the patients, I believe. They had a freely chosen posture of their feet and it was the same as normal in the cases that we looked at.

Dr. Dobbs: This was static position?

Dr. Hallett: In the static position with freely chosen foot posture, the normal subjects and the Parkinson's disease subjects chose the same base of support.

Dr. Panzer: Ours was during walking.

Dr. Noth: I think the conclusion that proprioceptive input is reduced with foam is not correct. What foam is doing is that the correcting movement is longer in amplitude before the proprioceptors are activated. So the whole time course of the correction is different with and without foam. At the end you have to reach the force to get your body over the center, so the proprioceptors have to be activated finally, but in a different time course.

Dr. Müller: I would fully agree that we get proprioceptive information in standing on foam as well, but I disagree that for small movements we really get the same amount of proprioceptive information. Have you ever stood on a thick piece of foam? I realized that I certainly had less control and less sense of my posture.

Dr. Noth: Yes, but there's another thing. Your movements are longer. So that's a very difficult subjective feeling. There's certainly a difference in your own opinion about force control or control of standing, but that doesn't tell you anything about the activation of the proprioceptors. And if you make a movement, the amplitude is larger, because it's no longer an isometric condition or a pseudoisometric condition, as you now activate your foot against another resistance.

Dr. Müller: This is certainly true. I would agree that this is not a pure variation or manipulation of the proprioceptive information coming into the system, but I even think that the response on foam or the response on a stable surface again gives us feedback coming from the proprioceptors and that is why earlier in this session it was pointed out that maybe no sway at all is not desirable because we want to get information; for that purpose, we basically need a little bit of sway to get information from the proprioceptors.

Dr. Hallett: Let me perhaps make a summary statement of this session. I think it is quite clear that patients with Parkinson's disease have a substantial problem with balance. They fall a great deal and it can be quantified to a certain extent clinically. However, it is clear from all the presentations that have been made that it is difficult to find an objective instrumental method for documenting that very well. We are all having a certain amount of difficulty. There are some minor successes, but there isn't anything obvious and easy right at the moment that will give this a very good quantification.

Tracking Measures of Movement

K.A. Flowers and M.R. Sheridan

Tracking devices are typically used to investigate voluntary movements of the upper limb, especially aiming movements. They are thus not directly concerned with reflexes, postural adjustments, involuntary movements, or whole-body movement synergies, but rather with the individually programmed or "fractionated" manipulative movements for which the primate hand and arm are specially adapted [15]. These involve "higher" brain circuits, i.e., those that link perceptual and/or cognitive systems to motor systems, whereby actions are related to plans and goals – the point where movement becomes behaviour. Tracking was one of the first techniques used to investigate the complex behaviour termed motor skill (or more appropriately perceptual motor skill) which accomplishes this. Its distinctive characteristics are that: (a) it involves a continuous adaptive interaction with the environment; (b) it requires an integration of perceptual, decision and motor processes; (c) it shows changes over time and with practice, i.e., learning.

Most tracking involves aiming at a target, sometimes directly (as in pointing tasks, e.g., pushing a bell), sometimes indirectly (such as moving a lever to control a cursor on an oscilloscope screen). Sometimes the target is only implicit, as in aiming in the dark or at a remembered target, but in this case it may be considered that the target is internal. Aiming implies spatial control, and most tracking tasks employ visual targets and cursors and measure spatial accuracy, but they can be used to measure non-spatial aspects of movement such as force generation where the hand itself does not move (Flowers and Sheridan, unpublished) or time to initiate movement [12].

In a typical tracking task (Fig. 1), subjects are presented with a visual display showing a target moving in one dimension (or possibly two) and a cursor whose movement is controlled by the subject using a manipulandum such as a lever. Originally the target moved continually (pursuit tracking) and the subjects' task was to make the cursor follow it as closely as they could, but more often nowadays the target moves in discrete jumps and the subject has to acquire it as quickly as possible whenever it moves (step tracking). The lever generates continuous voltage changes corresponding to its position in space. These can either be transformed (in real time or later from recordings) into moment-by-moment position data to portray the kinematics of the movement or used to derive other measures, such as lag (through cross-correlation) and error (through integration) or velocity and acceleration (through differentiation). Tracking thus offers a variety of quantita-

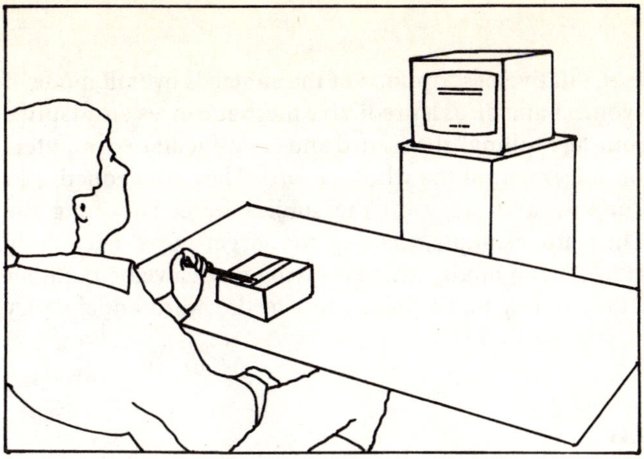

Fig. 1. A typical tracking test (see text for details)

tive measures which may be used to describe aspects of performance at several levels of analysis [10].

Tracking measures the overall performance of movements rather than their component muscular contractions, thus differing from physiological measures (although often closely related). They offer both quantitative and qualitative measures of performance which are not easily obtained by direct clinical observation and are not reducible to measures of muscular contraction. Their potential value to the clinician lies in their ability to delineate certain functional characteristics of the system as a whole and to allow inferences to be made about the component processes which underlie performance [4–7,11,13].

Measuring Performance in Tracking Tasks

Tracking studies may adopt either a deductive ("top-down") or an inductive ("bottom-up") approach. In the first kind of investigation, a model of the operator is postulated with appropriate measures of performance within the paradigm outlined, and any individual's performance judged accordingly. Early tracking studies, for example, were based on servo theory, and recent studies have adopted a programming theory or predictive control model; future studies may well apply a connectionist model. The crucial measures for comparison of subjects in this method are determined by the assumptions of the model; they may be direct measures, such as reaction time or error, or derived scores, such as frequency response or information-processing rate. Conversely, the inductive approach first measures various features of the subjects' output and then, from subject differences established simply by statistical comparison, derives higher-level functional measures and infers underlying mechanisms [14]. This means that tracking measures fall into three categories.

Paradigm Judgements

Paradigm judgements are qualitative descriptions of the subject's overall mode of performance, e.g., as a servomechanism, as a predictive mechanism, as an adaptive learner, etc. These arise from "eyeballing" the record and are difficult to computerise, as they are a matter of judgement of the whole record. They are deductive in nature and may in fact impose a strategy on the subject by constraining the conditions of the task. Thus, for example, making the target move irregularly forces subjects to perform in a servo mode, whereas giving them a velocity rather than a positional control device may make them use a feedforward anticipatory mode of control [1,2].

Parameter Measurements

Parameter (microscopic) measurements are quantitative measures of the kinematic features of the subjects' movement. They may be direct measures, such as reaction time to initiate discrete movements or amplitude and duration of movements, or they may be derived measures, such as velocity, acceleration, time to peak acceleration, etc. These allow direct comparison between subjects and groups and are theoretically neutral – any difference between scores could give rise to many interpretations at several levels of analysis. Thus, they offer the possibility of empirical quantitative comparisons between subjects which may be of clinical use and may give rise – through a process termed "reverse kinematics" [8] – to statistical measurements.

Statistical Measurements

Statistical (macroscopic) measurements are higher-level-derived measures of performance which describe or quantify hypothetical underlying mechanisms of movement generation and/or their functional parameters. They describe not individual features of movement, but general functional characteristics of the system, often based on combined or co-varying features of performance, e.g., error based on a combination of time and distance measures. Such scores may be inferred from parameter measures or measured directly, e.g., by integration. In pursuit tracking, such measures are mean lag/lead and frequency response [2,3,9]. In step tracking, such measures include mean error as a percentage of movement amplitude [4] or reaction time (RT) against index of difficulty [12].

A great advantage of these measures is that they often reflect functional efficiency better than lower level ones do, because they remain valid across a variety of changes in performance at different levels of the system. This is important in the assessment of complex skills because many factors can change at different levels during performance and we need to separate out changes and differences at the level of, say, the subjects' strategy from those at the level of movement execution, or vice versa. An example of this in relation to Parkinson's disease is shown in Fig. 2.

Figure 2 shows the records of two normal control subjects and two parkinsonian patients performing the step-tracking task of Fig. 1. The records show the tracks of ten movements from the standard starting position to a given target (two horizontal lines at the top of the screen between which the subject must halt the cursor). The striking thing about the control records is their consistency; clearly normal subjects produce very similar movements each time, even though other movements have intervened between each attempt. The parkinsonian records, however, show that patients with mild bradykinesia may show different kinds of abnormality. Patient A shows variability in timing of the movement, but ends up in the middle of the target each time, while patient B is relatively normal in the shape of the movement across time, but is wildly erratic in terms of endpoint accuracy.

Both these records are clearly abnormal, but if one measured only accuracy of movement, A would not appear so, while if one measured only movement duration, B would not. A derived macroscopic measure such as error plotted against duration of movement, however, would catch both these patients, especially if the variance of the error is shown, as neither patient could produce a curve of error across a range of movement durations similar to the normal control curve at all points. Where variability rather than overall trend is the crucial difference in performance, this would also be apparent, so that the graph would show not only the degree of abnormality for any subject, but also where and how changes in performance take place relative to the normal baseline.

Appropriateness of Tracking Measures for Clinical Use

We suggest, therefore, that measures of performance on skilled tasks such as tracking can provide a variety of data that may be of use in the investigation of motor disorders. So far such measures have not been used for clinical assessment, so the discussion must be limited to their potential usefulness. In assessing this, two questions need to be answered: (1) how good are they at measuring individual differences? and (2) what new information do they give?

Efficacy in Measuring Individual Differences

Up to now tracking studies (which have been mostly research investigations) have been used for group comparisons, with the results used to infer general changes or trends in performance which are supposedly typical of a given disorder compared to "normal" performance. For these purposes, only quantitative measurement and statistically significant differences are necessary. For clinical use, however, measures must be calibrated precisely enough to distinguish individual differences, so

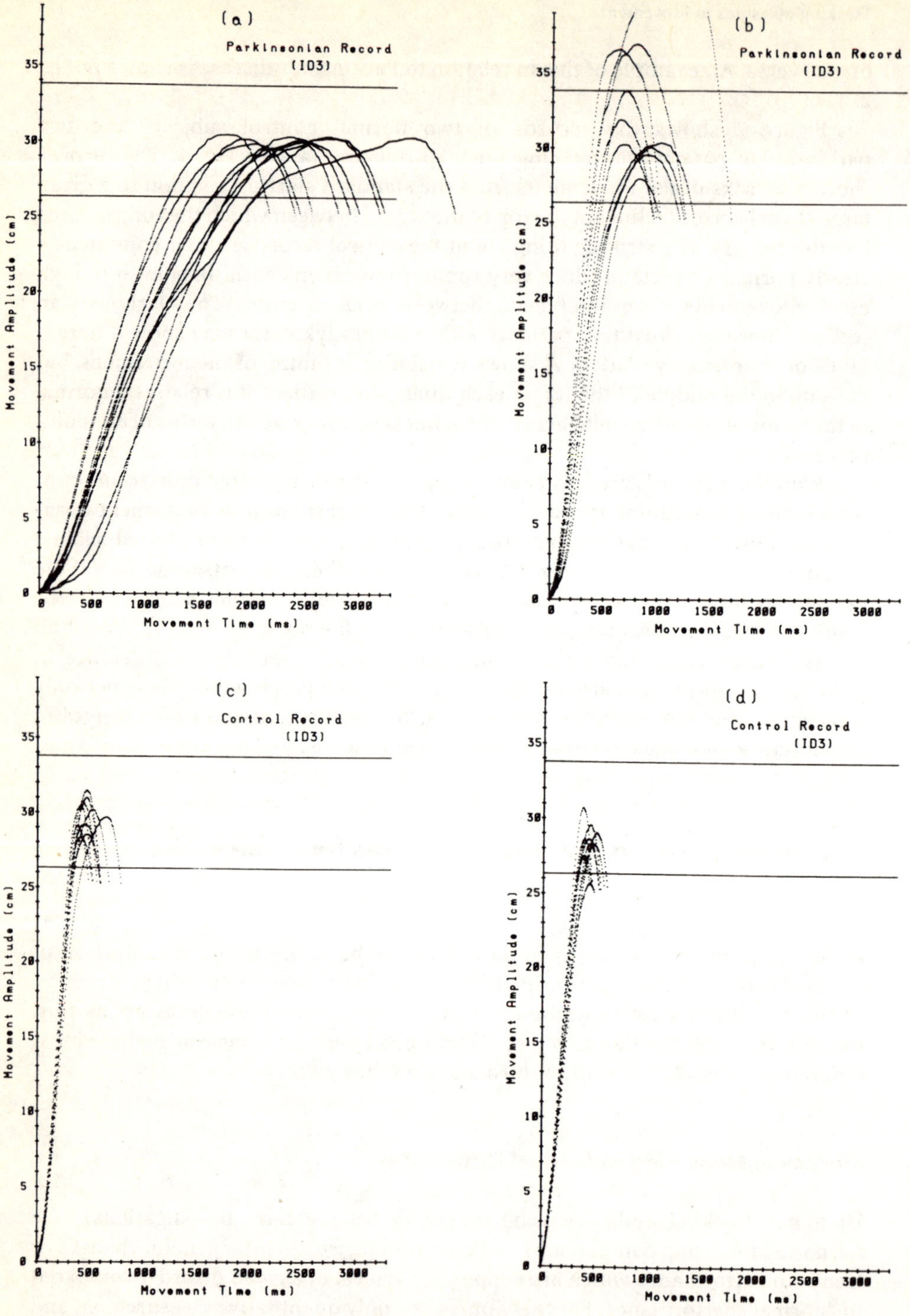

Fig. 2a–d. Records of two parkinsonian patients (**a,b**) and two normal control subjects (**c,d**) performing the step-tracking task of Fig. 1 (see text for details)

that norms and cut-off criteria can be established and critical diagnostic signs in the performance record established. This is a pre-requisite for standardisation of measures and their subsequent use in diagnosis, monitoring or correlation with clinical symptomatology.

The several measures available from tracking records differ in their potential to fulfil these requirements.

Paradigm Measurements

Paradigm measurements are difficult to envisage as direct clinical measures, as they tend to be all-or-nothing judgements and it is not yet clear whether the effect of a neurological disease shows up discretely or gradually, especially in the early stages. There is clearly room for some research into this question. Obviously if these measures showed a clear-cut difference between control and parkinsonian (or other neurological) subjects, they would be potential diagnostic markers which could be of great use clinically.

Parameter Measurements

Parameter (microscopic) measurements are quantitative and direct and thus potentially amenable to the establishment of such calibrated scales. To our knowledge, none have so far been established. Single parameter values, however, may be problematical, as has been shown above (e.g., Fig. 2), because patients may adapt to a developing impairment in different ways, which any one measure of performance may not pick up.

Statistical Measurements

Statistical (macroscopic) measurements allow comparison of subjects in terms of particular or overall functional characteristics, also with quantitative scores. They offer the possibility of better (because more stable and reliable) performance measures than have hitherto been used, and we suggest that the development of such measures would be well worthwhile. Again, though, there is as yet no calibrated scale for judging individuals this way.

New Information Provided by Tracking Studies

What new information do tracking studies give, as distinct from already existing measures (EMG, CT scans, etc.)? Motor skill tasks have several distinctive features. Firstly, they allow the investigator to regard control as a space–time continuum process and to measure both the kinematics of movement (which comprise the component processes of adaptive control: velocity, acceleration, timing effects and so on) and the macroscopic characteristics of performance, either of which may change as the result of nervous disease. The latter effects, especially, are not easily detectable by either clinical observation or physiological measures.

Secondly, they are uniquely suited in a way other tests and measures are not to measure: (a) adaptive changes over time; (b) the interaction between cognitive and perceptual motor skills; (c) secondary task effects and other higher level aspects of behaviour, all of which may play a vital part in the patient's condition and progress.

Thirdly, they are high-information tasks, thereby stretching the subject's mental and perceptual motor capacities to the maximum. This means that there is the potential for measures on skill tasks to pick up changes in efficiency of performance as soon as they occur, perhaps before they are severe enough to affect everyday activities. They may also be sensitive to changes in performance (either improvements or deterioration) caused by treatments such as drugs, physiotherapy, exercise or prostheses and may well have great potential use in monitoring these, thereby allowing, for example, better titration of drug dosages.

As an example of this last point, the evidence from Fig. 2 that the crucial effect in bradykinesia stems from variability in parkinsonian movements implies that any drug which is going to treat bradykinesia must act to reduce this movement variability; just increasing the force available to subjects may not be enough, because it is the *consistent control* of force that is lacking. A tracking task could be used to monitor drug effects here by measuring changes in error variance for a sample of aiming movements at different points in time. This may give a sensitive index of changes in the patient's motor control which would not be obvious to clinical observation, nor perhaps to physiological measurement (or at least not without having to take great pains).

Assessment Limitations

What are the limitations of perceptual motor skill measures? Firstly, measuring performance in only one or two dimensions may miss or minimise deficits showing up in three dimensions or in the integration of movement.

Performance measures in the relatively restricted area of voluntary upper limb movements will not of course indicate other kinds of difficulty such as postural or gait abnormalities. Nor will they measure involuntary movements, axial muscle function or simple muscle power directly. We do, however, have some (as yet unpublished) evidence that the measures of skill stand independently of other motor difficulties, e.g., tremor.

Another problem referred to above is that it is not yet certain whether changes in macroscopic variables are discrete (and therefore diagnostic markers) or gradual – in which case where are cutoff points for disorders? Nor is it clear whether paradigm judgements may be useful for classifying subjects in terms of their underlying nervous disorder or whether changes in strategies of performance have diagnostic value.

Also, a limitation at the moment is that it has not yet been demonstrated how performance measures relate to the difficulties of everyday life, i.e., their validity for predicting degrees of handicap in the activities of daily living [16].

The two last questions could easily be answered by further research, and their resolution would be well worthwhile.

Practical Criteria for Clinical Use

Practically, tracking tasks are very patient-friendly. They are usually regarded by patients as pleasant pastimes and, provided they do not tire the subjects' eyes or arm, are usually very stress-free. They are also relatively simple techniques to set up and run, use only conventional and inexpensive equipment and take relatively little time and effort to obtain their data. Skill tasks in general are relatively simple techniques, considering the variety and value of the data they generate.

References

1. Bartlett FC (1951) Anticipation in human performance. In: Ekman G, Husen T, Johansson G, Sandstrom CI (eds) Essays in psychology dedicated to David Katz. Almqvist and Wiksells, Uppsala
2. Craik KJW (1947/1948) Theory of the human operator in control systems. Br J Psychol 138:56–61, 142–148
3. Crossman ERFW (1960) The information capacity of the human motor system in pursuit tracking. Q J Exp Psychol 12:1–16
4. Flowers KA (1976) Visual "closed-loop" and "open-loop" characteristics of voluntary movement in patients with Parkinson's disease and intention tremor. Brain 99:261–310
5. Flowers KA (1978a) Some frequency response characteristics of parkinsonism on pursuit tracking. Brain 101:19–34
6. Flowers KA (1978b) Lack of prediction in the motor behaviour of parkinsonism. Brain 101:35–52
7. Gregory RL (1970) On how little information controls so much behaviour. Ergonomics 13:25–35
8. Jeannerod M (1988) The neural and behavioural organization of goal-directed movements. Oxford University Press, Oxford (Oxford psychology series no 15)
9. Poulton C (1952) The basis of perceptual anticipation in tracking. Br J Psychol 43:295–302
10. Poulton C (1974) Tracking skill and manual control. Academic, New York
11. Sheridan MR, Flowers KA (1990) Movement variability and bradykinesia in Parkinson's disease. Brain 113:1149–1161
12. Sheridan MR, Flowers KA, Hurrell J (1987) Programming and execution of movement in Parkinson's disease. Brain 110:1247–1271
13. Stark L (1968) Neurological control systems. Plenum, New York
14. Taylor FV, Birmingham HP (1948) Studies of tracking behavior. II. The acceleration pattern of quick manual corrective responses. J Exp Psychol 38:783–795
15. Trevarthen C (1978) Manipulative strategies of baboons and the origins of cerebral asymmetry. In: Kinsbourne M (ed) Asymmetrical function of the brain. Cambridge University Press, Cambridge
16. Tupper DE, Cicerone KD (1990) The neuropsychology of everyday life; assessment and basic competencies. Kluwer Academic, Boston

Discussion

Dr. Allum: I have just one comment to make about where you might find a large source of normal data. In the late 1960s, NASA spent a lot of money developing measures for pilot training and the work of McGrue et al. described in great detail measures in this area that you could use to quantify your results.

Dr. Dobbs: Would not the NASA results be telling you about elite people, not about normal people? We know a lot about elite athletes, but we don't know much about normal people.

Dr. Horstink: You talked about motor performance. There is a lot of cognitive processing in all those tracking tests, too. Can you tell me which part of your performance is cognitive and which part of your performance is motor, and can you discriminate between motor deterioration and cognitive deterioration?

Dr. Flowers: I think you can. I think you have to use proper experimental designs in which you systematically test people on different conditions and then use a sort of deductive process or subtractive process to show that the different levels of the system are working or not working. I think it is possible.

Kinematic Analysis of Complex Movements in Parkinson's Disease

R. Inzelberg, T. Flash, and A.D. Korczyn

The manifestations of Parkinson's disease (PD) are not only reflected in simple movements, but particularly in other functions of everyday life, including the execution of complex tasks such as handwriting or walking. The study of complex movements requires decomposition of the performance, allowing the analysis of specific constituents and elucidation of deficits at different levels of motor organization [16]. Several approaches have been used in the analysis of complex motor tasks in PD. This manuscript will mainly focus on the techniques used in these studies, trying to illuminate the advantages and limitations of quantitative methods when analyzing complex movements in PD, with special emphasis on kinematic measurements.

Benecke et al. [1] were among the first to study quantitatively the performance of two simultaneous movements of the upper limb in PD. Subjects were asked to squeeze the thumb and index finger and, either separately or simultaneously, to flex the ipsilateral elbow. PD patients moved considerably slower during simultaneous movements than when performing each movement separately. Interestingly, the degree of clinical akinesia correlated to this additional slowness observed in simultaneous performance. This work suggested that the superposition of separate motor programs is impaired in PD. Later, Benecke et al. [2] studied a similar paradigm in which the "flexion" and "squeezing" described above had to be performed sequentially. Different combinations of sequences were used, changing the order of "flex" or "squeeze" and the isometricity of each of them. Although each movement was slow when performed separately, a further decrease of speed was observed when movements were to be performed sequentially. In fact, each movement component was slower and the pause between them was prolonged in PD patients. In the sequential tasks, PD patients had longer interonset interval between the two movements than controls. The authors suggested that PD patients have difficulties in building motor sequences due to deficits in switching from one program to another.

Sternberg et al. [22] proposed a model of motor programming in normal humans which assumes that the abstract representation of a motor program for a learned sequence can be assembled and loaded into a motor "buffer." As the length of a sequence increases, so does the time required to read the motor buffer, resulting in an increase in reaction time (RT) of the first movement. Later, Rafal et al. [18] studied finger press sequences in PD. Overall, RT were slower in PD patients; however, RT increased as a function of the entire length of the sequence in PD patients and controls, as expected according to Sternberg's model in normal humans. They concluded that preprogramming according to Sternberg's model is possible, but slow, in PD. In another study, using a tapping sequence paradigm, RT increased linearly and significantly with the number of tappings in the sequence in healthy controls, but not linearly in PD patients [21]. Longer tap sequences were associated with increasing errors in PD. Similarly, Harrington and Haaland [13] studied sequences including different number of repetitions that also required different hand postures. For heterogeneous sequences, i.e., those which required not only repetitions, but also different hand postures, they observed a prolongation in RT with increasing sequence length, while in PD patients this prolongation was less prominent, implying worse preprogramming. For heterogeneous sequences, PD patients made more errors and were slower than controls when changing hand postures. These results implicated difficulties in the preprogramming of a complex task in PD. Some discrepancies between Rafal et al.'s [18] data and the above-cited studies can be attributed to differences in the experimental paradigms.

Cools et al. [4] coined the term "shifting aptitude" to describe the ability to rearrange the serial order of components according to the requirements of a behavioral task. They considered the deficit in sequential movements in PD to result from a decrease in shifting aptitude. This deficit could also be demonstrated both at a cognitive level, by difficulties in shifting between mental sets, and at a motor level, by switching between motor programs. Robertson and Flowers [19] used a sequential motor task in PD patients. Visual targets had to be reached in a determined order. Subjects were required to follow one sequence and then switch to another. While PD patients were generally able to produce each sequence on its own, they showed significantly more errors when shifting from one sequence to another. The authors assumed that shifting between motor sets is disturbed in PD, in parallel to cognitive shifting, and suggested that the deficit occurs at the level of a "junction box" which involves decisions and control of actions.

These studies, elegantly focusing on the programming of complex motor tasks in PD, were mainly based on the analysis of quantitative and qualitative parameters such as temporal variables (RT, movement time, interonset latencies) and different error categories. Thus, they mainly concentrated on the final product of the task, i.e., the actual limb movement or its electromyogram (EMG) counterpart.

In a simple reaching task, e.g., one in which a limb moves from one target to another, the paths generated by PD patients are as straight as those of control subjects [8,14]. However, the velocity profiles of such movements, analyzed by kinematic techniques, are obviously abnormal. In healthy controls, velocity profiles in a simple reaching task are smooth, bell-shaped, and symmetrical. In PD patients, they lack smoothness and symmetry, being composed of a shorter acceleration and a longer deceleration phases [8,14]. Unfortunately, however, there is a significant overlap between PD patients and controls. One might wonder whether this overlap could be due to technical problems. Findings in young adults, using the same paradigm, show significant differences between young and elderly normal subjects [14]. Thus, the similarities between the normal elderly and PD are probably due to age-induced changes in motor behavior.

Kinematic analysis, therefore, enables us to qualitatively analyze movements and to derive conclusions on hierarchically higher steps of motor planning, but it does not necessarily help in the diagnosis of PD, particularly in early stages of the disease.

Kinematic analysis can be used for the exact measurement of temporal variables, such as RT, movement time, time to peak velocity, time to peak acceleration, or kinematic variables, such as peak velocities or peak accelerations [8,14]. These measurements are of particular importance when complex tasks are used, since the determination of temporal variables is accompanied by special difficulties. In such a context, Flash et al. [6] studied normal young adults using a paradigm in which subjects were aiming to move their hand towards a visual target in the horizontal plane which was suddenly displaced. The hand started moving towards the first target and smoothly deviated to the second. This occurred although the target was displaced within the RT, i.e., before the onset of the movement towards the first target. The trajectory modification was smooth and, moreover, the RT to the change of stimulus showed no delays as compared to the RT to the first stimulus, suggesting that the two movement components were processed in parallel. Similar studies in PD patients and in the normal elderly show significant delays in the response to stimulus change, particularly in PD patients, confirming the known difficulties in switching motor programs in this disease [17]. According to these studies, kinematic analysis provides an exact method for measurements of temporal parameters of movements.

A possible application of kinematic analysis is the use of mathematical models that can describe normal motor behavior. A mathematical model was formulated by Flash and Hogan [5] that assumes that the system "attempts" to generate maximally smooth movements of the hand. Using this model, we studied PD patients and elderly controls [7]. The subjects had to move their hands in the horizontal plane from one visual target to another passing through a point. The results showed that PD patients qualitatively and quantitatively deviate from the behavior predicted by the model (which was developed for normal young adults) more than the healthy elderly. Many of the PD patients' trajectories included pauses between the two movement segments. In controls, the duration of both segments were roughly equal, regardless of the location of the point to be passed through, suggesting that the movement is planned as a whole. In PD patients, the duration of each movement segment was proportionate to its length, suggesting that PD patients do not plan a complex trajectory as a whole, but rather in separate segments, pointing to a deficit in the integration of motor programs in this disease.

The question still remains as to the exact value of kinematic analysis in clinical work and whether these techniques help to differentiate between PD and the healthy elderly. As discussed above, values derived from normal elderly subjects often overlap with those of PD patients. For example, a further look at other studies using a paradigm similar to ours [6] shows that RT to the target modification are similar to the RT to the first stimulus, both in normal young adults and in primates [10,11]. Normal elderly deviate significantly from young adults, and PD patients deviate even further in the same direction, albeit significantly overlapping with the normal elderly [15,17]. The studies of Benecke et al. [1,2], mentioned above as examples of simultaneous and sequential movements in PD, included a control group which was younger by about 10 years than the PD patients. Although this age difference was not significant, it could have contributed to the differences between the two groups. It is possible that in age-matched populations, the difference between control and PD subjects would be less prominent. For example, Harrington and Haaland [13] studied control subjects who were matched for age with PD patients and found a significant overlap in several parameters such as RT, errors, and interresponse intervals. Therefore, it is possible that some of the pathological observations in PD are related to normal aging, while others are due to "accelerated" aging of the motor system in this disease.

It is well known that motor performance deteriorates in the aging human. Welford [24] suggested that the deterioration with age of parameters such as RT is due to a combination of several mechanisms affected by aging and not necessarily dopaminergic failure. Thus, the delineation between the normal elderly and PD is often not possible in motor performance measurements.

Another problem emerging from quantitation of motion is the fact that the paradigm significantly influences the results. Simple changes in the task, such as the location of the target, can interfere with the results. We have previously shown [8] that in both PD patients and normal elderly performing an aiming task, longer RT are observed for more distally placed targets. Further evidence concerning the influence of the particular paradigm on the results of motor tasks comes from studies on complex bimanual movements in PD. While Benecke et al. [1] showed impairment of bimanual arm movements in PD, Stelmach et al. [20] could not replicate these observations. Instead, they observed that symmetrical and especially asymmetrical bimanual movements showed longer preparation and execution times than unimanual movements. Again, these differences were observed in both PD and normal elderly subjects. The disagreement between these findings and those previously reported is likely to derive from different task conditions. Goodrich et al. [12] studied simple (SRT) and choice RT (CRT) in PD and again established that it is indeed the SRT that is prolonged in PD, while CRT does not differ significantly between PD and normal age-matched controls. When using a more complicated paradigm, SRT of the normal group were prolonged and the differences between the two groups disappeared. Again, in this work the paradigm dictated the results. The large variability in the results in different task conditions precludes the definition of "normal limits" of motor performance, as are available in more established quantitative techniques in neurophysiology.

Beyond their use as research tools, quantitative methods might be useful for evaluating the effects of therapy in PD, for example to quantify the performance during "on" and "off" states [3] or following the course of a disease. Although most studies on PD report the stage of the disease of the examined subjects, there is insufficient information as to the effect of disease severity on kinematic parameters, and there has been no study which has specifically addressed this question.

This point is of prime importance when discussing the applicability of kinematic analysis to early detection of presymptomatic PD.

The necessity for objective measurement techniques as an ancillary to clinical evaluation has nowadays reached a state of international consensus. Some of these measures seem to be more practical for everyday life use [23]. Whether disease-specific patterns can be developed using these techniques and whether they can be used for differentiating PD from other parkinsonian syndromes remain issues for future research.

References

1. Benecke R, Rothwell JC, Dick JPR, Day BL, Marsden CD (1986) Performance of simultaneous movements in patients with Parkinson's disease. Brain 109:739–757
2. Benecke R, Rothwell JC, Dick JPR, Day BL, Marsden CD (1987a) Disturbances of sequential movements in patients with Parkinson's disease. Brain 110:361–379
3. Benecke R, Rothwell JC, Dick JPR, Day BL, Marsden CD (1987b) Simple and complex movements off and on treatment in patients with Parkinson's disease. J Neurol Neurosurg Psychiatry 50:296–303
4. Cools AR, van der Bercken JHL, Horstink MWI, van Spaendock KPM, Berger HJC (1984) Cognitive and motor shifting aptitude disorder in Parkinson's disease. J Neurol Neurosurg Psychiatry 47:443–453
5. Flash T, Hogan N (1985) The coordination of arm movements: an experimentally confirmed mathematical model. J Neurosci 5:1688–1703
6. Flash T, Henis E, Inzelberg R, Korczyn AD (1992a) Timing and sequencing of human arm trajectories: Normal and abnormal behavior. In: Thomassen AJWM, Rosenbaum DA, van Wieringen PCW (eds) Sequencing and timing of human movement. Elsevier Science, North-Holland, Amsterdam, pp 83–100
7. Flash T, Inzelberg R, Korczyn AD (1992b) Quantitative methods for the assessment of motor performance in Parkinson's disease. In: Rose CF (ed) Parkinson's disease and problems in clinical trials. Smith-Gordon, London, pp 87–106
8. Flash T, Inzelberg R, Schechtman E, Korczyn AD (1992c) Kinematic analysis of upper limb trajectories in Parkinson's disease. Exp Neurol 118:215–226
9. Georgopulos AP (1986) On reaching. Annu Rev Neurosci 9:147–170
10. Georgopulos AP, Kalaska JF, Massey JT (1981) Spatial trajectories and reaction times of aimed movements: effects of practice, uncertainty, and change in target location. J Neurophysiol 46:725–743
11. van Gielen CCAM, Van den Heuvel PJM, Van der Gon Denier JJ (1984) Modification of muscle activation patterns during fast goal directed arm movements. J Motor Behavior 16:2–19
12. Goodrich S, Henderson L, Kennard C (1989) On the existence of an attention-demanding process peculiar to simple reaction time: converging evidence from Parkinson's disease. Cogn Neuropsychology 6:309–331
13. Harrington DL, Haaland KY (1991) Sequencing in Parkinson's disease. Brain 114:99–115
14. Inzelberg R, Flash T, Korczyn AD (1990) Kinematic properties of upper limb trajectories in Parkinson's disease and idiopathic torsion dystonia. Adv Neurol 53:183–189
15. Inzelberg R, Plotnik M, Flash T, Korczyn AD (1992) Ability to switch between motor programs in Parkinson's disease before movement initiation and during execution. J Neurol 239[Suppl 2]:S82
16. Phillips JG, Muller F, Stelmach GE (1989) Movement disorders and the neural basis of motor control. In: Wallace SA (ed) Perspectives on the coordination of movement. Elsevier Science, North-Holland, Amsterdam

17. Plotnik M, Inzelberg R, Flash T, Korczyn AD (1992) Arm trajectory modification in Parkinson's disease. J Neurol 239[Suppl 2]:S81–S82
18. Rafal RD, Unhoff AW, Friedman JH, Bernstein E (1987) Programming and execution of sequential movements in Parkinson's disease. J Neurol Neurosurg Psychiatry 50:1267–1273
19. Robertson C, Flowers KA (1990) Motor set in Parkinson's disease. J Neurol Neurosurg Psychiatry 53:583–592
20. Stelmach G, Worringham CJ (1988) The control of aiming movements in Parkinson's disease. J Neurol Neurosurg Psychiatry 51:223–231
21. Stelmach GE, Worringham CJ, Strand EE (1987) The programming and execution of movement sequences in Parkinson's disease. Int J Neurosci 36:55–65
22. Sternberg S, Monsell S, Knoll RL, Wright CE (1978) The latency and duration of rapid movement sequences: comparisons of speech and typewriting. In: Stelmach GE (ed) Information processing in motor control and learning. Academic, New York
23. Watts RL, Mandir AS, Ahn KJ, Juncos JL, Zakers GO, Freeman A (1991) Electrophysiologic analysis of early Parkinson's disease. Neurology 41[Suppl 2]:44–48
24. Welford TA (1988) Reaction time, speed of performance, and age. Ann NY Acad Sci 515:1–17

Discussion

Dr. Corcos: In the task where you showed your velocity profiles which had quite a bit of noise on them – if you were to use patients who are primarily bradykinetic as opposed to those who are primarily tremulous, would you get the same or different results?

Dr. Inzelberg: I did not give the clinical details of the patients, but we observed the same results with patients who had no tremor clinically and only bradykinesia and rigidity. So it is not an artifact of tremor.

Dr. Hallett: You showed us that some of the abnormalities that you found in the Parkinson's disease patients might be ascribable to age, but surely some of the abnormalities actually were due to the disease. Which of the abnormalities that you saw really were parkinsonian?

Dr. Inzelberg: That's a difficult question to answer. Probably the delays in the movement times are due to parkinsonian behavior. We cannot say the same for reaction times, but considering the fact that the qualitative properties of movements disintegrated and also considering the velocity profiles, which are per se disturbed, I should say that these are the ones that are due to parkinsonism and not to age.

The Age Function of Normative Data for a Personal Computer-Based Test System for the Analysis and Quantification of Manual Movement Disability

J. Machetanz, C. Bischoff, B.-U. Meyer, J. Forster, and B. Conrad

Introduction

The exact evaluation and documentation of movement disabilities is an essential component of clinical work and research in the field of movement disorders. We have developed an inexpensive system for the evaluation of manual movement disability which can be run by medical assistants without any special training. While the specific aspects of the task implementations are discussed elsewhere [6], this paper deals with age-related changes of normative data.

There is some literature about age-related changes in various parameters measuring functional, pathological, biochemical, and imaging aspects. These include peripheral and spinal nerve conduction velocities [3,4], cognitive and sensory functions [11], and various structures of the brain as reflected by histology [9], magnetic resonance imaging (MRI) [10]; positron emission tomography (PET) [7]; and biochemical marker systems [8]. Taylor [15], Richter [13], Bischoff et al. [1], Sato et al. [14], and Reichlmeier et al. [12] found nonlinear effects of age on their target parameters (i.e., nerve conduction velocity, number of vestibular neurons, duration of the motor unit action potential, number and size of type II muscle fibers, and enzymatic activity). The results of these studies coincided in so far as clear nonlinearity began at the age of about 60. Taylor [15] compared a quadratic curve with the linear model and found a significantly better fit.

Methods

A total of 76 normal voluntary subjects (between 17 and 85 years; mean, age, 47.2 years; SD, 19.2) were assessed with a system testing manual motor ability. None of the subjects had any neurological or psychiatric deficits or was on any medication which is known to act on the motor or cognitive functions of the nervous system.

The test system [6] consisted of software that runs on MS-DOS and uses a standard computer mouse as the only input device for movement data. In this test system, the patient moves the mouse according to the instructions of a medical assistant who controls the test using the keyboard. The computer screen displays target and tracker symbols. The sample speed of the system is 100 Hz with a spatial resolution of 400 DPI. This is less than 0.07 mm.

In the test set used for the acquisition of normative data, there were four different types of tasks (paradigms): (1) pursuit tracking, (2) ballistic, (3) complex sequential, and (4) finger tapping. Individual researchers have used these paradigms in various implementations and the tasks have repeatedly been shown to be generally useful in the detection and quantification of movement disability due to movement disorders [6]. In pursuit tracking, a cross moved over the screen and the patient had to "capture" the cross with a tracker symbol (circle). In the ballistic task, a circle was displayed and a second circle "jumped" from the first circle to a new position which was 5 or 15 cm away. The patient had to move the tracker symbol as fast as possible to the new position as soon as he had visually recognized the jump. In the complex sequential task, the patient again had to move the tracker to visual targets (three or five targets). However, before being allowed to move to the next target he had to stop and click the mouse button. In finger tapping, the mouse button had to be repeatedly pressed down and released as fast as possible for 10 s with the wrist lying on the desk surface. In pursuit tracking the tracking pattern was varied between straight lines, sinusoids, zig-zag, and saw tooth. The straight line pattern preceded the other patterns as a practice task and was not analyzed. The complete test took between 30 and 40 min per subject.

A total of 44 parameters was calculated from the different tasks. After elimination of the practice trials (straight lines in tracking, any trials in which tasks were imperfectly understood), parameter means were calculated for each subject. For these means, linear regressions and a nonlinear approximation for a double linear algorithm which is described later were calculated.

Results

Of the 44 parameters analyzed, ten did not show a significant correlation with age (ANOVA $p > 0.05$), five were weakly correlated ($0.01 < p < 0.05$), and 29 reached significant levels ($p < 0.01$).

The representative parameter examples in Fig. 1 are fatigue (tendency to decrease amplitude during single sweeps), sequential movement time (mean movement time in the complex sequential tasks), lag vertical component (lag of the cross-correlation between the vertical target and tracker positions), tapping rate (in finger tapping), error horizontal component (absolute error of the horizontal component in tracking), discontinuity horizontal component (position changes in the horizontal movement component), best correlation (of the cross correlation between the horizontal target and tracker positions), and reaction time (in ballistic movements). Each data point reflects the mean of the motor parameter for one subject over all trials (at least six trials per data point). The smooth curves were calculated using LOWESS locally weighted regression and smoothing scatter plots [2].

Basically, three different types of age functions were observed: (1) with no significant age-related changes, (2) with an almost linear age-related change, and

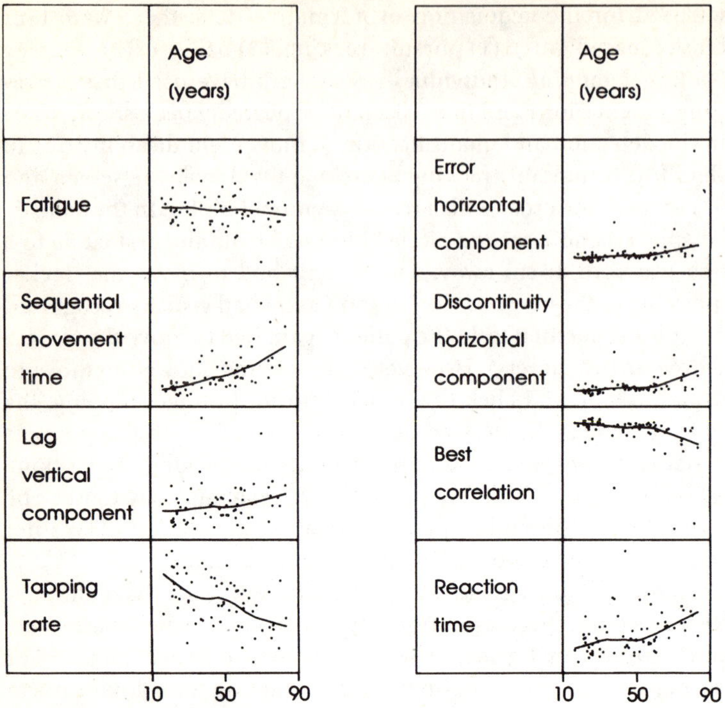

Fig. 1. Parameter examples for different types of age functions

(3) with age-related changes of different slopes among younger subjects and accelerated changes in older age. The best approach to describe the type 3 data is to divide the observed period of aging into two sections. Section 1 covers subjects younger and section 2 subjects older than about 58 years. Each section has an almost linear age function, but the slope of the age function of the second section is steeper. The transition between the two sections is smooth. In order to test whether this deviation from linearity reaches a significant level, data were separated into two groups according to the observed curve: the first group included data of subjects younger than 58 years and the second group all older subjects. For each group, a linear regression based on an absolute value loss function was calculated. The two linear models were compared with the real data of the total age span. Residuals were calculated and their absolute values were compared between the two models using a t test. Differences were highly significant for several parameters (for example, absolute horizontal deviation in tracking: t, –4.886, $p < 0.00001$; discontinuities of the horizontal component: t –5.357, $p < 0.000005$; maximum correlation of the vertical component in tracking: t, –5.670, $p < 0.000005$; root mean square error of the vertical component in tracking: t,–6.252, $p < 0.000005$).

When classifying all 44 parameters into types 1–3, type 1 (null-hypothesis slope = 0; linear regression ANOVA $p > 0.05$) was found in ten parameters. Type 2 (null-hypothesis slope = 0, linear regression ANOVA $p < 0.05$, and slope of subjects older than 58 was less than three times the slope of subjects younger than 58) was found in 25 parameters. Type 3 (linear regression ANOVA $p < 0.05$ and slope of subjects older than 58 was at least three times larger than slope of subjects younger than 58) was found in nine parameters.

In order to capture the observed age functions mathematically, we modeled a function that describes a double linear curve with a smooth transition:

$$\text{Parameter} = \text{constant} + \text{slope1} \times \text{age} + \text{slope2} \times \frac{(\text{age} - 58)}{1 + \exp(1 - 1 \times (0.3 \times \text{age} - 0.3 \times 58))}$$

The value of

$$\frac{(\text{age} - 58)}{1 + \exp(1 - 1 \times (0.3 \times \text{age} - 0.3 \times 58))}$$

is almost zero for age values much smaller than 58 years and is almost one for values much larger than 58. This part of the equation was introduced to give the variable slope 2 more bearing only after age 58 and to make the transition between the two linear sections smooth. Age 58 has been selected because visual inspection of the smoothed scattergrams repeatedly showed first deviations from linearity slightly before 60 years.

Note that the algorithm includes the other age functions that have been empirically observed (simple linear: slope 2 = 0; no age related change: slope 1 = 0 and slope 2 = 0). A graph of the algorithm is shown in Fig. 2.

Naturally, when comparing a simple linear model against the double linear model, the fit is better for the double linear model. However, when calculating

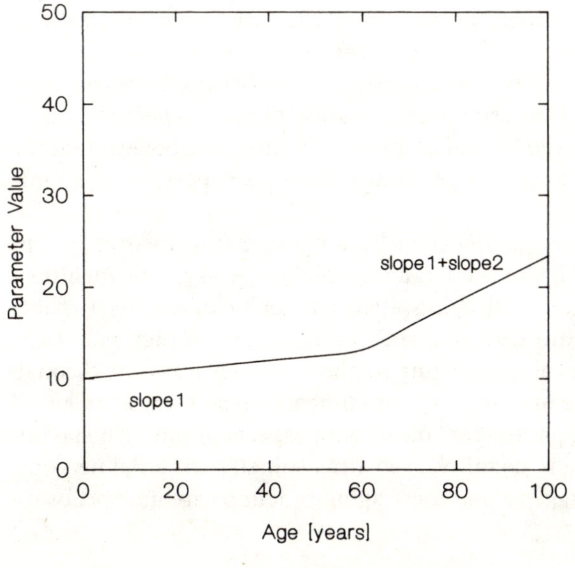

Fig. 2. Graph of the algorithm used to model the double linear curve of the type 3 age function. The variable values for the graph were as follows: constant = 10; slope 1 = 0.05; slope 2 = 0.2. The values were chosen arbitrarily so that the graph resembles actual data curves

parametric or nonparametric test statistics comparing the residuals between the sampled data and each of the two models, no significant differences were found for any of the motor parameters. This result can be explained by the large interindividual data dispersion.

When calculating the greatest error that might occur when using the simple linear model instead of the double linear model, the error would be between –0.2 and +0.6 standard deviation of the data set (compensated for age). These errors correspond to age effects between 20 and 60 years.

Discussion

Normative data were collected using a test system for manual motor ability. The primary goal of the present study was to establish an algorithm that sufficiently reflects the age function of motor abilities. A mathematical formulation of age function is important for two reasons: (1) it enables us to relate an individual patient's data to age-corrected norm values in order to quantify norm deviations and (2) patient populations of different diagnostic entities can be age corrected and then directly compared even if the age of the populations is clearly different (e.g., comparison of early onset and late onset cerebellar atrophies).

When trying to find an algorithm that reflects the age function, we first visually inspected various motor parameters as functions of age. While some parameters did not change with age, others changed linearly. A third group seemed to follow a double linear curve with two linear sections separated by a smooth transition at about the age of 58 years. Statistical analysis supported this impression in showing that the linear regression of the younger age group was significantly different from the linear regression of the older age group. However, due to large interindividual data dispersion, direct comparison of the data with a simple linear versus a double linear model did not show significant differences of the residuals. However, the double linear model fits the data better and the differences between the two models were up to –0.2 to 0.6 standard deviation of data dispersion, which corresponds to age effects between 20 and 60 years. We therefore believe that the implementation of the double linear model of age effects is superior to a simple linear model.

Moreover, the double linear model may be an interesting theoretical approach, because for the second linear section a variable (slope 2) can be identified which is characteristic for additional aging effects in older age. This variable can be directly correlated with results from corresponding functional (e.g., electrophysiological), pathological, or imaging methods. When scanning through the literature, one notes that age functions with nonlinearity beginning at an age of about 60 are not only found in parameters measuring aspects of motor behavior, but also in those corresponding to cognitive, sensoric, spinal, peripheral nervous, and muscular function. This suggests that these aging functions are not specific to the motor system and that they can probably be explained best on the level of the common structural elements. This would be on the cellular level or below.

References

1. Bischoff C, Machetanz J, Conrad B (1991) Is there an age-dependent continuous increase in the duration of the motor unit action potential? Electroencephalography and clinical. Neurophysiology 81:304–311
2. Cleveland WS (1979) Robust locally weighted regression and smoothing scatterplots. J Am Stat Assoc 74:829–836
3. Dorfman LJ, Bosley TM (1979) Age-related changes in peripheral and central nerve conduction in man. Neurology 29:28–44
4. Hume AL, Cant BR, Shaw NA, Cowan JC (1982) Central somatosensory conduction time from 10 to 79 years. EEG Clin Neurophysiol 54:49–54
5. Kondraske GV, Potvin AR, Tourtellotte WW, Syndulko KW (1984) A computer-based system for automated quantitation of neurologic function. IEEE Trans Biomed Eng 31:401–414
6. Machetanz J, Forster J, Bischoff C, Meyer B-U, Isenberg C, Conrad B (1993) A PC-based system for an objective quantification of manual movement disability for clinical and scientific purposes. J Biomed Eng 15:363–370
7. Martin WRW, Palmer MR (1989) The nigrostriatal system in aging and parkinsonism: In vivo studies with positron emission tomography. In: Calne DB et al. (eds) Parkinsonism and aging. Raven, New York, pp 165–171
8. McGeer L, McGeer E, Suzuki JS (1977) Aging and extrapyramidal function. Arch Neurol 34:33–35
9. McGeer PL, Itagaki S, Akiyama H, McGeer EG (1989) Comparison of neuronal loss in Parkinson's disease and aging. In: Calne DB et al. (eds) Parkinsonism and aging. Raven, New York, pp 25–34
10. Olanow CW, Holgate RC, Murtaugh R, Martinez C (1989) MR Imaging in Parkinson's disease and aging. In: Calne DB et al. (eds) Parkinsonism and aging. Raven, New York, pp 155–164
11. Pacaud S, Welford AT (1989) Performance in relation to age and education level: a monumental research. Exp Aging Res 15:123–136
12. Reichlmeier K, Ermini M, Schlecht HP (1978) Altersbedingte enzymatische Veränderungen im menschlichen Grosshirn-cortex. Aktuel Gerontol 8:441–448
13. Richter E (1981) Das Ganglion Scarpae im Alter. Laryngol Rhinol Otol 60:542–544
14. Sato T, Akatsuka H, Kito K, Tokoro Y, Tauchi H, Kato K (1984) Age changes in size and number of muscle fibers in human minor pectoral muscle. Mech Ageing Dev 28:99–109
15. Taylor PK (1984) Non-linear effects of age on nerve conduction in adults. J Neurol Sci 66:223–234

Discussion

Dr. Kraus: I see some problems with the third dimension and the use of the mouse. The resolution of mouse movement is one parameter you measured.

Dr. Machetanz: That's right. When a patient is not able to keep the mouse on the desk top, of course you can't do this. If you have a wildly hyperkinetic subject who always lifts the mouse, you can't assess him with this, at least not with the complete battery. That's right.

Dr. Kraus: So you can't measure everybody.

Dr. Machetanz: There are certainly limitations.

Dr. Rabey: What happens if you examine patients with a peripheral sensory neuropathy, for example, when they don't have an afferent nerve.

Dr. Machetanz: We have only examined a few. We didn't see any changes, at least not really relevant changes. They have direct visual feedback and those that we assessed did not have a problem.

Dr. Kraus: It's also a problem that patients are not familiar with the method, and therefore you have a very high interpersonal variability before you start. Younger patients are familiar with the mouse and the older ones don't know anything about computer methods.

Dr. Machetanz: Yes, that's right, and that's the problem with any computer test system you use. You can even have large practice trials to familiarize them with the system, but that's time-consuming; alternatively, you just take the very first value, and of course you also get all these factors.

Dr. Kraus: Therefore you have an undefined part of higher information processing.

Dr. Machetanz: That's true, but in comparing the subjects – for example, we had age-matched controls here – the patients are clearly different, although they have the same problems. You can see these effects, you are completely right. There are important cognitive factors.

Dr. Kraus: But it's unclear how high the part of recognition is, for example.

Dr. Machetanz: Certainly, you have vision in there, it's a big factor; you have cognitive abilities, but whenever you do these complex tasks you get these factors in your design.

Dr. Deuschl: But couldn't you just switch for example to a digitizing tablet instead of using the mouse and keep all the remaining things as they are?

Dr. Machetanz: The digitizing tablet has the same problems that Dr. Kraus mentioned. Again, it's a big cognitive task, and you have to become familiar with the complete system. The main disadvantage of the digitizing tablet is you have to purchase it: it has to be a standard digitizing tablet. The advantage of using a mouse is that you can go to any computer shop in the world and get a Microsoft mouse. It's the same everywhere.

Dr. Watts: Two suggestions. First, in order to give reliability in a given subject from one session to another, you have to have practice sessions, and I think that was the point unless you are looking at motor learning. If you do enough practice sessions, you should be able to achieve a performance level unless the task is too complex. Second, you probably have different levels of complexity of the task so that you can get something from everybody, even if they might have some element of dementia. If you have more simple tasks and then move on toward more cognitively complex tasks, you should then be able to use the method in any subject.

Quantitative Clinical Evaluation of Parkinsonism Based on Visuomotor Tracking and Tracing

S. Hocherman

Introduction

The motor deficits of patients with Parkinson's disease (PD) are evaluated periodically, in order that optimal pharmacological treatment be prescribed. To date, such an evaluation is based on crude observations of tremor, rigidity, and postural deviations, which together constitute a classification of patients into four categories on the Hoehn and Yahr scale [3]. In addition to clinical evaluation of patients with known PD, early detection of parkinsonism in new patients is gaining importance. New preventive treatments are becoming available, which may delay progression of the disease [5], and a decision whether to begin such treatment can no longer be based on crude clinical observations. Thus, a sensitive, reliable, and quantitative method for the assessment of parkinsonism is required.

The degradation of motor performance in PD patients has been documented in numerous papers. Increases in reaction time and movement time [6], inadequate electromyographic (EMG) activity during action [6], and segmentation of saccadic eye movements [7] have all been described. A deficit in motor planning, which is known to characterize this illness [4], is revealed by the inability of patients to perform open-loop movements for which visual guidance is not available [2]. On the other hand, closed-loop control is considered to be adequate, allowing tracing and tracking of slow visual signals [1].

The wealth of information regarding motor control in parkinsonism raises the question as to why this knowledge is not used to achieve better clinical evaluation. The present paper describes a new method which is designed to do just that. The visuomotor performance of patients is evaluated quantitatively, under conditions which include closed-loop and open-loop tracking, at several movement speeds and along paths which differ in complexity. In addition, the ability to trace the same paths, at an internally determined speed, is rated. Performance is evaluated separately along several dimensions, which include distance, velocity, and movement direction. The complete procedure produces a quantitative description of the subject's visuomotor performance, which is sensitive enough to discriminate between "on drug" stage I PD patients and age-matched controls and to follow the changes in an individual patient as the drug wears off. This system, together with some preliminary results of its utilization, is described below.

Methods

General Description

All tests are done using a computerized system which displays a trace model or a moving target circle on a computer screen. The screen display includes a subject-controlled pointer, whose position represents the location of a hand-held handle on the surface of a digitizing tablet. The handle and the hand holding it can not be seen by the subject. All tasks consist of tracing the model path or tracking the moving target circle with the subject-controlled pointer by moving the lever appropriately over the digitizing tablet.

Instrumentation

The system described is based on a personal computer (IBM PC -AT) which has a digitizing tablet (Numonics Grid Master) connected to it. The subject is seated in front of a 30 × 30 cm digitizing tablet at the lower chest level covered by a 3-mm-thick glass plate. The tablet's pen cursor is contained in a vertical handle that rests against the glass and is supported by a two-joint lever system, allowing free movement in the horizontal plan. A horizontal wood plate is fixed above the upper end of the lever, hiding it from the subject's view. A color monitor is placed on top of the wood plate, about 50 cm in front of the subject's face.

Location of the handle over the digitizing tablet is determined at a resolution of 0.05 mm every 10 ms. The output of a separate 1-kHz clock is read whenever a location is sampled, and these readings are stored together with the positional readings in the computer memory.

Tasks

Three different tasks are performed by each subject during the process of evaluation. All three tasks include movement along a horizontal line as well as along a sinusoidal path. Movement is always from left to right and covers a horizontal range of 20 cm.

Tracing

A tracing model (either a straight line or a sine wave) is displayed in white on the monitor screen. A circle 12 mm in diameter is displayed at the left end of the tracing model. The subject-controlled pointer is displayed on screen as a green spot. The subject is instructed to bring the pointer into the circle by moving the unseen handle with the tested hand. Upon entrance of the pointer into the circle, the latter disappears and a beep sound indicates that tracing should begin. From that point on, movement of the handle is shown on screen as a continuous green line, which the subject is asked to draw on top of the white tracing model. There are no requirements for movement speed and the trial is ended when the line reaches the right end of the model trace. Upon completion of a trial, the screen display is erased and a new trial begins. Each tracing model is used three times in three consecutive trials.

Tracking Along a Visible Model

Each trial begins by an initial display of the path model, with a 12-mm circle at its left end. Entrance of the pointer into the circle does not cause the latter to disappear. Instead, after the "go" signal, the circle begins to move along the model path at a preprogrammed speed. From here on, movement of the target circle has to be followed with the unseen handle, so that the subject-controlled pointer is maintained within its limits. In this task, the pointer remains a distinct green spot throughout the trial. If the circle is missed, i.e., the pointer is not positioned inside it, its movement stops until pointer contact is re-established. Tracking ends when the entire course is traversed, upon which event the screen is erased and a new trial with the same path model, but at a different speed, begins. Each path model is traversed three times at speeds of 4, 7, and 10 mm/s.

Tracking Along an Invisible Model

This task is identical to the above described task of tracking a visible model, except that the model path itself is not displayed during the entire trial. Thus, the trial begins when a target circle appears at the left side of the monitor screen and continues as this circle moves from left to right, with no display of its forthcoming trajectory. The same three movement speeds (4, 7, and 10 mm/s) are employed.

In all, the visuomotor performance of each subject is tested in six different sets of trials, with each set consisting of three separate trials. The entire procedure takes 15–30 min (depending on the subject) and does not wear out the tested person.

Data Acquisition and Analysis

The data recorded in each trial includes the XY position of the handle at every sampling point, together with the time (1 ms resolution) of sampling. In the tracing task, this amounts to saving the entire data stream. In the tracking tasks, the samples of handle position when the subject-controlled pointer is out of the target circle, i.e., when the target circle is stationary, are discarded. The data acquired during subject evaluation are analyzed off line and the following indices of performance are calculated:

Algebraic Error (AlgEr). The trace created by movement of the handle is subtracted from the model trace. The average difference and its standard deviation are computed.

Minimal Error (MinEr). The shortest distance which connects each sampled handle position to the model path is computed. This is done by finding the minimal root mean square of the $X^2 + Y^2$ difference between the sampled lever position and position along the path model. The computation is repeated for every sampled handle position and the results are then averaged to generate the MinEr and its standard deviation.

Vectorial Error (VctrEr). The vector of hand movement (direction and velocity) is calculated at every sampled handle position. This vector is broken into a component which parallels the model path vector (calculated for the point along the model path which is nearest to the sampled position) and into an error component which is perpendicular to the path vector. This error vector, which expresses deviation of handle movement from the required path, is then scaled by the size of the handle movement vector. The result is a local measure of the directional movement error, expressed as percentage of the total movement vector. Averaging these local measures produces the VctrEr of handle movement, which can range from 0% (movement parallel to the model path) to 100% (movement perpendicular to the model path). It should be recognized that the VctrEr is a true measure of the directional error and is not influenced by the distance between the actual and model paths (i.e., a 0% VctrEr will be found for a movement which exactly parallels the model path, but at some distance away from it).

Percentage of Movement Time During Which the VctrEr Exceeded 50% (T50%). This index measures the cumulative movement time during which the VctrEr exceeded 50% (movement away from the path more than along it) and expresses this time as percentage of the total movement time. It should be stressed that in the tracing task, movement time always equals the total trial time. However, in the tracking task, total movement time does not include periods during which the target circle is missed and thus may be shorter than the total trial time.

Number of Interruptions (Nints). This index is relevant only to tracking, because it constitutes a count of the number of occasions during a trial on which the subject-controlled pointer has deviated out of the target circle.

Speed Error (SpdEr). This index is again specific to tracking. It expresses the average difference between the speed with which the target circle and the handle move along the tracking path.

Results

A comparison between the performance of stage I and II PD patients and that of age-matched controls reveals highly significant differences between these groups,

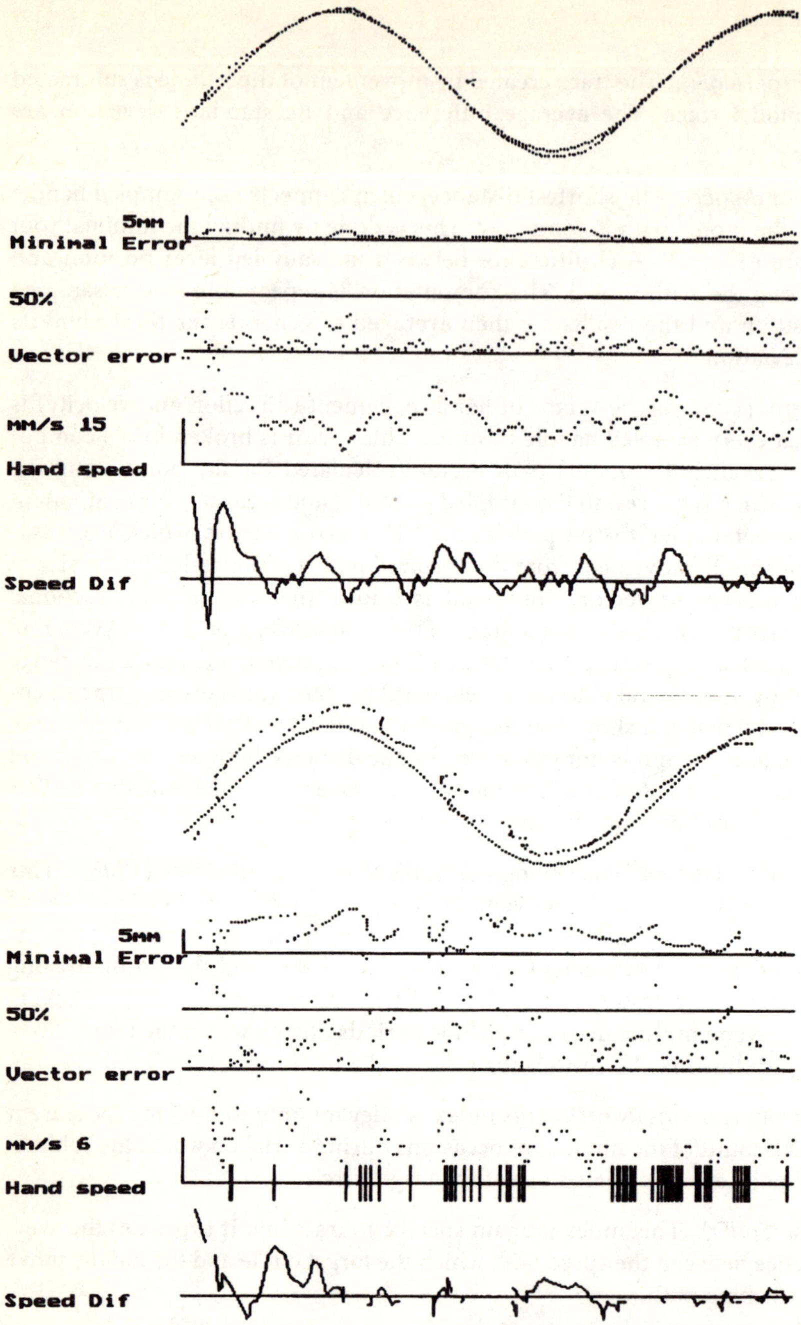

Fig. 1. Tracking along a sine wave path by a control subject (*top*) and by a Parkinson's disease (PD) patient (*bottom*). The path model and the path traversed by the hand are shown at the upper part of each section. The instantaneous values of the minimal error (MinEr), vectorial error (VctrEr), hand speed, and difference between the velocities of the hand and target circle are shown in the corresponding traces. The *small vertical bars* on the hand speed trace denote points along the path where an interruption occurred

with all performance indices. Figure 1 shows the performance of a control subject (top) and that of a PD patient (bottom) in the tracking task. The uneven tracking of the patient stands in obvious contrast to the smooth performance of the control subject. This difference is typical, but clinical rating needs to include the results of all tests. The following results have already been determined in a pilot study:

1. Patients at an early stage of the disease (stage I or II), in "on" condition, still have greater MinEr than age-matched controls in tracing as well as in tracking tasks. In tracing tasks, they differ from controls mainly in having a significantly greater VctrEr while tracing a sinusoidal path than when tracing a straight path. In tracking tasks, they are characterized by greater T50% values, regardless of the tracking speed, and by a speed-dependent Nints.
2. More severe patients show larger MinEr and VctrEr in tracing tasks and are grossly impaired during tracking tasks. In the latter tasks, performance may be too impaired to allow reliable quantification, in which case evaluation must rely mainly on scoring in the tracing task.
3. The MinEr index provides the most sensitive distinction between controls and PD patients. However, it is less sensitive to differences between patients, which may be best emphasized by use of the VctrEr, T50%, and Nints.
4. The ability of PD patients to specify the direction of upcoming movements is impaired even when visual feedback is allowed and no speed is required. This impairment is apparent in sine wave tracing, but is noticeable even in straight line tracing.

Discussion

The present paper describes a methodology for quantitative evaluation of impairments in motor control which characterize parkinsonism. To be effective, such a method must be sensitive enough to detect early symptoms at a preclinical stage. It must have a wide range of operation, so that changes in patients with advanced disease would still register, and it must be practical enough to be implemented in a regular clinical setting. The present system meets all these requirements by combining different tests which apply to different aspects of motor control. In parallel, the scoring system relates differentially to various aspects of central motor programming, which together allow quantitative evaluation of disease severity.

Acknowledgments. The author is greatly indebted to Prof. M. Youdim, without whose encouragement and support this publication would not be possible. The invaluable help of Dr. J. Aharon in providing access to her patients is acknowledged.

References

1. Berardelli A, Accornero N, Argenta M, Meco G, Manfredi M (1986) Fast complex arm movements in Parkinson's disease. J Neurol Neurosurg Psychiatry 49:1146–1149

2. Flowers KA (1976) Visual "closed loop" and "open loop" characteristics of voluntary movement in patients with parkinsonism and intention tremor. Brain 99:269–310
3. Hoehn MM, Yahr MD (1967) Parkinsonism: onset, progression and mortality. Neurology 17:427–442
4. Marsden CD (1982) The mysterious motor function of the basal ganglia: the Robert Wartenberg lecture. Neurology 32:514–539
5. Tatton WG, Greenwood CE (1991) Rescue of dying neurons: a new action for Deprenyl in MPTP parkinsonism. J Neurosci Res 30:666–672
6. Teasdale N, Phillips J, Stelmach GE (1990) Temporal movement control in patients with Parkinson's disease. J Neurol Neurosurg Psychiatry 53:862–868
7. Warabi T, Yanagisawa N (1988) Changes in strategy of aiming-tasks in Parkinson's disease. Brain 111:497–505

Kinematic Properties of Upper Limb Movement Trajectories

H. Hefter, J.D. Cooke, S.H. Brown, P. Weiss, H. Kuhlmann, and H.-J. Freund

Introduction

Since the beginning of this century, unidirectional goal-directed movements of the upper extremity have been extensively studied (e.g., [23]). Early on, movements were divided into the intuitively satisfying classes of "fast" and "slow." This classification found support in the apparent differences of the electromyographic (EMG) activities associated with these movements (e.g., [9,23]). Subsequently, many workers have studied the relationship between muscle activation and the characteristics or kinematics of the resulting movements. For the most part, relations were sought between the magnitudes, durations, and relative timing of phasic EMG bursts and such movement characteristics as movement amplitude and duration (e.g., [2]). These two kinematic properties of movement were studied because it seemed reasonable that they were important in determining the central program for movement. In addition, however, they were the only movement characteristics which were amenable to experimental manipulation. That is, one could ask subjects to make movements of different sizes or at different speeds. From such experiments it was concluded that movements of a wide range of properties are generated by modification of a common motor program. For example, a linear relation between movement peak velocity and amplitude is seen in movements ranging in amplitude from 1° to over 60° (Fig. 1). Thus, relationships between movement parameters are preserved, although the movements may be produced by different motor units with different discharge characteristics.

The Bell-Shaped Velocity Profile

In part, this regular relation between movement size and speed arises because of the tendency to make movements having a standard temporal structure. Movement velocity is smooth and bell-shaped, with approximately the same time spent in acceleration as in deceleration. Such profiles have been observed in single joint movements in the horizontal plane (e.g., [19]) as well as in single joint, vertical

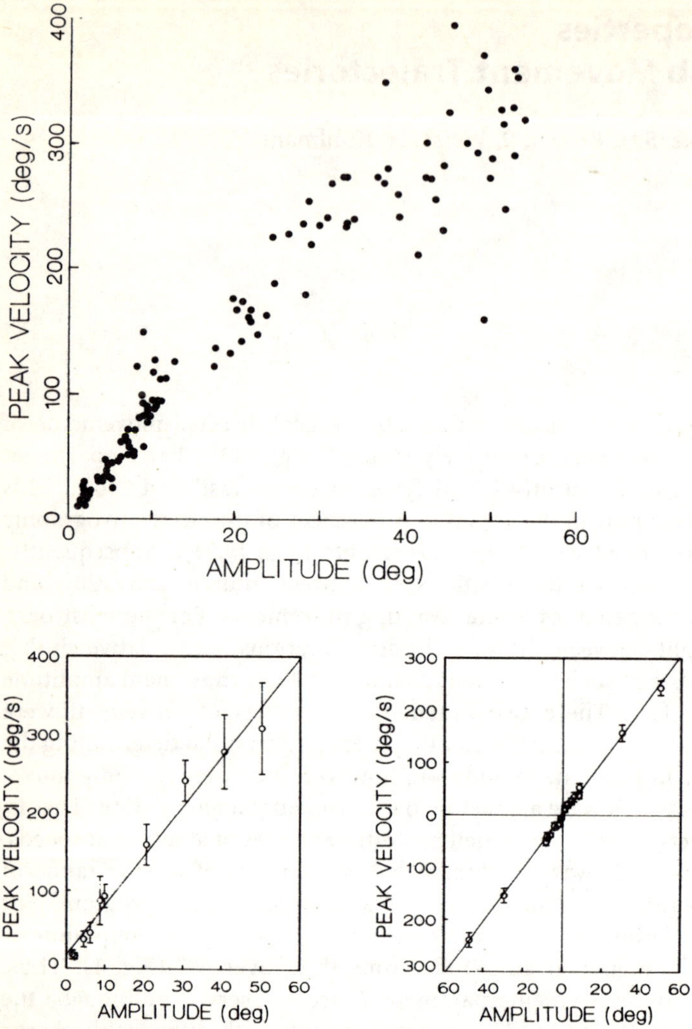

Fig. 1. The *upper* part reveals peak velocities of more than 90 forearm flexions of a normal subject performed at different movement amplitudes. Mean values of the same data are presented in the *left lower* part. The linear relationship between peak velocity and amplitude over a range of 60° is evident. In the *right lower* part, mean peak velocities of flexions and extensions are presented for another normal subject. The linear relationship between peak velocity and amplitude is preserved over a large amplitude range for extensions and flexions

movements [1], multijoint movements [14,21], speech movements [18], and movements of the vocal folds [15]. This velocity profile remains "invariant" under scaling in both amplitude and duration [7,14,19]. This invariance has been taken as indicative of an underlying organizing principle in the central planning [20] of the commands for movement (e.g., [10,12,17]).

The "Triphasic" EMG Pattern

The commands for movement have been extensively studied using the EMG. Since the time of Wacholder and Altenburger [23] it has been recognized that "fast" movements are produced by a regular sequence of phasic activity in the opposing muscle groups. This regular pattern, consisting of agonist (AG1), antagonist (ANT), and second agonist (AG2) bursts, is known as the "triphasic" pattern. Given the presumed importance of movement amplitude and speed in movement planning, many studies have been made on the relationship between these kinematic parameters and the characteristics of the phasic components of the triphasic pattern (e.g., [2,8,11,16]). Recently, however, it has been shown that the triphasic pattern mainly encodes the acceleratory characteristics of the movement. Using phase plane tracking, Brown and Cooke [3] showed that the triphasic pattern is modified to produce movements which do not have the bell-shaped profile. Changes in the relative durations of acceleration and deceleration are associated with marked changes in EMG, even though movement duration, amplitude, and peak velocity remain constant (Fig. 2).

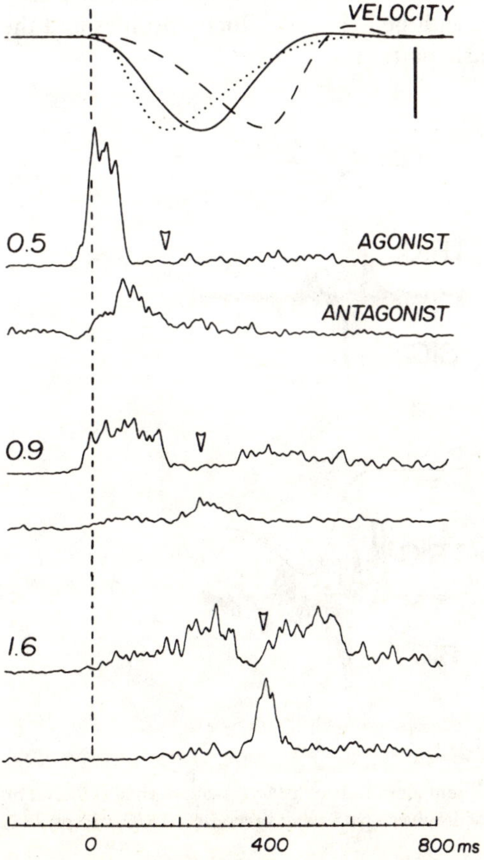

Fig. 2. Variation of the symmetry ratio (acceleration duration divided by deceleration duration) of elbow flexions from 0.5 to 1.6 modifies the underlying electromyogram (EMG) pattern considerably

The "Quadraphasic" EMG Pattern and Symmetric Velocity Profile

While movement-related EMG activity has often been termed triphasic, there are, in many movements, four distinguishable periods of phasic activity (Fig. 3). There is often an early period of antagonist activity which, while noted by many investigators, has been little studied. The explanation of this quadraphasic EMG pattern arose from the demonstration that phasic EMG during single joint movements encodes the acceleration–deceleration characteristics of the movement. Cooke and Brown [6] investigated movements made at constant velocity. Such movements are initiated by a "pulse" of acceleration followed by a period of movement at constant velocity (zero acceleration) and terminated by a pulse of deceleration. In such movements, acceleration is developed by the initial agonist burst (AG1). This acceleration is terminated by the early antagonist burst (ANT1). Deceleration is initiated by an antagonist burst (ANT2) and terminated by a second agonist burst (AG2). Thus, acceleration and deceleration are produced by paired activity of the opposing muscles. When the duration of the constant velocity phase of movement was progressively decreased (Fig. 4), the acceleration and deceleration pulses merged to form the pattern associated with bell-shaped velocity profiles and the EMG bursts merged to form the triphasic pattern.

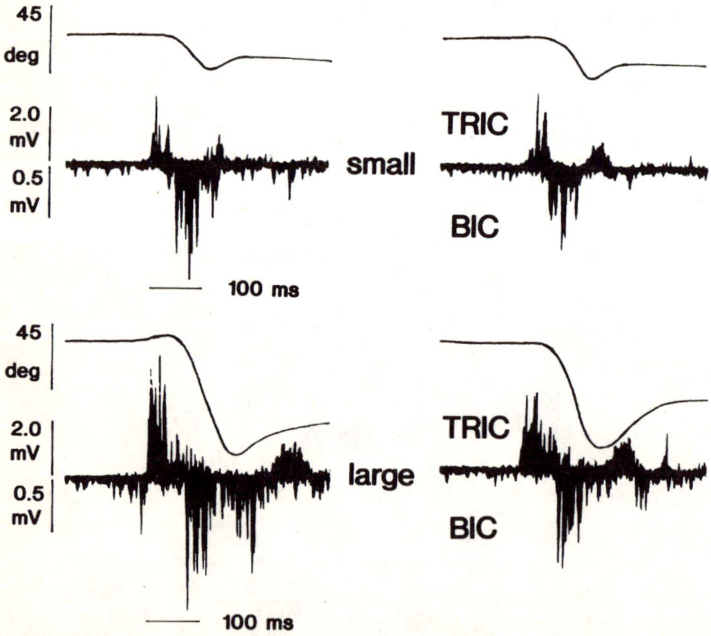

Fig. 3. Four single rapid elbow extensions of different amplitude of a 35-year-old normal subject. For the largest movement (*left lower part*) a clear quadraphasic pattern was recorded. *TRIC*, triceps; *BIC*, biceps

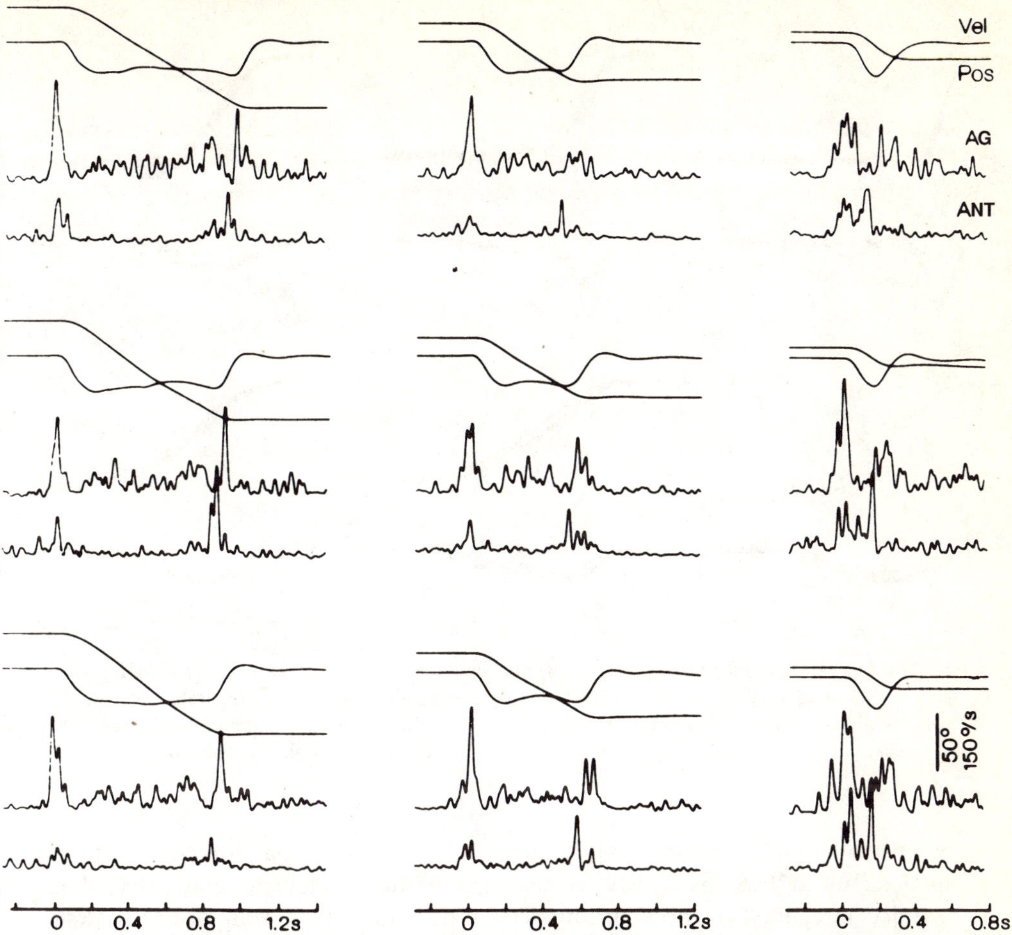

Fig. 4. Tracking of a constant velocity profile yields two pairs of electromyogram (EMG) activity: an agonist and antagonist burst pair for the acceleration and an antagonist and agonist burst pair for the deceleration. With decrease of the duration of the constant velocity plateau, the "quadraphasic" pattern merges into the well-known "triphasic" pattern. (This type of constant velocity tracking needs a considerable amount of training until it can be performed successfully). Velocity (Vel), position (Pos)

Thus, the symmetrical velocity profile seen in many movements arises as a consequence of an underlying organization in which acceleration and deceleration are both produced by paired muscle activities, the roles of the agonist and antagonist being reversed. The symmetry of the velocity profile thus arises from the symmetry in the organization of the acceleration and deceleration.

Velocity Profiles in Parkinsonian and Cerebellar Patients

Clinically, this explanation of the symmetry of the velocity profile of movements is supported from studies on cerebellar patients. Such patients have disturbed

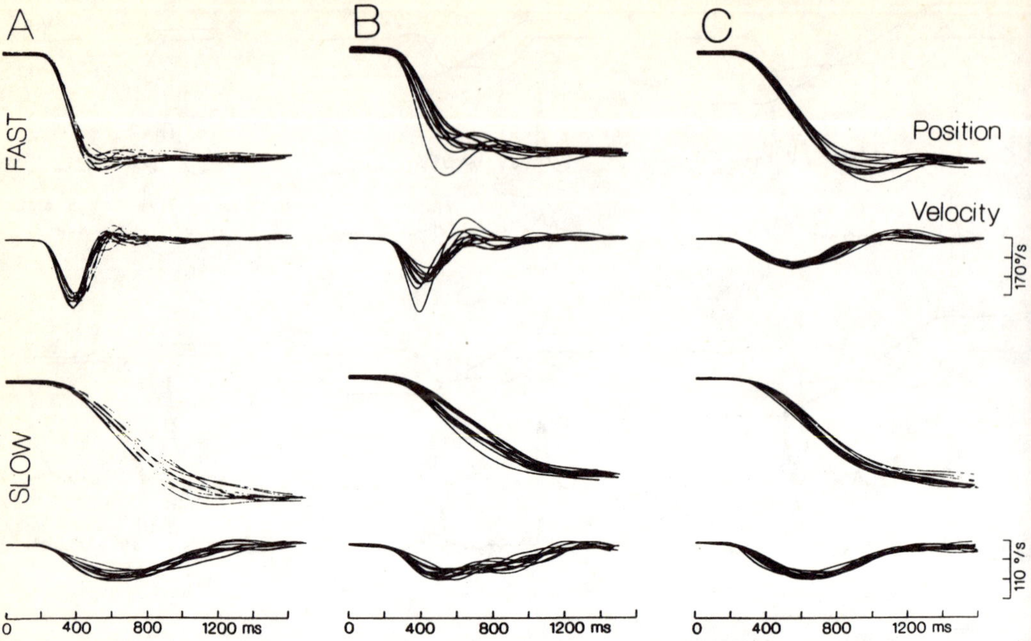

Fig. 5A–C. Comparison of fast (*upper traces*) and slow (*lower traces*) forearm flexions in a normal subject (**A**), a cerebellar patient (**B**), and a parkinsonian patient (**C**) of comparable age. In the parkinsonian patient and the normal subject, the velocity profiles look fairly symmetric, whereas in the cerebellar patient the profiles appear to be asymmetric, especially in the slow movements

agonist–antagonist relations [4]. In contrast, parkinsonian patients who perform movements at least as slowly as cerebellar patients may not have disturbed agonist–antagonist relations or impairment of the relative timing of EMG bursts [22]. Analysis of the symmetry ratio (relative times spent in acceleration and deceleration) in these two patient groups shows that it is movement amplitude dependent in cerebellar patients, whereas it is amplitude independent in both Parkinson's patients and normal subjects. This is illustrated in Fig. 5.

As noted previously, symmetric velocity profiles are not only observed during single joint movements, but also during a variety of more complex movements such as reaching and grasping. Such movements are illustrated in Fig. 6. During a pointing movement of the entire arm to a target, the finger tip performs a movement trajectory with a symmetric profile of the tangential velocity. Such a bell-shaped velocity curve with only two changes of curvature minimizes the energy demands in comparison to other profiles with more changes of the curvature [12,17]. In contrast to the single joint case, how the motor system realizes such velocity profiles during complex multijoint movements is not known. Such movements constitute the majority of our standard repertoire and an understanding of their generation is crucial to understanding the motor dysfunctions resulting from various disease processes.

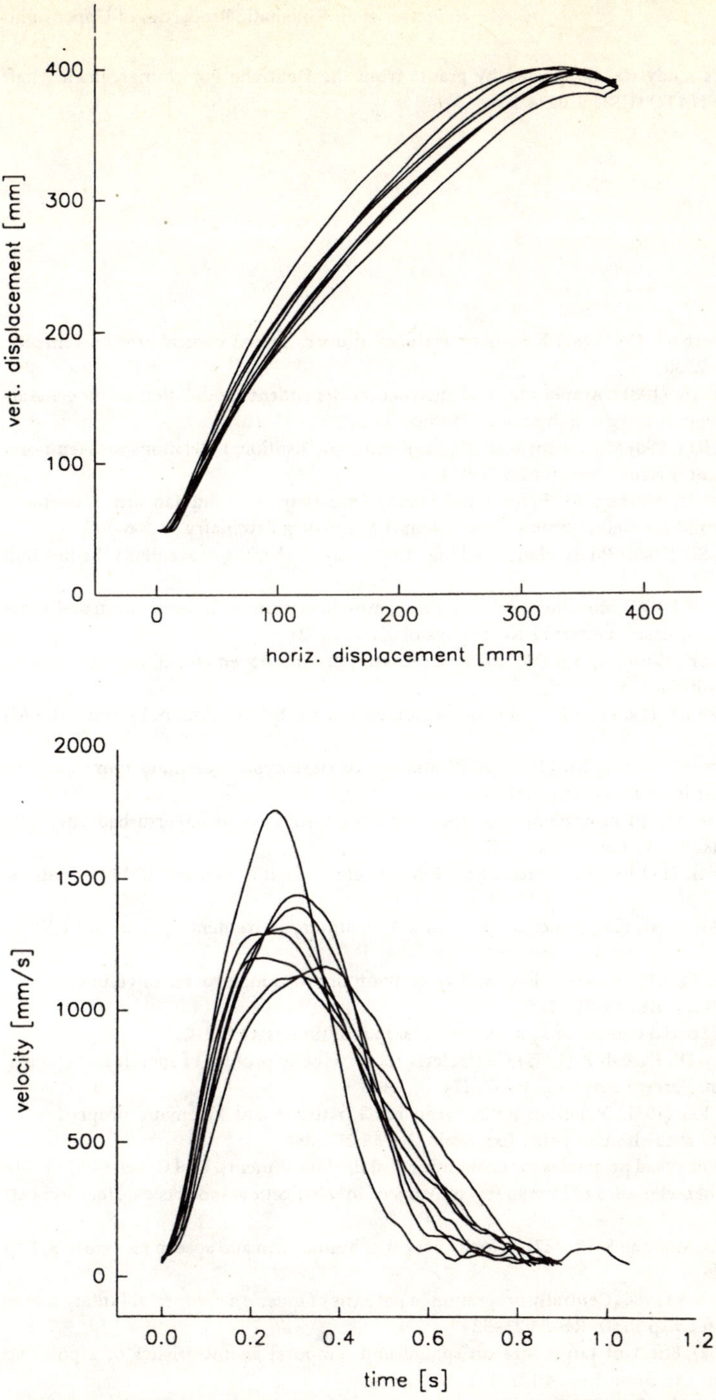

Fig. 6. The trajectories of the finger tip of a normal subject during pointing to a target (*upper part*) are generated with rather symmetric tangential velocity profiles (*lower part*). Trajectories were recorded using a Selspot II-system

Acknowledgment. This study was supported by grants from the Deutsche Forschungsgemeinschaft (SFB 194, A5) and the NATO (CRG 910234).

References

1. Atkeson CG, Hollerbach JM (1985) Kinematic features of unrestrained vertical arm movements. J Neurosci 5:2318–2330
2. Brown SH, Cooke JD (1981) Amplitude- and instruction-dependent modulation of movement-related electromyogram activity in human. J Physiol (Lond) 316:97–107
3. Brown SH, Cooke JD (1990) Movement-related phasic muscle activation: I. Relations with temporal profile of movement. J Neurophysiol 63:455–464
4. Brown SH, Hefter H, Mertens M, Freund H-J (1990) Disturbances in human arm movement trajectory due to mild cerebellar dysfunction. J Neurol Neurosurg Psychiatry 53:306–313
5. Cooke JD, Brown SH (1986) Phase plane tracking: a new way of shaping movements. Br Res Bull 16:435–437
6. Cooke JD, Brown SH (1990) Movement-related phasic muscle activation. II. Generation and functional role of the "triphasic" pattern. J Neurophysiol 63:465–472
7. Cooke JD, Brown SH, Cunningham DA (1989) Kinematics of arm movements in elderly humans. Neurobiol Aging 10:150–165
8. Hallett M, Marsden CD (1979) Ballistic flexion movements of the human thumb. J Physiol (Lond) 294:33–50
9. Hallett M, Shahani BT, Young RR (1975) EMG analysis of stereotyped voluntary movements in man. J Neurol Neurosurg Psychiatry 38:1154–1162
10. Hasan Z (1986) Optimized movement trajectories and joint stiffness in unperturbed, inertially loaded movements. Biol Cybern 53:373–382
11. Hoffmann DS, Strick PI (1990) Step tracking movements of the wrist in humans. II. EMG analysis. J Neurosci 10:142–152
12. Hogan N (1984) An organizing principle for a class of voluntary movements. J Neurosci 4:2745–2754
13. Lestienne F (1979) Effects of inertial load and velocity on the tracking process of voluntary limb movements. Exp Brain Res 35:407–418
14. Morasso P (1981) Spatial control of arm movements. Exp Brain Res 42:223–227
15. Munhall DG, Ostry DJ, Parush A (1985) Characteristics of velocity profiles of speech movements. J Exp Psychol Hum Percept Perform 11:457–474
16. Mustard BE, Lee RG (1987) Relationship between EMG patterns and kinematic properties for flexion movements at the human wrist. Exp Brain Res 66:247–256
17. Nelson WL (1983) Physical principles for economies of skilled movements. Biol Cybern 46:135–147
18. Ostry DJ (1986) Characteristics of human jaw movement in mastication and speech. Neurosci Lett Suppl 26:S87
19. Ostry DJ, Cooke JD, Munhall KG (1987) Velocity curves of human arm and speech movements. Exp Brain Res 68:37–46
20. Sanes JN, Jennings VA (1984) Centrally programmed patterns of muscle activity in voluntary motor behavior of humans. Exp Brain Res 54:23–32
21. Soechting JF (1984) Effect of target size on spatial and temporal characteristics of a pointing movement in man. Exp Brain Res 54:121–132
22. Teulings H-L, Stelmach GE (1991) Control of stroke, size, peak acceleration, and stroke duration in parkinsonian handwriting. Hum Mov Sci 10:315–334
23. Wacholder K, Altenburger H (1926) Beiträge zur Physiologie der willkürlichen Bewegung. X. Einzelbewegungen. Pflugers Arch 214:642–661

Discussion

Dr. Hallett: I would like to make a comment emphasizing one of the points that you made in that the task you ask the particular subject to do really determines exactly what they actually do. One of the differences between the results that Brown and Cooke got in relation to the movement parameters in patients with cerebellar disease versus the results that I got with a number of workers including John Rothwell and the work that J. Hore and H.C. Diener did was that in the cerebellar patients, we found a larger acceleration time compared to deceleration time in both of those two studies compared to the work of Brown and Cooke. We tried to look at what could possibly be the reason for the differences in the study and my eventual interpretation was that the differences were really related to the nature of the task, that while you have said that the task was to do it as quickly as possible, the accuracy demands in that task were still relatively high. That may be the reason for the particular differences, so I think that the actual task demanded is very important and what people actually do is very different depending upon all the little details of the requested action.

Dr. Hefter: I can only agree with that. You have to carefully control how you instruct people. You should do that in a standardized way. I think that is very important and has been shown by a variety of studies.

Use of Quantitative Assessment in Evaluating Patients with Neural Transplants

J.C. Rothwell

Introduction

One of the main inclusion criteria for the Swedish/UK Parkinson's disease transplant programme is that the patients should have severe hypokinesia and rigidity [7,8]. The aim of our physiological evaluation programme was to select an objective method of measuring hypokinesia which would be consistent with the clinical evaluation of the patient and which would be sensitive enough to detect any changes in performance after transplantation.

We selected the flex and squeeze task developed by Benecke et al. [2,3], which consists of a combination of four different simple and complex arm movements: (1) flexion of the elbow alone, (2) squeeze of an isometric force transducer in the hand alone, (3) simultaneous performance of flex and squeeze and (4) sequential performance of squeeze followed by elbow flexion. The inclusion of simultaneous and sequential movements in these tasks is important. Although patients with Parkinson's disease are impaired when performing simple movements about one joint alone (e.g., [5]), the speed of these movements generally is not well correlated with the clinical status of the patient. For example, Benecke et al. [2] showed that the speed of a simple self-paced elbow flexion movement did not correlate well with the degree of clinically assessed akinesia in a group of ten patients with Parkinson's disease. Even within a single patient, performance on these tasks changed little with the clinical state of the patient. In a later study, Benecke et al. [4] investigated five patients with Parkinson's disease "on" and "off" their normal L-dopa therapy. The speed of elbow flexion increased in the "on" condition, but only marginally, and never reached normal values. Much better correlations with clinical status were seen when performance in simultaneous and sequential movements was analysed.

During simultaneous or sequential tasks, normal subjects perform the individual components of flex and squeeze at the same maximum speed as they do when they perform each task alone. In addition, the interonset latency (IOL, the time from the beginning of the squeeze component to the beginning of the flexion component of the movement) in a sequential task is usually of the order of 240 ms. Normal subjects can decrease the IOL further, but only at the expense of a decrease in the speed of the second (elbow flexion) movement

[1]. Given the usual instructions of the task, that subjects should move as fast as possible, all normal subjects seem to prefer to execute the individual movements as fast as possible at the expense of a slight prolongation of the interonset latency. Patients with Parkinson's disease have additional difficulties in performing complex movements, over and above those predicted from analysis of each single movement alone (see classical description by [11]). In the simultaneous flex and squeeze task, the speed of both components of the movement are slowed. In the sequential task, the speed of the second movement is often slowed and the interonset latency prolonged. As in normals, the speed of the second movement depends to some extent on the interonset latency. Benecke et al. [2] showed that the extra slowing in simultaneous movements (compared with the speed of each single movement performed on its own), as well as the interonset latency in sequential movements, was well correlated with the clinical state of the patient. In addition, the change in these parameters when patients were studied "on" their therapy as compared with their movements studied 12 h after withdrawal of therapy was much greater than the change in each simple movement made alone.

Benecke et al. [2] considered two other combinations of complex arm movements: elbow flexion plus an isotonic movement of the fingers (rather than the isometric squeeze) and flexion of one arm coupled with squeeze movement of the other arm. Although both these combinations were affected in patients with Parkinson's disease, the largest changes were seen in the unilateral flexion plus isometric squeeze task which was chosen here.

We also considered several other possible physiological tests to perform in addition to the flex and squeeze tasks. These were simple and complex visual reaction times, ballistic wrist flexion movements (e.g., [5]), long-latency stretch reflexes in wrist or thumb flexor muscles (e.g., [9]), anticipatory postural responses in leg muscles (e.g., [12]) and *bereitschaftspotentials* (e.g., [6]). However, we were limited in the time available to study each patient. All were evaluated in the early morning, 12 h after overnight withdrawal of their L-dopa therapy, and tests had to be performed on both the left and right sides of the body. Most patients are uncomfortable and irritable after withdrawal of therapy, and in order to obtain reliable results, it is necessary to perform evaluation in the shortest time possible. Because of this, we concentrated on the flex and squeeze task, although data was collected on reaction times and *bereitschaftspotentials* in some, but not all of the patients. Stretch reflexes and postural anticipatory reflexes were not examined, because these have an intrinsically high variability and are not well correlated to the clinical state of the patient. Rothwell et al. [9] showed that the long-latency stretch reflex in wrist and thumb muscle was increased in rigid patients with Parkinson's disease, but that there was an enormous spread of values between patients with similar degrees of clinical rigidity. The same conclusion was reached by Traub et al. [12] when they examined anticipatory postural responses in leg muscles of unstable parkinsonian patients.

Methods

Subjects were seated comfortably with their right arm abducted to 90° at the shoulder and their semipronated forearm resting on a lightweight manipulandum which was pivoted so as to be co-axial with the elbow joint. The angular position of the elbow was monitored by a sensitive potentiometer attached to the pivot. At the end of the manipulandum, and adjusted according to the length of the forearm, was a U-shaped bar of aluminium which could be grasped between the thumb and the finger. A strain gauge was mounted on one of the vertical arms of the U, so that the force of squeeze could be monitored. Subjects were asked to perform four different tasks: (1) flex the elbow joint as rapidly as possible in their own time through an angle of 15° from a starting angle of 135° flexion ("flex" task); (2) squeeze the strain gauge as rapidly as possible in their own time up to a force of 30 N ("squeeze" task); (3) execute both tasks simultaneously as rapidly as possible in their own time ("simultaneous" task); (4) perform an isometric squeeze up to 30 N followed as rapidly as possible by elbow flexion through 15°; the elbow flexion was not to start before the target force of 30 N had been achieved ("sequential" task). The four tasks were performed in a cyclic order. Both elbow position and the amount of grip force were displayed as two vertical bars 2 cm in length on an oscilloscope screen 60 cm in front of the subject. Each individual performed about five practice trials of each of the four tasks; thereafter, ten single trials of each type were collected. Measurements were made on each single record using the computer visual display unit. From the data of Benecke et al. [2], we selected four measurements which were both the most reliable from trial to trial and subject to the greatest changes with variations in the clinical status of the patient. These were: (1) time taken to perform the elbow flexion movement alone, (2) time taken to perform elbow flexion in the simultaneous task, (3) time taken to perform elbow flexion in the sequential task and (4) the IOL between the onset of squeeze and the onset of flex in the sequential task. The duration of movement was estimated by visual inspection of the velocity signal (onset to first zero crossing).

The most important aspect for these tasks is to secure optimal performance by the patients in all the movements. Strong encouragement must therefore be given at all times. In addition, speed of movement, rather than accuracy must be emphasised. In our experiments, we allowed up to ±50% over/undershoot from trial to trial of the target movement.

Results

Two groups of two patients with Parkinson's disease have now undergone foetal neural transplants into the striatum of one hemisphere. The first two patients were operated in 1987 [7]. Although there were no significant postoperative complications, there was no major therapeutic benefit as judged either by the patient, the clinical neurologists or performance of simple and complex arm movements.

A minor improvement in performance of flex and squeeze movements contralateral to the graft was seen in patient 2 (Fig. 1) 6 months postoperatively, at a time when there seemed to be a slight increase in the percentage of daily time spent in the "on" state from 43%–47% to 57%–63%. The improvement in performance of the sequential task was much greater than that seen for elbow flexion on its own.

The second two patients were operated using a modified technique in which the transplantation catheter was smaller in diameter. Both patients showed a gradual and significant amelioration of parkinsonian symptoms (most marked in patient 3) starting at 6 and 12 weeks after grafting, respectively, reaching a maximum stability at approximately 4–5 months; the patients remained relatively stable thereafter for a 1-year follow-up period. There was clinical improvement in the amount of time spent in the "on" phase and a reduction in the number of daily "off" periods. There was less bradykinesia and rigidity during the "off" phase, which was mainly, although not solely on the side contralateral to the graft. Repeated positron emission tomographic scans in these patients showed increased uptake of fluorodopa in the grafted striatum in both patients, whereas non-grafted striatal areas showed unchanged or reduced fluorodopa uptake [10]. The interpretation is that foetal mesencephalic grafts can survive transplantation into diseased parkinsonian brains and exert significant and sustained functional effects.

The results for the flex and squeeze task are illustrated in Fig. 2 for patient 3, who had a left-sided implant. Also included is a graph showing the results of conventional clinical measurements of the speed of pronation/supination wrist movement. For the sake of clarity, normal data is not included on this graph; the

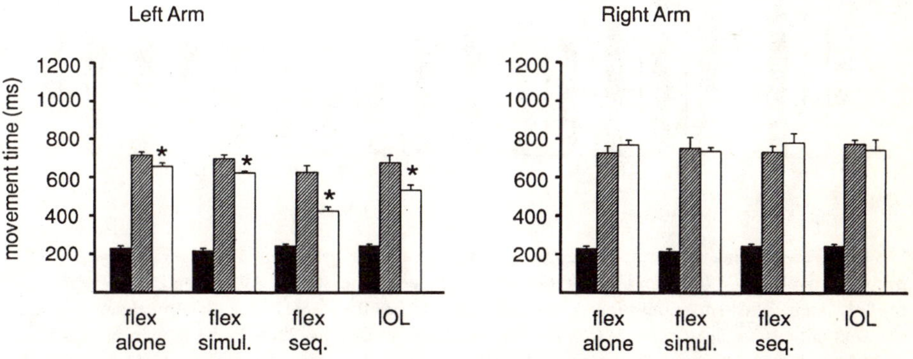

Fig. 1. Results from the flex and squeeze task in patient 2 on the right and left sides pre-operatively (*hatched bars*) and 6 months post-operatively (*open bars*). Average data from a group of eight age-matched normal subjects (*solid bars*) are included for comparison. Histograms plot: (a) time taken for elbow flexion movement on its own (*flex alone*), (b) time taken for elbow flexion when performed at the same time as the squeeze (*flex simul.*), (c) time taken for elbow flexion in the sequential task (*flex seq.*) and (d) the interonset latency between squeeze and flex in the sequential task (*IOL*). All of the movements were self-paced and made as rapidly as possible. Data are means ±SEM. *Asterisks* indicate significant pre-operative versus post-operative differences ($p < 0.05$). All movements were made in the "off" sate

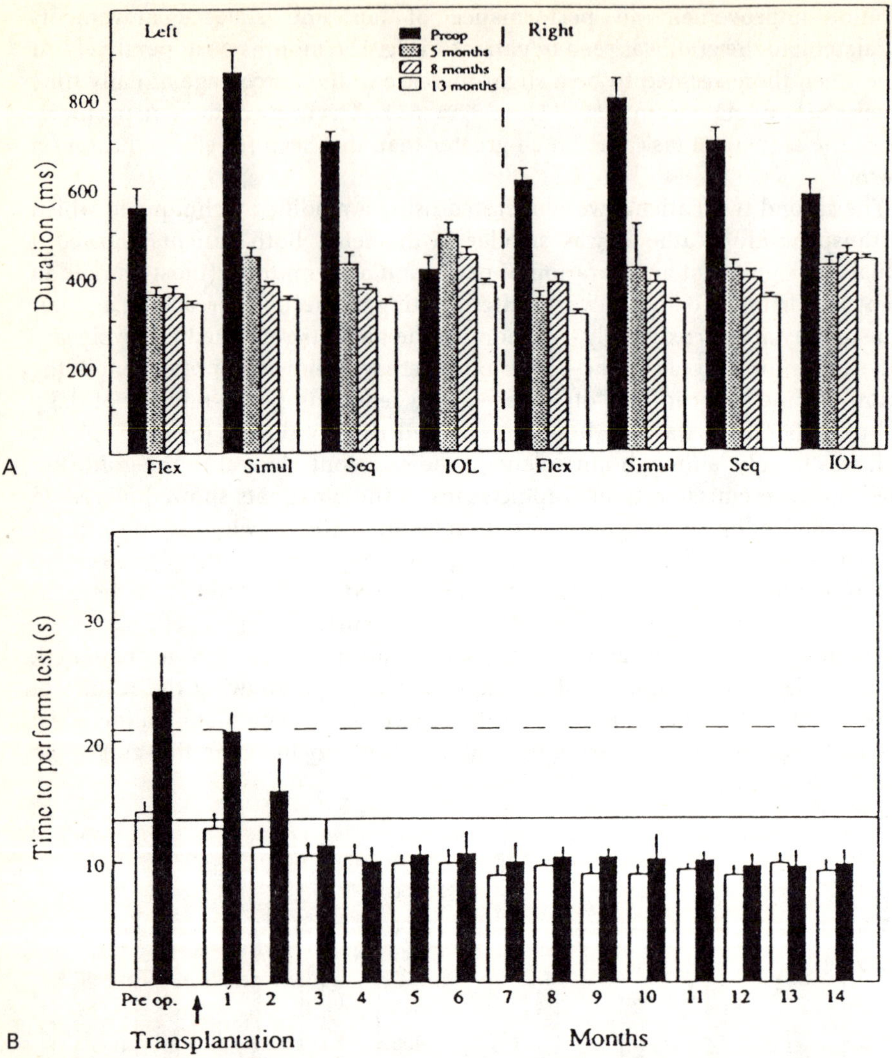

Fig. 2. **A** Performance of simple and complex arm movements by patient 3 on the right and left sides pre-operatively (*solid bars*) and at 5, 8 and 13 months post-operatively. All movements were made in the "off" state. The histograms plot: (a) the time taken to flex the elbow (*Flex*), (b) time taken to flex the elbow at the same time as squeeze (*Simul*), (c) time taken to flex the elbow in the sequential task (*Seq*), and (d) the interval between the onset of squeeze and flex in the sequential task (*IOL*). Data are means ±SEM. All movement times were improved ($p < 0.05$) 5 months after surgery except for the IOL on the left side. This improvement was sustained at 8 and 13 months. **B** Time taken to perform 20 pronations/supinations with the left (*open bars*) and right (*solid bars*) in the "off" state. From the second month after transplantation, this task was performed more rapidly than pre-operatively. The improvement was bilateral, but was more pronounced on the right side (contralateral to the graft). From [8] with permission

normal values, however, can be obtained from the example in Fig. 1. These results are in striking comparison to the data from the previous patient. There was a clear increase in the speed of elbow flexion movements in the simple, simultaneous and sequential tasks on both sides post-operatively. In addition, there was a decrease in the IOL on the right hand side, which was contralateral to the graft. These results compare very well with clinical measurements of pronation/supination movements, which also show improvement (particularly on the right side) 2–3 months post-operatively.

Conclusions

Measurements of movement time in simple and complex arm movements can provide a useful objective measure of parkinsonian bradykinesia. The measurements correlate with clinical assessment in patients who have undergone foetal nigral transplants.

Acknowledgements. This work was a collaborative effort with many colleagues, in particular Dr. Benecke, Dr. Thompson and Dr. Day. Mr. R. Bedlington was technically indispensable.

References

1. Benecke R, Rothwell JC, Day BL, Dick JPR, Marsden CD (1986a) Motor strategies involved in the performance of sequential movement. Exp Brain Res 83:585–595
2. Benecke R, Rothwell JC, Dick JPR, Day BL, Marsden CD (1986b) Performance of simultaneous movements in patients with Parkinson's disease. Brain 109:739–757
3. Benecke R, Rothwell JC, Day BL, Dick JPR, Marsden CD (1987a) Disturbance of sequential movements in patients with Parkinson's disease. Brain 110:361–379
4. Benecke R, Rothwell JC, Dick JPR, Day BL, Marsden CD (1987b) Simple and complex movements "off" and "on" treatment in patients with Parkinson's disease. J Neurol Neurosurg Psychiatry 50:296–303
5. Berardelli A, Dick JPR, Rothwell JC, Day BL, Marsden CD (1986) Scaling of the size of the first agonist burst during rapid wrist movements in patients with Parkinson's disease. J Neurol Neurosurg Psychiatry 49:1273–1279
6. Dick JPR, Rothwell JC, Day BL, Cantello R, Buruma O, Gioux M, Benecke R, Berardelli A, Thompson PD, Marsden CD (1989) The Bereitschaftspotential is abnormal in Parkinson's disease. Brain 112:233–244
7. Lindvall O, Rehncrons S, Brundin P et al. (1989) Human foetal dopamine neurones grafted into the striatum in two patients with severe Parkinson's disease. Arch Neurol 46:615–631
8. Lindvall O, Widner H, Rehncrona S et al. (1992) Transplantation of foetal dopamine neurones in Parkinson's disease: one year clinical and neurophysiological observations in two patients with putaminal implants. Ann Neurol 31:155–165
9. Rothwell JC, Obeso JA, Traub MM, Marsden CD (1983) The behaviour of the long latency stretch reflex in patients with Parkinson's disease. J Neurol Neurosurg Psychiatry 46:35–44
10. Sawle GV, Bloomfield PM, Brooks DJ et al. (1992) Transplantation of foetal dopamine neurones in Parkinson's disease: positron emission tomography (18F)-6-L-fluorodopa studies in two patients with putaminal implants. Ann Neurol 31:166–173

11. Schwab RS, Chafetz ME, Walker S (1954) Control of two simultaneous voluntary motor acts in normals and in parkinsonism. Arch Neurol Psychiatry 72:591–598
12. Traub MM, Rothwell JC, Marsden CD (1980) Abnormal anticipatory postural responses in Parkinson's disease and other akinetic-rigid syndromes, and in cerebellar ataxia. Brain 103:393–412

Discussion

Dr. Korczyn: Congratulations on your laborious efforts and your success in showing that some of the complex arm movement analyses are clinically relevant. The question is whether they really are relevant. The fact that you show a correlation with what you as a clinician see is of interest, but it does not address the issue of whether it also correlates with, say, activities of daily living (ADL). After all, most of us here are both clinicians and neuroscientists, and although we are interested in neuroscience, we basically need to know how the patients function, whether they do any better, and whether your sequential analysis correlates with the ADL better than with anything else.

Dr, Rothwell: I think that's a very reasonable point and you've noticed that we haven't done that correlation, which is very reasonable. I think, in fact I'm quite sure if we were to work it out, if we were to have given the patients a sort of inventory of ADL, it would have correlated quite well in these particular cases. I know that because certainly for this last patient that I showed you, he's doing so well that in fact now he's not taking any medication at all. He spends far more of his time "on": 90% of his time is "on" every day, whereas before it was 50% "off". Although we haven't done a proper analysis, I think it would be true.

Dr. Korczyn: What you measure is movement time first, pure movement time; it does not contain the reaction time and so on. What people complain of when they say that they are slow or what we notice when we examine them and say that they have bradykinesia is that when we tell them to do something or they want to do something, it takes them a long time. So this is not only the actual movement time, but also the preparatory phase, which then includes the reaction time plus many other things. I think that's what you show: that the difference is not really due to – or not restricted to or even mainly due to – the movement slowness per se but also includes a lot of other things that go wrong in patients with Parkinson's disease. Can you tell us something about the treatment of the patients? Have these patients been treated with levodopa? I remember you said they were off drug when you tested them, but there could be some residual effect of drugs if they have been taken prior to it. Have they been stable on their therapeutic drug?

Dr. Rothwell: The Swedish program is very strict on this. They're stable on their medication for 1 year preoperatively and then subsequently postoperatively, I think, except for this last patient, who's now being withdrawn from his medication after 2 years.

Dr. Horstink: I'm not surprised that clinical rating of akinesia did not correlate to simple movements, single simple movements, because as far as I know the clinical rating of akinesia is also based on sequential or more complex movements. So how did you measure your clinical rating? I suggest that there are sequential or repetitive or complex movements and no simple movements?

Dr. Rothwell: That's right. They're complex. It's not me who measures them, it's someone else; it involves doing complex movements, e.g., pronation/supination. They are not simple movements, because of course they don't correlate, so it's not surprising.

Dr. Deuschl: I wonder if you would agree with the following statement: "If you want to investigate a patient, you first have to define the clinical symptom and then you have to be with your measure as near to that clinical symptom as possible; then you will succeed." Is that the way to do instrumental tests?

Dr. Rothwell: That's what we want to innovate, and that's what we wanted to do with these particular tests. We wanted some sort of measurement which would reflect what the clinician thought was happening, because if we have a measurement that the clinicians don't agree with, then you won't really get very far with them when you're trying to do a cooperative study. We're trying to look at what the clinician is trying to assess and see whether we can measure it. That was the main aim of our study.

Dr. Panzer: You said that the measurement you showed didn't seem to respond well to dopa and you correlated that with the akinesia clinical rating. I think we really need to address: bradykinesia and akinesia are, clinically rated, different things. Akinesia is not necessarily responsive to L-dopa, as some people have noted here in the last 2 days, and bradykinesia may often be confused with other things such as rigidity. I think we could spend some very valuable time in reaching an agreement on what we mean when we say akinesia, hypokinesia, bradykinesia; if we had some uniformity of terminology, we would be more knowledgeable about how these things respond. There is as yet no agreement upon terminology. People use the same terminology for different things and different terminology for the same thing.

Measurement of Diadochokinesia

P. Klotz and P.H. Kraus

Introduction

Diadochokinesia is a fast oscillating movement of the agonist–antagonist type. It is interesting for assessment because it shows disturbances early. The disturbance of this movement was first described by Babinski in 1907 (cited after [3]) as "dysdiadochokinesia."

Dysdiadochokinesia is not a well-defined entity, it is a label for different disturbances of this kind of movements. Dysdiadochokinesia is the common end of different disturbances between different parts of the nervous system and, for example, of muscles and joints. As seen in clinical investigation, different cause show at least partially distinguishable, different disturbances in diadochokinetic movements.

Therefore, it should be of interest to investigate diadochokinesia for developing different parameters which describe this complex movement more clearly. Our intention was to gain a better understanding of the as yet unclarified central control mechanisms of fast motor performance.

Research Design and Methods

There are different designs to measure diadochokinesia with instrumental methods, e.g., video recording or accelerometric assessment [2,4]. We decided to measure the movement mechanically and to process received data on a personal computer.

The disadvantages of this method include:

- Quasi laboratory testing conditions, i.e., we do not assess the natural movement, but only a nearly natural movement course
- Reduction of movement to a one-dimensional sampling criterion
- Reduction of the multiple degrees of freedom in the movement in the different joints

The advantages of this design are:

- Low costs in comparison to telemetric or video detection

- Reduced variability of movement and improved reliability of assessment by hardware control of the kind of movement
- Clearly arranged and easy to understand assessment of a movement quite close to natural conditions

Instrumental Design

The experimentee has to hold two balls in his hands almost as if holding an imperial orb, but holding the arms in a position quite similar to that adopted in clinical examination. This design assures comparability to clinical examination and reduces the degree of freedom in the shoulder joint and the cubital joint to nearly zero; it is also well defined for all experimentees. Rotational movement is limited by the flexibility of the radiocarpal joint. The total rotational angle of this joint is about 180°.

The arrangement of balls is adjustable for different height and width of the shoulders of the examinee and has to be adjusted for every test subject. Clinical impression is sufficient to make the adjustment.

Measurement of Movement

As in clinical examination, forced diadochokinetic movements are susceptible to early fatigue because of the presumably only weak oscillator in the assessed muscular system, so only a short time measurement is possible; this short time is, however, all that is needed. We decided to detect the movement during 5 s, i.e., for normal controls about 14 movement cycles. We started with detection after the movement had found its equilibrium, about 1–2 s after starting the movement. To obtain more information about the basic oscillation conditions, we assessed simultaneous movements of both hands together and afterwards diadochometry of first the right and then the left hand in a single-handed task under the same conditions.

Results

This assessment of diadochokinesia, as well as clinically well-known parameters, also provides information not detectable or obtainable in clinical rating. These parameters differentiate between patients and controls.

Frequency of Movement

As standard parameters, we processed the raw data for receiving information about the frequencies of movement cycles. The results are presented in Table 1. As

Table 1. Frequency of diadochokinesia in different samples (Hz)

	Controls n = 31	Parkinson's disease patients n = 32	Cerebellar ataxia patients[a] n = 20
Both hands together			
Left hand	2.757 ± 0.704	1.952 ± 1.006	1.543 ± 0.599
Intraindividual SD	0.194 ± 0.102	0.266 ± 0.254	0.123 ± 0.083
Right hand	2.877 ± 0.786	2.082 ± 1.071	1.589 ± 0.558
Intraindividual SD	0.184 ± 0.097	0.276 ± 0.286	0.120 ± 0.083
One-handed			
Left hand	2.823 ± 0.723	2.156 ± 1.101	1.605 ± 0.520
Intraindividual SD	0.230 ± 0.221	0.287 ± 0.359	0.139 ± 0.159
Right hand	2.976 ± 0.686	2.353 ± 1.280	1.593 ± 0.600
Intraindividual SD	0.218 ± 0.102	2.208 ± 1.545	0.121 ± 0.054

[a] Hereditary ataxia types Friedreich, Menzel, Holmes; cerebellar atrophia.

Table 2. Amplitude of diadochokinesia in different samples (degrees)

	Controls	Parkinson's disease patients	Cerebellar ataxia patients[a]
Both hands together			
Left hand	91.293 ± 20.451	63.525 ± 33.032	103.356 ± 15.223
Intraindividual SD	8.055 ± 3.659	8.186 ± 4.360	6.372 ± 3.855
Right hand	84.957 ± 17.211	60.293 ± 32.805	96.868 ± 16.347
Intraindividual SD	6.754 ± 5.270	7.184 ± 3.028	6.969 ± 3.361
One-handed			
Left hand	97.992 ± 20.593	73.824 ± 32.260	109.324 ± 14.378
Intraindividual SD	7.053 ± 5.121	7.241 ± 3.513	7.575 ± 7.926
Right hand	87.681 ± 22.199	66.019 ± 29.704	107.640 ± 20.659
Intraindividual SD	6.596 ± 2.569	7.567 ± 6.189	7.240 ± 4.859

[a] Hereditary ataxia types Friedreich, Menzel, Holmes; cerebellar atrophia.

expected from clinical experience, controls are faster than parkinsonian patients, who in turn are faster than patients with cerebellar ataxia. The frequencies for both hands together are not different. In the single-handed task, the dominant hand (in our sample the right hand) is slightly faster than the other hand. As we can see, parkinsonian patients have a broader range of frequencies intraindividually. The reason for this is probably the disturbed oscillator.

Amplitude of Movement

The amplitudes of diadochokinetic movements as presented in Table 2 show reduced values for the parkinsonian group. For all groups there are no differences between coordinated and single-handed tasks and no difference in intraindividual variability of amplitudes in the movement cycles.

Ratio of Frequencies of Simultaneous to Single-Handed Tasks

For the simultaneous task, we calculated the ratio of frequencies by dividing the frequency of the left hand by the frequency of the right hand; we computed the data for the single-handed task in the same way. The ratio of the frequencies of both hands for the simultaneous task is nearly exactly 1.0 in all tested groups. This is probably the effect of coordination between the supposedly different oscillators. This effect becomes most noticeable in the parkinsonian group when compared to the single-handed task. The values of the ratio for the single-handed task are 1.09 ± 0.13 for controls, but 1.10 ± 0.49 for parkinsonian patients and 1.01 ± 0.18 for patients suffering from cerebellar ataxia.

Shape of Movement and Phase Shift

Using a high degree of oversampling rate, we are not only able to detect frequency rates, amplitudes, and their variances, but also characteristics such as phase shift and shape of movements.

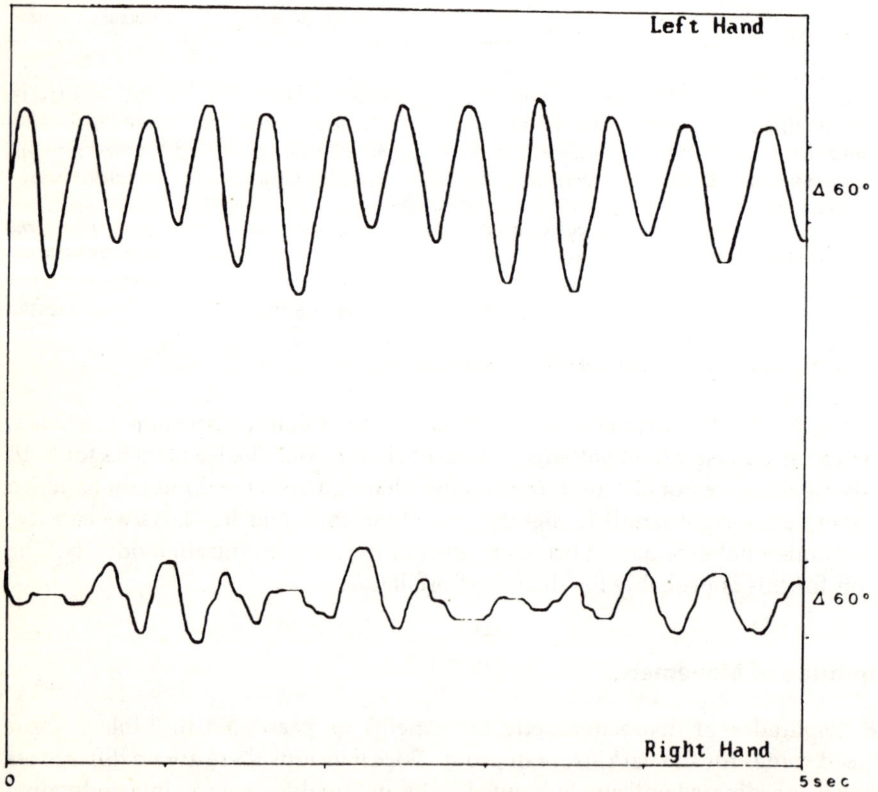

Fig. 1. Diadochokinetic movements of a 52-year-old parkinsonian patient. For details, see text

Figure 1 shows a diadochokinetic movement. Time is displayed on the x-axis and the degrees of movement are displayed as y-axis. The results shown are those for the simultaneous task performed by a male 52-year-old parkinsonian patient. The patient was suffering from a severe right accentuation and dyskinesias. First, it is shown how a severely disturbed oscillator (right hand) is triggered to reach a small amount of synchronization to the leading left hand. The shape of movement of the left hand is nearly sinusoidal, as would be expected for normal controls in both hands.

Second, the shape of movement of the right hand has changed. Because of hypokinesia, the amplitude is reduced. Here there is a slower ascent and plateaus are detectable at the turning points of movement; sometimes the movement stops between the turning points and is re-established by a new start. The movement looks quite irregular. The plateaus at the turning points have two functions: on the one hand, they are needed for a new impulse to move in the other direction and on the other hand, they constitute the necessary delay for re-establishing synchronization of movement with the left hand.

Conclusion

From the results of measurement of diadochokinesia, it seems that controls may have reached their transition frequency for ergodic movement, while values for patients remain below this frequency. These results are in agreement with the theoretical and practical results of Bunz and Haken [1] for similar movements.

Patients with Parkinson's disease and hereditary ataxia have reduced frequencies compared to controls and different shapes of movement compared to controls or the respective other disorder.

References

1. Bunz H, Haken H (1987) Quantitative theory of changes in oscillatory hand movements – application of methods of synergetics. In: Rensing L, an der Heiden U, Mackey MC (eds) Temporal disorder in human oscillatory systems. Springer, Berlin Heidelberg New York, pp 102–109
2. Evarts EV, Teräväinen H, Calne DB (1981) Reaction time in Parkinson's disease. Brain 101:167–186
3. Holmes G (1939) The cerebellum of man. Brain 62:1–30
4. Okada M, Okada M (1983) A method for quantification of alternate pronation and supination of forearms. Comp Biomed Res 16:59–78

Discussion

Dr. Hefter: You can simulate hemi-parkinsonian patients by putting weight on one side of a normal subject and you get the same results on normal subjects. So this is a general coupling phenomenon of oscillators. I would be cautious about saying that there are two different oscillators. For example, when you perform swinging of a manupendulum of different lengths on each side, you find a medium swing rate for both sides. So there is a complex interaction of the network on both sides. Quite extensive work has been done by Kelso and colleagues on that aspect.

Dr. Klotz: But surely it's true that though there aren't two exactly separated oscillators, there are still two different components which are seen.

Dr. Horstink: I can agree with the coordination of timing of manual movements, because we once tested patients who had to write with one hand and to squeeze with the other hand; when they had to write the letter "E," they squeezed faster than when they had to write a whole word at once. So the rhythm of the one hand is influenced by activity and rhythm of the other hand.

Dr. Lücking: Did you get any information during your investigation of diadochokinesia about what causes the movement to be slowed down and then stopped, sometimes after three or four and sometimes after ten turning movements?

Dr. Klotz: We are not absolutely sure. It could be that the oscillator is disturbed and then the ballistic movement is changed and started a new; parkinsonian patients, for example, have problems in starting movement – they have problems in restarting this ballistic movement. I'm not absolutely sure if that's right, however; it's only a hypothesis.

The Complexity Effect as an Indicator for the Parkinson Plus Syndrome

M. Ruß and P.-A. Fischer

Given the manifest slowing of motor functions in parkinsonian patients, it would seem only logical to measure reaction time and to take this as a basis for developing a scoring system to assess the pathological impairment caused by the disease. This has, of course, been done before, yet with contradictory results, since the nature of the stimulus–response situation affects the behavioral response in parkinsonian patients in a quite distinct manner [1]. Cognitive and motor elements are confounded in the reaction time, and separating the one from the other calls for sophisticated methods of mental chronometry [6,7]. Parkinsonian patients have particular problems with motor reactions if the situation is effort-demanding and self-directed, movements have to be initiated and organized in space, or the necessary movements are sequential, simultaneous, complex, or without visual feedback [2,3]. While other cerebrally impaired patients with focal or diffuse lesions and, notably, demented display marked deficits of varying degrees in all reaction tasks, parkinsonian patients are, under certain conditions, perfectly able to react in the same way as normal controls, providing the degenerative disease process does not exceed the nigrostriatal system and no additional cerebral lesions ("Parkinson plus" (PLUS)) exist [4,9–11]. In the following, we shall examine whether an instrument-based reaction test which, while stress-inducing, also constitutes an action situation a typical parkinsonian patient is able to cope with can enable us to distinguish between an uncomplicated Parkinson's syndrome (PD) and PLUS reliably, validly, and with an acceptable amount of time and effort.

Method

Patients

Parkinsonian patients (n = 133) were compared with normal controls (NC) and demented in terms of their reaction performance. Educational levels in the groups, classified on a scale of four on the basis of profession and intelligence as measured, were not unevenly distributed in the chi-squared test. Equally, there were no significant differences with regard to sex distribution.

NC (n = 79) consisted of healthy volunteers and outpatients without any organic-pathological abnormalities aged between 38 and 86 (mean = 56.1; SD =

12.8); there were 53 men and 26 women. The AD/MID group ($n = 62$) was made up of 26 patients with Alzheimer's disease (AD) and 36 patients suffering from multi-infarct dementia (MID) aged between 35 and 82 (mean = 63.5; SD = 12.4); there were 36 men and 26 women, all demented according to the DSM-III criteria.

The parkinsonian group consisted of 95 patients with a simple PD and 38 patients with PLUS aged between 35 and 82. The mean age in PD (52 women and 43 men) was 59.1 (SD = 9.8), and in PLUS (36 men and 26 women), 67.6 (SD = 9.7) years. In the group as a whole (PD and PLUS), the number of patients with stages I–V on the Hoehn and Yahr scale was 28, 52, 42, 10, and 1, respectively.

The duration of the disease ranged from 1 to 15 years (mean, 5.0; SD, 4.2). The mean L-dopa dosage (Madopar) administered to the treated patients was 617 mg (SD = 210); 60 patients were untreated. The average score on the Webster Rating Scale was 11.0 (SD = 4.9). Symptoms were more pronounced on the right side in 58 patients, on the left in 49, and equally pronounced on both sides in 26. A total of 80 were of the rigid-akinetic type, 30 were assigned to the tremor-dominant type, and 23 patients were of a mixed type. There were slight, yet significant age differences between the four groups ($F = 11.03$; $df = 3/270$; $p < 0.001$). NC and PD did not differ in the single contrast analysis (Newman-Keuls Test), yet PLUS and AD/MID were significantly older than NC.

Procedure

Using a commonly available reaction-testing unit (Wiener Reaktions- und Determinationsgerät, Schuhfried Ltd., Mödling, Austria), the reaction time was measured at five levels of progressively increasing task complexity. At level 1, patients had to react to a yellow light signal by pressing a button with the index finger of their choice and at level 2 to a combination of the yellow lamp with an acoustic signal (choice reaction). At level 3, ten lamps lit up in five different colours in an irregular sequence. The reaction took the form of a finger touch to a key in the corresponding colour. At level 4, two right–left signals were added, with the right or left pedal being activated using the corresponding foot when the signal lit up. At level 5, patients also had to distinguish between sounds of differing pitch. In response to a high tone, a key marked "H" had to be pressed and in response to a low tone, a key marked "T." At each level, the test lasted about 1 min.

From the individual times recorded at each level, the mean value was determined. In addition, the complexity effect (variable CE) was calculated for each subject. CE is defined as the tangent of the slope of the linear regression line determined by the reaction times at levels 1–5. Following the reaction test, all subjects completed an intelligence test, the Standard Progressive Matrices (SPM) as defined by Raven [8].

Experimental Results

The reaction times as measured in the comparative groups at the five levels of task complexity rise systematically with the complexity and severity of the cerebral

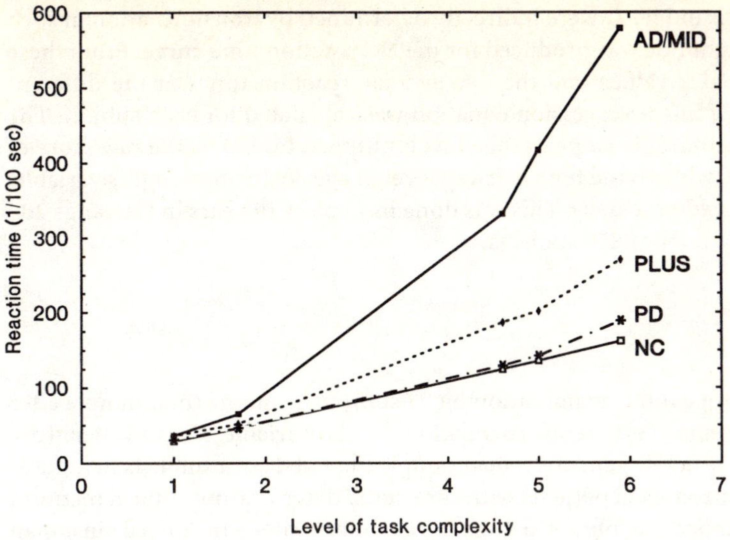

Fig. 1. Reaction time (age-adjusted means) and task complexity in the comparative groups normal controls (*NC*), Parkinson's disease (*PD*), Parkinson plus (*PLUS*), und Alzheimer's or multi-infarct dementia (*AD/MID*)

disease (Fig. 1). In the analysis of variance (ANOVA) with a between-groups factor (NC, PD, PLUS, AD/MID) and the repeated measures factor complexity (five dependent variables, reaction times at levels 1–5), significant effects are produced for groups ($F = 73.3$, $df = 3/269$; $p < 0.001$), complexity ($F = 327.7$, $df = 4/1076$; $p < 0.001$), and groups × complexity ($F = 49.9$, $df = 12/1076$, $p < 0.001$). Single contrasts tested against NC are significant only for PLUS ($F = 14.8$, $df = 1/269$; $p < 0.001$) and AD/MID ($F = 177.2$, $df = 1/269$; $p < 0.001$), not however for PD ($F = 0.82$, $df = 1/269$; $p = 0.36$). There is a marked difference in the effect of complexity on reaction time across the groups (Fig. 1). In the variable CE, defined as indicator for this effect, group differences exist ($F = 97.0$, $df = 3/269$; $p < 0.001$). The mean CE values (*T* scores) are 60.1 (SD = 8.3) in NC, 55.4 (SD = 9.1) in PD, 47.4 (SD = 9.1) in PLUS, and 35.1 (SD = 9.4) in AD/MID. In the Newman-Keuls test (post hoc), group differences to NC are significant throughout.

Scoring System

Scaling and Norming

The complexity effect was scaled using an additive factor model of information processing [6] and working on the assumption that there is a linear rise in NC reaction time as complexity increases. The five scale values (1.0, 1.7, 4.7, 5.0, 5.9) of complexity (x-axis in Fig. 1) were indirectly determined by transformation in such a way that a straight line was produced for the NC reaction time curve. From these theoretically based x-values and the five average reaction times at the different levels (y-values), a linear regression equation was calculated for each subject. The value of the tangent of the slope of this line, multiplied by 100, is the raw score of the variable CE. Owing to the high existing level of age correlation in this variable, age-norming proved necessary. This was done in steps of 10 years in the range 20–80 years in a data pool of 850 subjects.

Reliability

We were able to repeat the examination on 73 subjects from the total sample after a period of 2–5 years. Test–retest correlation for the variable CE is $r = 0.60$ ($p < 0.001$). As this very heterogeneous repeat sample included both subjects in a stable condition and neurological patients with constantly deteriorating clinical pictures, one could not expect to obtain a higher reliability value. In 20 parkinsonian patients forming part of this group who had, over the repeat examination period, shown no major change in terms of their disease, a far higher reliability value was obtained. Here, correlation between first and second examination was $r = 0.87$ ($p < 0.001$).

Criterion Validity

Within the total parkinsonian group, there is a significant correlation between CE and both the stage of the illness on the Hoehn and Yahr ($r = -0.35$) and Webster Rating Scale ($r = -0.45$). There is no substantial link to the duration of the disease ($r = -0.08$; n.s.), the duration of the treatment ($r = -0.12$; n.s.), or the L-dopa dosage ($r = -0.11$; n.s.). The most marked correlation is between CE and the intelligence level in the Raven Test ($r = 0.60$; $p < 0.001$). If we examine the effects of the factors most affected side (left, right) and dominance type (akinesia-dominant, tremor-dominant, mixed), the ANOVA yields no significance for side ($F = 0.01$, $df = 1/105$; $p = 0.93$) or type ($F = 1.3$, $df = 2/129$; $p = 0.26$).

The distribution of the age-normed variable CE in the groups NC, PD, and PLUS (Fig. 2) reveals a distinct overlap between NC and patients with a simple PD. Clearly set off from the rest is, however, the PLUS group. A cut-off value of CE at $T = 50$ produces maximum separation of groups PD and PLUS. To further estimate the validity of CE for the separation of PD and PLUS, the hit rate and correlations with clinical symptoms of PLUS were determined. At a cut-off of $T = 50$, 74% of clinically diagnosed parkinsonian patients were correctly assigned to the PD or PLUS groups using CE (Fig. 2). Pathological findings in the additional instrument-based examinations (CT, EEG, VEP, Doppler ultrasound, tilting table) and the clinical examination (e.g., ataxia, gaze paresis, pyramidal tract signs, orthostatic dysregulation) are signs of secondary cerebral diseases or signs that the degenera-

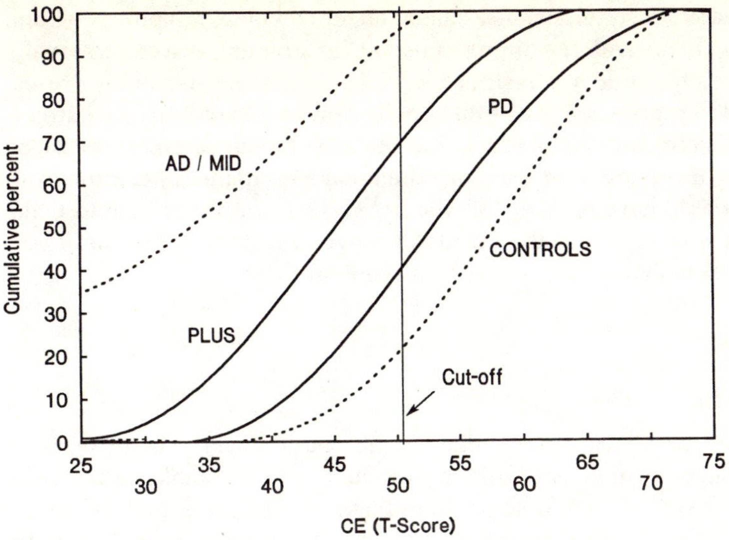

Fig. 2. Cumulative distributions of the age-normed complexity effect *CE* (*T* scores) in normal controls (*NC*), Parkinson's disease (*PD*), Parkinson plus (*PLUS*), and Alzheimers's and multi-infarct dementia (*AD/MID*) groups

tive process in the parkinsonian patients exceeds the nigrostriatal system [4,5]. In the total parkinsonian group, there is a correlation ($r = 0.30$; $p < 0.01$) between CE and EEG background activity. Following the formation of "findings normal" and "findings pathological" groups, the CE differences (ANOVA) in cranial computer tomography ($F = 11.0$, $df = 1/96$; $p < 0.001$), EEG ($F = 11.8$, $df = 1/179$; $p < 0.001$), pyramidal tract signs ($F = 5.6$, $df = 1/118$; $p < 0.02$), and gaze paresis ($F = 90.8$, $df = 1/117$; $p < 0.01$) are significant. In all other symptoms (here excluding dementia), there is (in view of the small sample sizes) no significance. If the number of PLUS signs from the examinations routinely carried out on all parkinsonian patients is correlated with CE, a significant link emerges ($r = 0.40$; $p < 0.01$). ANOVA also demonstrates that the number of plus signs has a significant effect on the variable CE ($F = 4.6$, $df = 4/113$; $p < 0.002$). Occurring most frequently here were pathological CT and EEG findings.

Face Validity

The reaction test meets with unqualified acceptance on the part of the parkinsonian patients, who see it as one that is both meaningful and designed to tackle the heart of their problems. The examination causes slight stress, yet often also gives rise to a certain degree of satisfaction since patients can – to their own surprise – perform more or less normally. It shows them the potential they are able to draw on under the set conditions, despite their motor impairments. The necessary movements are not simultaneous, sequential, or complex. A motor program, memorized beforehand and remaining constant, is stimulus driven, externally guided, and takes place under visual feedback. The examination can also reveal something about the propensity of motor actions to malfunction when stress-inducing demands are made upon them. The situation can, in certain respects, be compared to that of driving a car. Patients often make spontaneous comments to this effect. One would have to examine whether CE is an indicator able to make valid predictions with regard to the quality of movement in everyday life. There seems to be sufficient evidence to support this assumption.

Conclusions

A graded reaction test was used to examine whether the gradual rise in the reaction time, scaled and age-normed as cognitive variable CE, is a suitable measure for distinguishing patients with a simple PD from those with PLUS. Using an optimal cut-off, it proved possible to correctly assign 74% of parkinsonian patients; the test-retest reliability of CE was $r = 0.87$. Validity tests by means of correlations with PD parameters, clinical/instrument-based findings, and intelligence would suggest that CE can be interpreted as an indicator of cerebral intactness and general intellectual performance. In instances where Parkinson's disease is linked to a system-exceeding disease process and accompanying mental deficits, the complexity effect as defined above can prove useful as a measure of the cognitive compensation reserves of the motor-impaired parkinsonian patient, as an indicator for PLUS, and possibly as a predictor for the quality of movement in everyday situations.

References

1. Benton A (1986) Reaction time and brain disease: some reflections. Cortex 22:129–140
2. Brown RG, Marsden CD (1990) Cognitive function in Parkinson's disease: from description to theory. Trends Neurosci 13:21–29
3. Dubois B, Boller F, Pillon B, Agid Y (1991) Cognitive deficits in Parkinson's disease. In: Boller F, Grafman J (eds) Handbook of neuropsychology, vol 5. Elsevier Science, Amsterdam, pp 195–240
4. Fischer PA (1986a) Long-term course in Parkinson's syndrome and cerebral polypathy (Parkinson plus). Adv Neurol 45:235–238
5. Fischer PA (1986b) Progression und Polypathie beim Parkinson-Syndrom. In: Fischer PA (ed) Spätsyndrome der Parkinson-Krankheit. Editions Roche, Basel, pp 67–82
6. Meyer D, Osman AM, Irwin DE, Yantis S (1988) Modern mental chronometry. Biol Psychol 26:3–67
7. Rafal RD, Posner MI, Walker JA, Friedrich FJ (1984) Cognition and the basal ganglia. Separating mental and motor components of performance in Parkinson's disease. Brain 107:1083–1094
8. Raven JC (1985) Standard progressive matrices. Lewis, London
9. Ruß M, Fischer PA (1988) Reaktionszeitmessungen bei Parkinson-Kranken: der Komplexitätseffekt als Parkinson-plus-Indikator. In: Fischer PA (ed) Modifizierende Faktoren der Parkinson-Therapie. Editiones Roche, Basel, pp 149–160

10. Ruß M, Fischer PA (1989) Reaktionszeit und Aufgabenkomplexität: der Komplexitätseffekt als ein neuropsychologischer Indikator für den Schweregrad der zerebralen Beeinträchtigung. Z Diag Diff Psychol 10:145–153
11. Ruß M, Fischer PA (1990) Vergleichende testpsychologische Untersuchungen zur intellektuellen Leistungsfähigkeit von Parkinson-Kranken. Nervenarzt 61:88–93

Discussion

Dr. Spieker: Do you think that it is possible with this test to predict whether newly diagnosed parkinsonian patients will subsequently develop a "Parkinson plus" syndrome, because this distinction can usually only be made after a couple of years of disease?

Dr. Ruß: The test is not for prediction: these patients already have a Parkinson plus syndrome.

Dr. Flowers: I think David Marsden and his group have suggested that parkinsonian patients can sometimes be divided into two groups: one with patients that predominately have a motor problem and one with patients with a cognitive problem, according to which parts of the brain and all the basal ganglia are affected. I wondered if you'd correlated your cognitive results with any motor disturbance to see if you can confirm that you can divide them into groups, or is it always the motor symptoms that correlate with the cognitive ones? I think that's a very interesting question, a general question for the whole problem of classifying patients and predicting how they're going to progress.

Dr. Ruß: My motor variables are Purdue pegboard, finger tapping, and foot tapping, and a correlation of these variables with all my cognitive variables is very low in general.

Dr. Flowers: So you might confirm the idea that there could be two groups of patients progressing in two different areas independently?

Dr. Ruß: Yes. In my personal experience it's absolutely true.

Dr. Flowers: In which case we need to have two separate measures for patients and not just call them parkinsonian because they have one of a heterogeneous collection of symptoms?

Dr. Lücking: Is it justified to call a patient a Parkinson plus patient if he has a lot of cognitive dysfunction? Because if you remember Alexander's proposal with the different circuits of the striatum and putamen, this is really on the line of a slowly progressive incapacity of a lot of circuits in this area which could always be together, always be a Parkinson syndrome, without any need for a plus diagnosis.

Dr. Ruß: Having done this work, I think you can say that Parkinson's disease patients developing severe cognitive impairments are Parkinson plus patients. There's something more in the brain than in the typical Parkinson's disease.

Dr. Lücking: You can always restrict it to the nigrostriatal deficit?

Dr. Ruß: I don't believe you can.

Dr. Lücking: Because all these circuits need the dopamine of the substantia nigra, and then they go to the dorsolateral prefrontal and the lateral orbifrontal and are connected.

Dr. Ruß: Maybe. But in my variables it's fully unrelated to the dopamine treatment, unrelated to the dosage and unrelated to whether patients were treated or untreated. Sixty patients were untreated, and when I compare the treated and untreated patients, there's no difference. That's the case for most other cognitive variables, too.

Quantitative Assessment of Akinesia in Parkinson's Disease

C.H. Lücking, A. Hufschmidt, and J. Wiesenfeldt

Despite the progress made in the instrumental analysis of motor behaviour, the diagnosis of Parkinson's disease is still basically a clinical one. The most sensitive signs are the diminishment of involuntary or subconscious movements such as facial expression or the natural change of position of some part of the body every few seconds [2]. This component played an eminent role in early clinical descriptions, and it tends to be forgotten under the influence of the more recent research on voluntary movement.

What, then, is the possible role of motor tests, if not for diagnosis? The first answer is that they can help physicians to understand in more detail the disability of their patients. It is not sufficient to state that a patient is severely akinetic. Instead, one has to assess to what degree the subdeficits of which akinesia is composed are expressed in an individual patient. The second answer is that motor tests can help to reveal the pathophysiology of akinesia. Thus, the first part of this paper will concentrate on the relation of motor test scores to the clinical state, and its second part on some results of patho-physiological analysis.

Relationship Between Manual Test Scores and Clinical State

Methods

Motor function was assessed by a test battery:

1. Auditory reaction time (auditory RT) (parameters, median and minimal RT out of ten trials)
2. Visual RT (parameters, median and minimal RT out of ten trials)
3. Visual delay (i.e., mean visual RT minus mean auditory RT)
4. Goal-directed movement, externally triggered (acoustic signal – reaching out 50 cm and pressing button; parameters, RT and movement time)
5. Goal-directed movement, self-triggered (no start signal; parameter, Movement time)
6. Diadochokinesia (turning a knob to and fro by pronation/supination of the hand as fast and as widely as possible for 10 s; parameter, mean absolute angular velocity)

7. Tracking (following a slowly moving target horizontally over a computer screen with a tracking cursor by turning a potentiometer; parameter, tracking error, i.e., integrated absolute distance between target and response bar)

The clinical assessment was based on the Unified Parkinson's Disease Rating Scale (UPDRS). For statistical purposes, a number of subscores of the UPDRS was defined to combine the scores of closely related motor functions (Table 1). In addition, each patient was assessed by a mini-mental state examination.

Results

Predictive Value of Motor Test Scores for Clinical Scores

Multiple regression was performed with motor test scores including the parameters "age" and "duration of illness" as independent variables and each of the UPDRS subscores in turn serving as a dependent variable. This procedure measures the influence of every independent variable on the dependent variable (beta weights) and the fraction of the total variance of the dependent variable which is explained by all independent variables together (R^2 value). The best correlation between functional test and clinical scores was for simple hand movement (Fig. 1). The R^2 value of 0.71 indicates that 71% of the variance of the clinical score can be

Table 1. Subscores of the Unified Parkinson's Disease Rating Scale (UPDRS)

Subscore	UPDRS scores (item)
Gait	
Falling	13
Walking	15
Gait	29
Handwriting	8
Complex movements	
Dressing	10
Hygiene	11
Turning in bed	12
Rising from chair	27
Speech	
Reported	5
On examination	18
Tremor	
Reported	16
At rest, on examination	20
Hand movements	
Finger taps	23
Hand movements, open/close	24
Rapid alternating movements	25
Facial expression	19

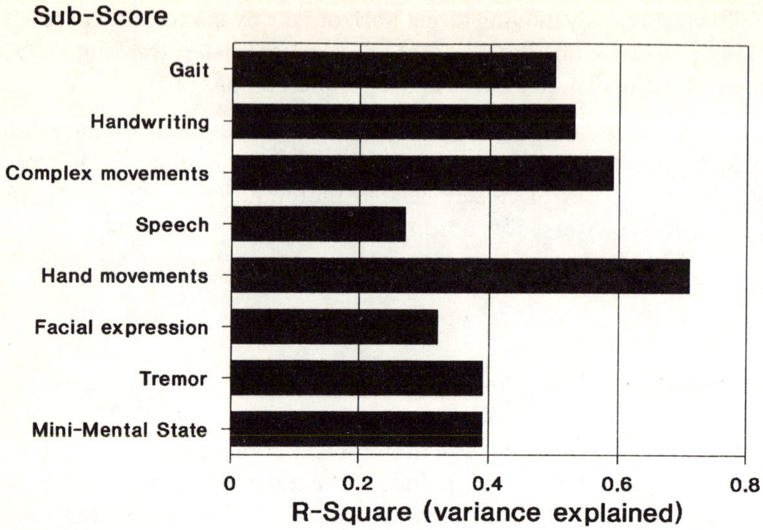

Fig. 1. Predictive value of some instrumental tests of manual motor function for clinical subscores of the Unified Parkinson's Disease Rating Scale. The R^2 values plotted as *bars* represent the fraction of the variance of the dependent variable (here clinical scores) which can be explained by all independent variables (here test scores) together

explained by quantitative tests. The beta weights of this regression (not plotted) indicate that diadochokinesia and duration of illness have a significant influence on the clinical score. The value of the test battery to predict the amount of micrographia is less than for simple hand movements: only 53% of the variance of the clinical score "handwriting" are explained by the tests scores. There is a significant contribution of auditory reaction time to the handwriting score. We have no good explanation for this link. It is probably due to an abstract subdeficit in akinesia such as a decrease of motor initiative.

Remarkably, the motor scores can also to some degree predict the disturbance of complex movements, although all the tests are based on hand movements, whereas the score for complex movements contains almost exclusively multisegmental movements of the whole body. This suggests that manual functions can to some degree be used as an indicator for the function of other body segments. As a diagnostic tool, they cover obviously more than just one limited aspect of the whole motor disturbance.

Influence of Age and Duration of Illness on Motor Performance

All the clinical scores except "facial expression" were significantly correlated with duration of illness (Table 2). This is what one would expect in a progressive disease. Interestingly, the situation is different for the motor tests (Table 3). There was a significant influence of age on most of the parameters, which was sometimes

Table 2. Influence of age and duration of illness on subscores of the Unified Parkinson's Disease Rating Scale (38 patients with Parkinson's disease)

Subscore	Correlation with age	Correlation with duration of illness
Gait	*	***
Handwriting	n.s.	****
Complex movements	n.s.	***
Speech	n.s.	***
Tremor	n.s.	***
Hand movements	n.s.	***
Facial expression	n.s.	n.s.

n.s., not significant.
* $p < 0.05$; ** $p < 0.01$; *** $p < 0.005$; **** $p < 0.001$.

Table 3. Influence of age and duration of illness on some motor tests (80 patients with Parkinson's disease)

Parameter	Correlation with age	Correlation with duration of illness
Auditory RT	*	n.s.
Visual delay	n.s.	*
Goal-directed movement	*	n.s.
Diadochokinesia	***	**
Tracking	****	*

n.s., not significant.
* $p < 0.05$; ** $p < 0.01$; *** $p < 0.005$; **** $p < 0.001$.

even stronger than the correlation with duration of illness. This suggests that either the normal age-related decrease in motor capacity is accelerated under the influence of parkinsonism or that the impact of the disease on motor function is a different one in young and old parkinsonian patients.

In order to examine this phenomenon more closely, patients were matched so as to form two age groups balanced for their duration of illness. Group I contained 17 patients under the age of 70 (mean age, 58.8 years), and group II eight patients aged 70 years or more (mean age, 73.8 years). The mean duration of illness in group I was 5.6 years, and in group II, 5.4 years. The absence of a significant difference in duration of illness was confirmed by the Wilcoxon test for independent samples ($p = 0.6178$). The control group of normal elderly subjects was also divided into groups containing individuals below (mean age, 59.5 years) and above the age of 70 (mean age, 75.8 years), respectively.

There were significant differences between younger and older parkinsonian patients for auditory ($p < 0.005$) and visual reaction time ($p < 0.01$), movement time (externally triggered movement; $p < 0.05$), tracking ($p < 0.005$), and for the

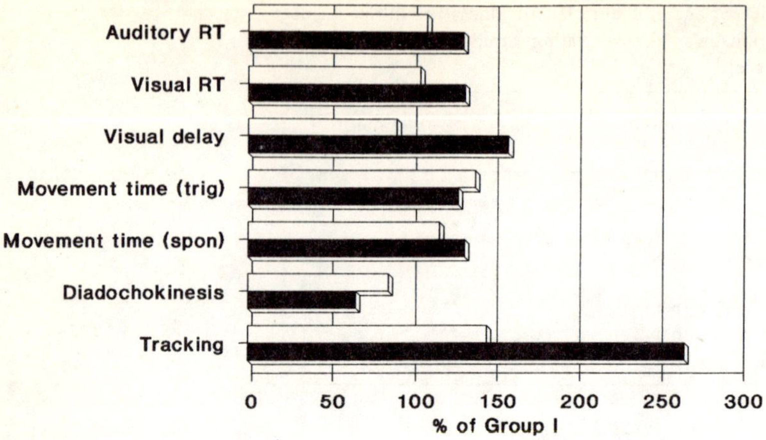

Fig. 2. Age-dependency of motor test scores in patients with Parkinson's disease (*black bars*) and healthy elderly subjects (*white bars*). Group I <70 years, group II ⩾70 years. The bars represent the percentual increase or decrease of motor test scores in the older group (I) in relation to the younger group (II) for patients and controls. The parkinsonian patients in the two groups were matched for duration of illness (5.6 and 5.4 years, respectively)

mini-mental state test ($p < 0.005$; Fig. 2). In the control group, in contrast, all differences found between the two age groups were nonsignificant. The mini-mental state test was not assessed in the control group. The parameter with the most remarkable difference was tracking error, which was increased in the old-age group by a factor of 2.66 in parkinsonian patients and only by a factor of 1.46 in normal subjects. However, due to the small number of subjects, the two-way interaction for tracking error between age group and diagnosis was below the 5% level of significance. Still, these data suggest that in patients with Parkinson's disease, aging exerts an aggravating influence on some motor functions which is stronger than the one seen in healthy individuals. It appears that the motor system of patients above the age of 70 is more susceptible to the functional damage caused by Parkinson's disease.

Pathophysiological Considerations

Tracking performance has been shown to be a most sensitive indicator of akinesia [1]. This finding prompted the question as to which component of the task represents the main difficulty for parkinsonian patients. In the tracking task used in our previous study, an extremely slow (9.3°/s) rotational hand movement was required. Thus, velocity was obviously not critical, considering that the patients were quite well able to execute single movements at much greater velocity if asked to do so. In a follow-up experiment, therefore, we performed a more detailed analysis of the potential sources of tracking error.

Methods

The experiments were performed on 12 patients with Parkinson's disease and 17 normal controls. The experimental set-up was the same as described above. The target movement to be tracked, however, was a pseudorandom pattern generated by superimposition of several sine waves. The pattern was presented in 32 identical trials of 12.8-s duration each, with target and response signals being sampled at intervals of 50 ms. Tracking error was again defined as the integrated absolute distance between target and response position. To allow comparison with other tracking tests, the tracking error scores were normalized to the error in a test trial in which the subject performed no movement at all. The following descriptive parameters were computed for every trial: amplitude gain, velocity gain, time lag between target and response, the fraction of phases where no movement at all was performed, and the fraction of directional errors (movement in the wrong direction). Time lag was assessed by cross-correlation of target and response signal. The gain parameters as well as the amount of directional errors were computed on curves corrected for time lag.

Results

Tracking error, as in the previous study, was significantly ($p < 0.05$) larger in the patient group. Significant differences (Table 4, columns 1 and 2) were also found for amplitude gain ($p < 0.01$), velocity gain ($p < 0.05$), and the "no movement" parameter ($p < 0.02$). Interestingly, the parameters "time lag" and "directional errors" exhibited no significant difference between parkinsonian patients and controls, confirming that a delay in reaction time was not likely to be responsible for most of the tracking error.

Table 4. Group differences between normal subjects and patients with Parkinson's disease (PD) and results of multiple regression of the descriptive parameters on tracking error as a dependent variable

Parameter	Group differences		Multiple regression (beta weights)	
	Control	PD	Control	PD
Tracking error (%)	53	66*	–	–
Amplitude gain	0.76	0.58***	–0.058	–1.233****
Velocity gain	0.81	0.63*	0.168	0.712***
Time lag (ms)	165	217	0.699***	0.522
No movement (%)	26	34**	0.192	0.033
Directional errors (%)	6.5	11.1	0.239	–0.103

Note that the significance levels given for multiple regression indicate the probability by which the regression coefficient (not listed here) is different from zero and *not* a group difference.
* $p < 0.05$; ** $p < 0.02$; *** $p < 0.01$; **** $p < 0.005$.

The main focus of the study was to assess the contribution of these parameters to tracking error. Therefore, multiple regression was performed with tracking error as the dependent variable and the descriptive parameters as independent variables. In normal subjects, time lag was the only parameter which had a significant influence on tracking error (Table 4, column 3). Conversely, in parkinsonian patients, tracking error correlated very closely with amplitude gain and less with velocity gain (Table 4, column 4). Both of these parameters were decreased. This suggests that parkinsonian patients have a poor tracking performance because they are not able to adjust their movement amplitude and, to some degree, their movement velocity to the requirements of the task. The decrease of amplitude gain was visible even in the original plots of target and tracking movements. One could argue that the patients were unable to perform movements of 40° amplitude required in this task. However, in control experiments it could be shown that all of them could perform a movement of more than 100° amplitude on command. Two possible reasons for this behaviour are conceivable.

1. The task gives the subjects a chance to move less than necessary without actually breaking the rules. Therefore, it could be sensitive for a deficiency of motor initiative.
2. The patients may perform an amplitude/phase lag trade-off by trying primarily to keep their phase lag small and accept a decrease of movement amplitude for this reason.

In order to find out which of these two explanations is correct, a second experiment was performed in which tracking velocity was reduced to 50% in every second trial. This caused an increase of amplitude gain of about 40% in the patient group, suggesting that the patients indeed make larger movements when movement velocity is less critical. They obviously use less of their adaptive strategy when the reason for this strategy (temporal pressure) is removed. Therefore, the patients appear to be overrun by the temporal stress under which the task is performed, without exhibiting a remarkable time lag in their tracking movements.

References

1. Lücking CH, Hufschmidt A, Deuschl G (1990) Electrophysiological methods in the early diagnosis of Parkinson's disease. In: Dostert P et al. (eds) Early markers in Parkinson's disease. (New vistas in drug research, vol 1) Springer, Vienna New York, pp 49–57
2. Meyer CH (1982) Akinesia in parkinsonism. Relation between spontaneous movement (other than tremor) and voluntary movements made on command. J Neurol Neurosurg Psychiatry 45(7):582–585

Discussion

Dr. Kraus: Did you take into consideration the fact that you had to adjust your level of significance when calculating for each item its own multiple regression? And did you try to estimate how much the variance overall is which both methods – instrumental testing and scoring – evaluate in parallel?

Dr. Lücking: I am sure that our statistics did that.

Dr. Kraus: It's not very easy; there is no simple method for doing it.

Dr. Lücking: I believe what we did that with our statistics and I was convinced that all these aspects were really exact.

Dr. Inzelberg: How many patients were involved?

Dr. Lücking: We scored about 80 patients, and in some subscores only some of them, but here we tested more than 100 patients.

Dr. Korczyn: You showed the number of pauses as a function of the speed, and it turns out that it's very similar in patients with Parkinson's disease and in controls. Can you comment on that?

Dr. Lücking: Most of these patients for the tracking task are mildly affected patients; there are some near the values of normal subjects.

Dr. Korczyn: But they have more pauses, don't they?

Dr. Lücking: They have more, and the most sensitive was the tracking; you saw that they could even have more power in slow movement target and can adapt to this different velocity of the target, but if the velocity is too high – and this is clearly in contrast to normals – then they made all these errors. What we saw was the amplitude gain reduction and the velocity gain.

Dr. Korczyn: But without pauses?

Dr. Lücking: Without pauses!

Dr. Korczyn: When you showed this example, it seems that there is a delay in the onset as the first movement was clearly out of phase and then the movement itself was exactly in phase. Can you give an explanation of that?

Dr. Lücking: They hesitated in starting and then they jumped too: I think this could really be an initiative block or lack of initiative of movement, but when they realized they had jumped, they could follow immediately.

Dr. Korczyn: So the initiation was worse than the tracking itself.

Dr. Lücking: But even in normals there is a phase lack in the beginning.

Dr. Korczyn: Were they trained by the time you've done this? This was not the first experiment?

Dr. Lücking: There's a good training effect for normals, but there is no training effect or at least only a small training effect in parkinsonian patients.

Dr. Potvin: For part of your analysis here you divided your Parkinson's disease patients into two groups – one 70-years-old and older and the other group below 70 – and you found some significant differences, especially with regard to tracking, and then made some strong inferences. My concern is that you only had eight patients that were over 70 years old. How convinced are you that those eight patients are representative of all Parkinson's disease patients over 70? I'm concerned that the sample size is too small here. Would you like to comment on that?

Dr. Lücking: I agree. It is a good point and we should sample more than eight patients, but as a statistical probe it seems to be enough to make this statement. I think you are right, though; we should add to this number of patients.

Dr. Rabey: The comparison between the difference in the subscales in the Unified Parkinson's Disease Rating Scale and some features was made in all the Parkinson's disease patients together. My question is whether there is the same weight of the separate items when you separate different stages of the disease? If you consider the comparison, for example, for stage I versus stage V, are the parameters still the same?

Dr. Lücking: We didn't make a clear difference between mildly, moderately, and severely affected patients. Most of these patients are mild to moderate, because it needs some motor capacity and attention to do the tests, but it's not enough to classify these different groups.

Motor Performance Test after Schoppe and Clinical Rating Scales – A Comparison

H. Przuntek, P.H. Kraus, and P. Klotz

Introduction

In 1985 we began to plan and organize a long-term trial to compare the benefit of levodopa monotherapy and that of a combination therapy of levodopa and bromocriptine in de novo patients suffering from Parkinson's disease.

Main target criteria were designed to establish changes in motor function including complications of long-term therapy (fluctuations, dyskinesias, and dystonia). Considering the experiences of former studies [1], a large number of patients was necessary. Therefore, we had to choose a multicenter design. This design is disadvantageous because of increased interrater variability, which is additionally increased by changes of some rater teams over the long period of time. In consequence, we had to look for an additional method of assessment which had high objectivity and also had maximal resolution in the range "healthy" to "mildly affected."

At time of planing the study design, the Webster rating scale [6] was established as a practicable standard. For the above-mentioned objective method, the motor performance test after Schoppe [2,5] was chosen, for which the main test criteria had already been examined. Furthermore, the Zung self-rating scale for depression [7] and a self-rating scale of every day activities were used among others. Fluctuations, dyskinesias, and dystonia were assessed by additional items.

The present paper deals only with those components of the data set which are of special interest for the comparison of clinical rating scales and motor performance tests.

Methods

Over 4 years the patients were recruited, examined, and treated by 101 experienced, practicing neurologists. Patients were cross-checked half-yearly in 27 Parkinson centers, where patients were also assessed by instrumental methods. The initial number of patients was 664; in the course of the long-term trial, this number decreased by patients dropping out.

The motor performance test after Schoppe assesses fine motor skills in several subtests which have to be carried out separately for the right and left hands, as described by Schoppe [5].

Plugging. The subject is required to transfer 25 pins (diameter 2.5 mm, length 5 cm), individually and as quickly as possible, from a rack into a series of appropriate holes (diameter 2.8 mm) in a contact board. This test measures the time interval between plugging in the first and the last pin.

Tapping. The subject is required to tap on a contact board with a contact pencil as rapidly as possible. This test measures the number of contacts during two time intervals of 16 s each. As a measure of alteration of speed (e.g., caused by fatigue), we use the difference between the two numbers as an additional parameter.

Steadiness. The steadiness 4.8 mm test was performed in the smallest hole of the series in the board without support for the arm in action. A contact pencil had to be held for 32 s vertically in a hole with a diameter of 4.8 mm without touching either the rim or the bottom of the hole. This test measures the number and duration of contacts. The steadiness 8.5 mm test was performed in the same manner using a hole of 8.5 mm diameter.

Aiming. In this test, the subject has to hit 20 contacts with the contact pencil. The test measures the total time required to perform the test, number of hits, number of misses, and duration of misses.

Tracing. In the test line tracing, the patient has to follow a grooved path as exactly as possible with a stylus. This test measures the total time required to perform the test, number of errors, and duration of errors.

Results

The study results are published elsewhere [3,4]. The data material allows on the one hand cross-sectional comparison between the different methods for each visit and, on the other hand, it is possible to compare the course of the results of the different methods over time.

Cross-sectional correlation between the motor performance test and the Webster rating scale (Table 1) for each examination gives a conclusive description which is stable over time. For example, the Webster item "tremor" and the results of "steadiness" of the motor performance test correlate significantly, as do the Webster sum score and the complex motor performance subtest "plugging." Plugging shows significant correlation with all items of the Webster rating scale. The items in the motor performance test for tapping have only a nearly zero correlation with any Webster item.

Table 1. Correlation matrix between Webster items and motor performance test items for initial examination

Motor performance	Webster Rating Scale items										
	Bradykinesia	Rigidity	Posture	Arm swinging	Gait	Tremor	Facial expression	Seborrhea	Speech	Independence	Sum
LFF	0.145**	0.146**	0.163**	0.93	0.194**	0.168**	0.072	−0.067	0.092	0.127*	0.183**
LFFD	0.211**	0.167**	0.285**	0.237**	0.387**	0.096	0.168**	0.022	0.195**	0.333**	0.339**
LFGD	0.269**	0.236**	0.204**	0.241**	0.239**	−0.026	0.156**	0.058	0.132**	0.242**	0.287**
S1F	−0.045	−0.052	−0.032	−0.110	0.035	0.273**	−0.090	−0.105*	−0.099	−0.045	−0.046
S1FD	0.086	0.008	0.121*	0.092	0.197**	0.161**	0.052	0.020	0.054	0.127*	0.146**
S4F	0.050	0.015	0.067	0.039	0.102*	0.260**	0.006	−0.019	0.030	0.041	0.093
S4FD	0.058	0.032	0.063	0.063	0.186**	0.085	0.040	0.043	0.048	0.138**	0.120*
AIF	0.055	−0.060	0.109*	0.014	0.070	0.241**	0.014	−0.022	0.041	0.074	0.080
AITR	0.052	−0.004	0.038	−0.041	0.051	0.243**	0.005	0.010	0.058	0.089	0.073
AIGD	0.211**	0.172**	0.236**	0.133**	0.326**	0.112*	0.146**	0.059	0.161**	0.326**	0.300**
TP1	−0.022	0.013	−0.020	0.028	−0.088	−0.068	0.028	0.102*	−0.012	−0.051	−0.015
TP2	0.007	0.018	−0.017	0.031	−0.073	−0.034	0.043	0.117*	−0.001	−0.036	0.007
TPSUM	−0.008	0.015	−0.019	0.030	−0.082	−0.052	0.036	0.111*	−0.007	−0.044	−0.004
UMGD	0.350**	0.316**	0.349**	0.324**	0.477**	0.173**	0.274**	0.141**	0.318**	0.487**	0.513**

A total of 549 patients were examined; motor performance tests carried out were line tracing, steadiness, aiming, plugging, and tapping.
Line tracing: LFF, number of errors; LFFD, duration of errors; LFGD, total time for task. Steadiness: S1F, number of errors for small hole; S1FD, duration of errors for small hole; S4F, number of errors for bigger hole; S4FD, duration of errors for bigger hole. Aiming: AIF, number of errors; AITR, number of correct hits; AIGD, total time for task. Tapping: TP1, number of hits in first interval; TP2, number of hits in second interval; TPSUM, number of hits for total task. Plugging: UMGD, total time for task.
One-tailed significance $^{*}p = -0.01$; $^{**}p = -0.001$.

It has to be considered that results of both methods are affected by errors which together diminish the correlation. There is no analytical method for multivariate correlation of all ten Webster items with all 26 items of the motor performance test over the present nine visits. For the question of correlation over time, we have to compare the shape of the course of the single items.

As expected, changes are reflected most markedly by the sum score of the Webster rating scale because of additional effects of internal consistency (Fig. 1). The items of the Webster rating scale and the items of the motor performance test (Fig. 2) give an impression of the course of therapeutic effect over time and progression of disease. As can be seen, for some items in both assessment designs there are different courses compared to the overall description. The mean course of disease seems to be more accurately reflected by the Webster items.

For interpretation, the fact that there are large interindividual differences in fine motor performance has to be taken into account. Furthermore, age dependency is well examined and should be taken into consideration for evaluation.

The course of subtest plugging is well correlated to the Webster sum score: under therapy we observed a marked improvement within the first 6 months, while after 1.5 years, despite adequate therapy, a deterioration begins, which over the course of 4 years reaches the region of the initial level.

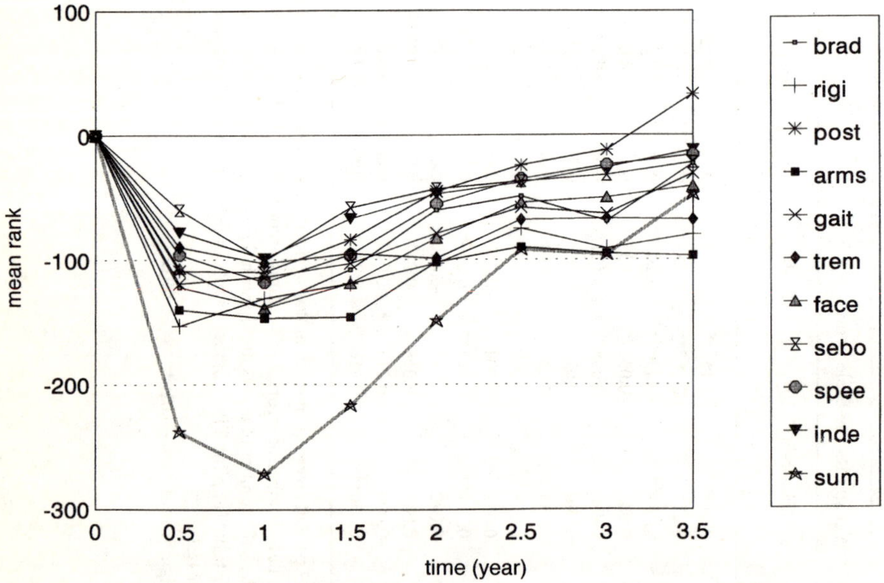

Fig. 1. Course of the therapeutic effect over time and progression of disease. Items of Webster Rating Scale. For the initial (pretreatment) period, $n = 549$. The ordinate scale shows the mean rank normalized to the pretreatment period. *brad*, bradykinesia; *rigi*, rigidity; *post*, posture; *trem*, tremor; *sebo*, seborrhea; *spee*, speech; *inde*, independence; *arms*, arm swinging; *sum*, overall Webster sum score

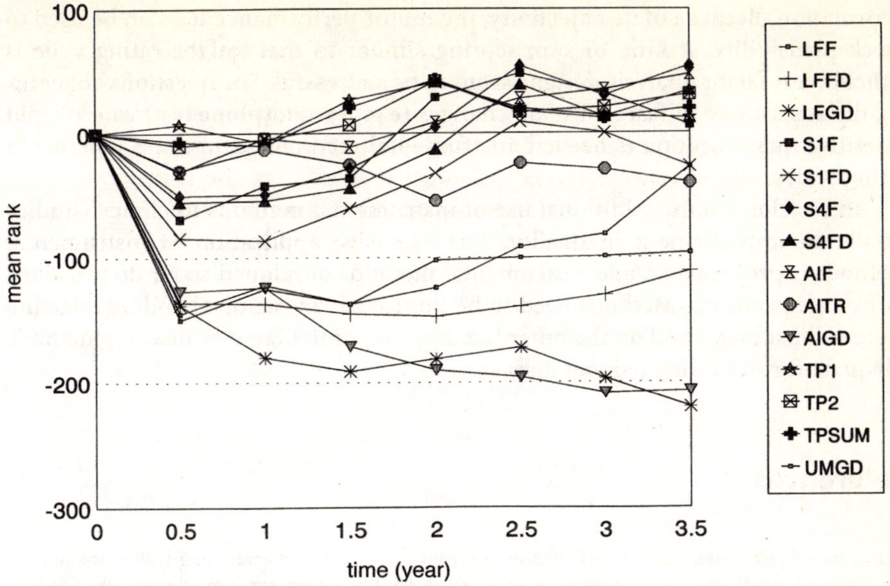

Fig. 2. Course of therapeutic effect over time and progression of disease. Items of the motor performance test after Schoppe. For the initial (pretreatment) period, $n = 549$. The ordinate scales show the mean rank normalized to the pretreatment period. For explanation of abbreviations, please see footnote to Table 1

In contrast, other parameters of the motor performance test (e.g., line tracing) after the start of therapy show an improvement without following the deterioration as documented by the rating scale.

Tapping items in the motor performance test show no interpretable changes during the study course. This has to be taken into consideration in assessing the usefulness of tapping, since this test or variations of it are used as part of newer scoring systems.

As far as the resolution of the motor performance test is concerned, it should be noted that this test was especially constructed for differentiation within normal motor performance. Compared with the rating scale, one advantage is the projection to a quasi continuous spectrum of values, but the real resolution is not the smallest difference between neighboring values but has to be estimated by retest examinations. In our case, this "confidence interval" is a function of the value (Kraus, Fortmeier, Klotz, unpublished data).

In principle, the parameters for retest reliability are good (Kraus, Fortmeier, Klotz, unpublished data; repetitive design, 249 parkinsonian patients, retest correlation about 0.9 for most of the items). A similar examination of retest reliability by fast repetitive clinical examination is not practicable.

After extensive examination of our data, including calculation of factor models, we conclude that the motor performance test is less specific than the rating scale and does not include all parkinsonian phenomena, but gives additional information. Because of its objectivity, the motor performance test can be used to check plausibility. A kind of sum scoring similar to that for the rating scale is difficult, but factor analysis designs seem to be successful. For questions concerning the assessment of fast and small changes (e.g., apomorphine test) where rapid repetitive quantification is needed, instrumental methods seem to be superior to rating scales.

In conclusion, the additional use of instrumental methods in clinical studies entails an improvement in quality. The exclusive application of instrumental methods is problematic, and instrumental methods developed so far do not allow sufficient specificity. Methods need to be improved: on the one hand by selecting more valid subtests and on the other hand by more intelligent evaluation methods adequate for multidimensional disease.

References

1. Fischer PA, Przuntek H, Majer M, Welzel D (1984) Kombinationsbehandlung früher Stadien des Parkinson-Syndroms mit Bromocriptin und Levodopa. Ergebnisse einer multizentrischen Studie. Dtsch Med Wochenschr 109:1279–1283
2. Hamster W (1980) Die Motorische Leistungsserie, Handanweisung. Schufried, Mödling
3. Przuntek H, Welzel D, Schwarzmann D, Letzel H, Kraus PH (1992a) Primary combination therapy of early Parkinson's disease. Eur Neurol 32[Suppl 1]:36–45
4. Przuntek H, Welzel D, Blümner E, Danjelczyk W, Letzel H, Kaiser HJ, Kraus PH, Riederer P, Schwarzmann D, Wolf H, Überla K (1992b) Bromocriptine lessens the incidence of mortality in L-Dopa-treated parkinsonian patients: prado-study discontinued. Eur J Clin Pharmacol 43:357–363
5. Schoppe KJ (1974) Das MLS-Gerät: Ein neuer Testapparat zur Messung feinmotorischer Leistungen. Diagnostica 20:43–46
6. Webster DD (1968) Clinical analysis of the disability in Parkinson's disease. Mod Treat 5:257–282
7. Zung WWK (1965) A self-rating depression scale. Arch Gen Psychiatr 12:63–70

Discussion

Dr. Rabey: You mentioned that tremor was not correlated to plugging?

Dr. Przuntek: Tremor was a little bit better correlated to plugging than, for example, line tracing. Plugging is influenced by tremor.

Dr. Panzer: Do you consider bradykinesia to be a subset of akinesia or related to rigidity?

Dr. Przuntek: I assume we have to differentiate between two types of akinesia; one type could be bradykinesia and the other dysrhythmicity of movement.

Dr. Fahn: Each of the 27 centers had one of these devices, so they could all use them identically and everybody was trained how to do this?

Dr. Przuntek: Yes. They were trained and they know how to do it.

Dr. Fahn: You can also train a technical assistant to do clinical rating scores, too.

Dr. Przuntek: Yes, that's true, but I think it's simpler to train them with this machine.

Round Table Discussion 2: Instrumental Methods

Dr. Korczyn: Are there any questions?

Dr. Fahn: First of all, I want to thank the organizers, and I also have a comment: I think one of the things most of us came here to learn is whether there is some simple objective test that we could do in addition to our clinical ratings – if we are going to test a new drug, for example, or compare two drugs – whether there is a more objective method. I would like the members in this room to take a vote on what should be recommended for, say, somebody who had an instrumentation, someone who has nothing right now, and someone who gets started with one. What would be the conclusion of this conference? That's what I would consider a scientific conclusion.

Dr. Korczyn: In a democracy you go by the majority, but the majority is not always right, you know. With that in mind, let me ask how many of you think that instruments are an improvement in the terms that we are discussing now – not in research, but in the study of a new drug – do you think that clinical evaluation is superior to instruments? Can you use clinical evaluation alone? As a result of our poll, I think there is about an equal number of those who say that we need a combination of instruments and clinical evaluation and those who say that clinical rating should be sufficient on its own, and very few think that instrumentation is extremely important. Now, do you want to break down the clinical ratings?

Now, of those of you who have presented their methods of instrumentation, is anybody of the opinion that in order to do drug studies, you should also use other instrumentation that you've heard about here?

Dr. Rabey: Before you continue – I remember what you said yesterday, Dr. Fahn I think that we need to be fair to ourselves. You were referring to patients who had the same score using the Unified Parkinson's Disease Rating Scale (UPDRS), but who felt that they needed the rescue drug. That means that the methodology we are using for scoring is not sufficient. We are missing something. I still feel that I belong to the group that thinks clinical evaluation is very important, but I also feel that there is something missing in the way I am evaluating my patients.

Dr. Fahn: That's why I asked the question. Which method should be used? Is there one test that I can use as a way of following a patient objectively.

Dr. Rabey: I was commenting, for example, on Hoehn and Yahr staging. Everyone was criticizing the fact that it only stages the disease, but later on today a lot of presentations referred to the staging by Hoehn and Yahr, for example. So if it is so wrong, why is it so good? The point is – and this is my comment to Dr. Klotz – that maybe we need to try to apply one of the simple methodologies and find out whether there is any correlation with daily performance and what the deviation from the normal standard for this specific task is.

Dr. Klotz: Yesterday you said that we should not always take total UPDRS, and I think it's the same for the instrumental methods. I have to check in advance what I am really interested in, what the real target is that I have to investigate and the method I should choose.

Dr. Fahn: If, say, you want to compare one drug versus another drug and placebos in a double-blind study, besides measuring the clinical things blinded, is there some test, a global test –

Dr. Korczyn: But there is no such thing, there can't be. If you treat a person for tremor, it's different from treating a person for gait instability. You cannot have one instrumentation test, even if in theory one such test existed, that will answer both questions. There is a different question when you treat a patient for a condition that they already have now as opposed to prophylactic treatment.

Dr. Przuntek: If you want to test tremor, for example, within a very short time, then I would recommend the test presented by Dr. Scholz from Tübingen today. If you would like to know something about bradykinesia and akinesia, I think that the tracing test and also the aiming test are really very good; in early stages, they are better than clinical evaluation.

Dr. Hallett: I was going to say something similar to what is being said right here at the moment: that Parkinson's disease is a multifaceted disease. Clinically, in the rating scale there are perhaps 100 or 150 items or however many it is, and there would have to be multiple instrumental tests, too. I think that what we have heard here is that there are a number of different instrumental tests that look at different facets of Parkinson's disease. They were often compared to clinical tests and many of them seem to be very good for what they were designed for. Some of them don't seem to be so good, for example in the area that I was talking about in relation to postural tests. The tests there don't seem to be very good at the moment. However, there are a number of tests for tremor that seem very good, and there are lots of tests for slowness of movement, many of which were very good indeed. The question that you're really asking now and that we haven't really looked at involves taking the 15 or 20 tests that have been brought forward for bradykinesia and comparing them with each other to see which of them might be the best. Using any one of them might be a useful addition to the clinical battery for all the reasons that we have been talking about; you then end up having scales which are continuous and which can be easily done. I don't think that we really came to any conclusion about which of these tests is the best, but perhaps that would be where to proceed next. If there's going to be a logical continuation of this meeting, it would be to look at all of the tests, compare them with each other, and perhaps make some sort of decision about which aspects of them are the best; then we could find an answer to your question. But at the moment I'm not sure that we can answer your question, although we have a lot of raw data here. In order to reach an answer it would take another day or so of debate, comparing the tests to make a final decision.

Dr. Watts: I wish strongly reiterate what Mark Hallett just said. The comment I wanted to make is that you really need a battery, and a good place to start is with the cardinal motor symptoms of Parkinson's disease: bradykinesia, tremor, rigidity, and posture. In our laboratory we can measure three of those, but we cannot measure gait, balance, and those kinds of things well because it's a difficult undertaking, as Mark Hallett's presentations showed, among others. I think that's where we need to move, because there is no one test, as there is no part of one disability rating scale. But I think if we could quantify these four cardinal motor features and take them to 1 ms and a very precise measurement, it stands to reason that's going to be a good extension of our clinical abilities.

Dr. Korczyn: Of course. Although you need clinical relevance, it's not just instrumental accuracy that you're looking for. You have to have clinical relevance.

Dr. Deuschl: Basically I want to emphasize what Dr. Hallett said. I think concerning instrumentation we are now at the same point we were at about 5 years ago before construction of this Unified Parkinson's Disease Rating Scale. Out of the number of tests we have, we now have to select the tests which really measure the major things which we want to measure. These are these three symptoms and we need to measure them separately. Once we have done this, we will have to do the same that is now necessary for the rating scales. We have to reduce them to a reasonable test which can be done in a short time. I think in the long term some instrumentation is useful, because it gives us an objective and linear measurement of symptoms, which is useful.

Dr. Korczyn: So everybody says that we should have instruments for each of these parameters, but Les Findley says not for tremor?

Dr. Findley: No, I would say you've got to validate these measurements against disability. You're giving drugs against disability, and just because you can measure it doesn't mean it's significant.

Dr. Korczyn: That's what I meant by clinical relevance.

Dr. Hallett: I will come back to that same point. I'm not sure that just because the three cardinal manifestations of Parkinson's disease are bradykinesia, rigidity, and tremor that those are the three things that we in fact want to look at here. I think that tremor and rigidity may end up being relatively low down on the list. Bradykinesia and all of its ramifications is probably the most important, and if we're looking for instrumental tests, that's going to be the area that will probably be the most useful.

Dr. Korczyn: As you said, bradykinesia may have many manifestations: moving an arm may have very little to do with being able to turn in bed, which may be very important for a person with Parkinson's disease.

Dr. Panzer-Decius: I would like to just reiterate something I said earlier, which is that I think one of the key things that we can do in addressing this issue is to find out what in fact we want to measure. Is there axial bradykinesia or akinesia different from bradykinesia of the limbs? Maybe the reason that some of the different test paradigms have shown different results is exactly that. When we say akinesia, are we all trying to measure the same thing? I think that this is a very important aspect.

The second part of what I'd like to say is again that the functional role may in fact help us solve the issue of disability. If we can make tests that are more relevant to disability, then this may help us, because maybe it doesn't matter whether it is axial or related to the extremities, it matters how it affects which particular activity the person has to do or is concerned with.

Dr. Streifler: We seem to agree upon the necessity of combining both clinical assessment and instrumental tests for specific areas and specific functions, but we have another aim in this meeting: early detection. Now early detection is certainly a problem with clinical assessment, and which one of the instrumental methods should be used in order to come closer to the possibility of detecting as early as possible? This is one point one should stress, and if it has not been stressed enough in this meeting, maybe it should serve as a direction for a coming meeting.

Dr. Korczyn: Yes, presymptomatic examination should, by definition, use instrumentation or a biochemical marker or whatever. So you are right in stressing this, thank you.

Dr. Fahn: I'd like to follow up on what Mark was saying. I agree with him that you don't need to test all the cardinal findings if you want to find a narrowed-down instrumentation test available. I would also agree that bradykinesia is a key one and it seems to me from listening to everybody's papers that simple movement time may be adequate for early detection. I would also like to say that tremor should probably be measured, because these other tests don't measure it. For the third test, if we are going to have a third one, I would not pick rigidity at all, because I think it has a minor role in terms of disability in Parkinson's disease, and posture instability is such a late phenomenon that by then patients are on drugs anyway , so it's a different issue. What I would like to suggest maybe as a third thing to measure is complex movement of some sort, by which I mean the difficulty the Parkinson's disease patient has in doing the simultaneous or the sequential test. We need a simple kind of test, not instrumentation costing $20 000 that you have to do in a certain room, but some other kind of test that you can do in the office setting or maybe with a simple computer, if you're going to do the movement time as well. So these are the three things that I, as an outsider who never uses instruments at all, would like to see developed. Maybe we have to get the people concerned to sit down together and hammer it out.

Anonymous: I think if one wants to push the idea of movement time very hard, one also has to look at each patient and then pose the question of whether there is one joint which is more impaired than any other joint. So I think that you didn't use toe tapping because it was clearly going to show the problem, whereas heel tapping might not. If we look very carefully at patients, their joints, and their impairment and then look at the tasks, we have a better chance than if we give every patient the elbow flexion task alone.

Dr. Korczyn: Yes, although not all patients may behave in the same way, and for some patients we know that axial structures suffer first, so the more proximal joints may be affected earlier than distal ones.

Dr. Lange: Speaking from my experience with Huntington's disease patients, I find it's very convenient to videotape them for monitoring, also for drug effects. They can be videotaped in a specific position, the videotapes can be rated by other observers who are blind to treatment and to the phase when the picture was taken. For early detection in Huntington's disease, you have to rely on neurophysiological testing and imaging techniques; you also need cognitive testing, and that has to be standardized.

Dr. Korczyn: Dr. Fahn, I hear somebody saying that the UPDRS is not good enough because there is an inter- and intrarater variability, that when somebody tests a patient now and in 3 weeks they will rate them differently. That's why it was suggested you need a videotape. Now you are a great supporter of videotapes, you brought it to the fore, I think, in movement disorders at least. Is it true that you cannot depend on the UPDRS as it is?

Dr. Fahn: Well, first of all the interrater reliability which I showed was actually quite good; it was based on videotape exams, so everybody had the same thing to look at. But that's only a way of testing validity with a lot of people; even if a lot of people examine the same patient, there's too much variability because the patient may have a good phase with one examiner and not with another, at a different time or on a different day or whatever. So you've got to use a video if you're going to validate any of these, I think.

Dr. Korczyn: But the question was if it should be done in everyday testing in clinics when you test a patient for drug studies, etc.

Dr. Fahn: I don't think you really need to – it's too time-consuming for somebody to sit down and score them again from a video rather than just scoring them in the office, especially if you're doing it blinded. You could do this if you wanted a safety device and you want to have several people give you scores and then average them out. If you really wanted to be perfect, that may be the way to do it; that way you get multiple examiners at the same time. But otherwise it is too time-consuming. I think it's good, and anyway we like to videotape every patient just for documentation of what they have, and some day if you go back and look at them, there is a lot of information you can get from the videotape besides just following the severity of the disease, which is of course another useful aspect.

Dr. Korczyn: Right. So there is another use for videotapes and I think Dr. Plotnik suggested that since we are all talking about the functioning of the patient at home, it should be very easy with the instruments that are now available to videotape the person getting out of bed in the morning and doing whatever they do, getting dressed and making breakfast and so on, and then to see what this correlates to in our examination. So I think this is an interesting idea that was brought forward.

Dr. Steg: Of course we need test batteries, but it was agreed upon that bradykinesia is something essential. We agreed that complex movements are extremely important in this context. You called for some methods cheaper than $20 000. Well, how about a stopwatch applied to a complex movement? A battery of well-chosen complex movements could be recorded by stopwatch for purposes of drug testing, but if you want to analyze the ADL stability, you have to have more complex equipment. So it might be the right to use a stopwatch and in the background have some more elaborate equipment.

Dr. Fahn: The CAPIT (the Core Assessment Program for Intracerebral Transplantations for quantitating the severity of Parkinson's disease before and after transplantation) came up not with the UPDRS, but a time test – I think it was how many taps you can do in a certain period of time; there are four things.

Dr. Hallett: Yes, there are four things: one is the time taken to stand up, walk a certain distance, turn, come back, and sit down; another is how long it takes to do individual fractionated finger movements; the third is an examination of movement of both arms; and the final is doing a repetitive pronation–supination, trying to establish limb symptoms, trying to get at distal/proximal symptoms and trying to achieve reasonable balance. The idea behind the core assessment was that anybody anywhere in the world could do that couple of clinical evaluations off and on, and no matter what treatment you're doing, you can compare some objective measures and the clinical disability rating scale and so forth. I think that what Prof.

Steg said is a step in the right direction – if we can do them, anybody can do them, but we ought to develop technology that can take us beyond that in the future.

Dr. Korczyn: How good was the intercorrelation between these four tests? Because as you say, some are proximal and some are distal; this, of course, raises the question of whether we need all of them?

Dr. Hallett: We haven't looked at that specifically, but they measure different aspects of our motor repertoire.

Dr. Korczyn: But there could still be a very good correlation between them.

Dr. Hallett: That's right. Especially the limb-related aspect of the movement.

Dr. Fahn: The DATATOP (Deprenyl and Tocopherol Antioxidative Therapy of Parkinsonism) study did two time tests with it. One was the step/second test, which was originally part of Webster's scale, I think – somebody recommended it, but I can't remember if it was Webster or not. In the step/second test, you have to walk for a certain time and the observer measures how many steps you have taken and how long it took. The other time test was the peg board test, where you have to put the pegs into the hole as a time test. Now as it turns out, in these early milder cases of Parkinson's disease patients, the step/second test wasn't very good because they did pretty well. It wasn't sensitive enough, let's put it that way. The peg board test showed a little better correlation and you can differentiate between degrees of severity, so that may be something else that needs to be looked at, particularly with different severities of the disease, but they would be bradykinesia tests.

Dr. Steg: I would suggest that it is important that movements are as natural as possible, fitting into the ordinary daily scheme of living. Otherwise you get laboratory artifacts and learning effects and so on. But it should be possible to design some such tests.

Dr. Korczyn: Clinical relevance!

Subject Index

Springer-Verlag and the Environment

We at Springer-Verlag firmly believe that an international science publisher has a special obligation to the environment, and our corporate policies consistently reflect this conviction.

We also expect our business partners – paper mills, printers, packaging manufacturers, etc. – to commit themselves to using environmentally friendly materials and production processes.

The paper in this book is made from low- or no-chlorine pulp and is acid free, in conformance with international standards for paper permanency.

Printing: Mercedesdruck, Berlin
Binding: Buchbinderei Lüderitz & Bauer, Berlin